I0797196

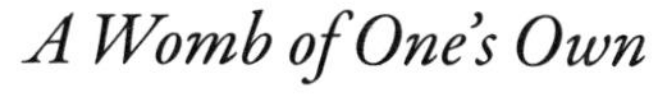

A Womb of One's Own

The publisher and the
University of California Press Foundation
gratefully acknowledge the generous support of the
Ahmanson Foundation Endowment Fund
in Humanities.

A Womb of One's Own

LOST HISTORIES OF CHILDBIRTH IN ANCIENT ROME

Tara Mulder

UNIVERSITY OF CALIFORNIA PRESS

University of California Press
Oakland, California

© 2026 by Tara Mulder

All rights reserved.

Library of Congress Cataloging-in-Publication Data

Names: Mulder, Tara, author
Title: A womb of one's own : lost histories of childbirth in ancient Rome / Tara Mulder.
Description: Oakland, California : University of California Press, [2026] | Includes bibliographical references and index.
Identifiers: LCCN 2025036250 (print) | LCCN 2025036251 (ebook) | ISBN 9780520398740 cloth | ISBN 9780520398757 ebook
Subjects: LCSH: Childbirth—Rome—History—To 1500 | Pregnancy—Rome—History—To 1500 | Midwives—Rome—History—To 1500 | Women—Health and hygiene—Rome—History—To 1500
Classification: LCC RG513 .M85 2026 (print) | LCC RG513 (ebook)
LC record available at https://lccn.loc.gov/2025036250
LC ebook record available at https://lccn.loc.gov/2025036251

Manufactured in the United States of America

GPSR Authorized Representative: Easy Access System Europe, Mustamäe tee 50, 10621 Tallinn, Estonia, gpsr.requests@easproject.com

35 34 33 32 31 30 29 28 27 26
10 9 8 7 6 5 4 3 2 1

For my grandmothers,
Annie Laurie and Carolyn Ann,
and for the midwives

CONTENTS

ILLUSTRATIONS

NOTES ON HERBAL AND MEDICAL TERMINOLOGY, TRANSLATIONS, AND DATES

This book includes references to many plants, processes, and tools used in herbal medicine, as well as various types of medical instruments and procedures. It also contains specialized vocabulary related to pregnancy and childbirth. While I often define these terms as I go, I have also included a glossary at the back of the book. Please refer to it as needed.

The passages from ancient texts in this book were all originally written in Ancient Greek or Latin. Unless I indicate otherwise, I have done the translations myself. In the bibliography under "Ancient Sources" I have, where it is possible to do so, indicated available English translations. Otherwise, the sources given are in the original language.

The dates in this book straddle the year 0. For time periods before the year 0, I use BCE (before the Common Era) and for those after I use CE (Common Era). If a date is unmarked, it is CE.

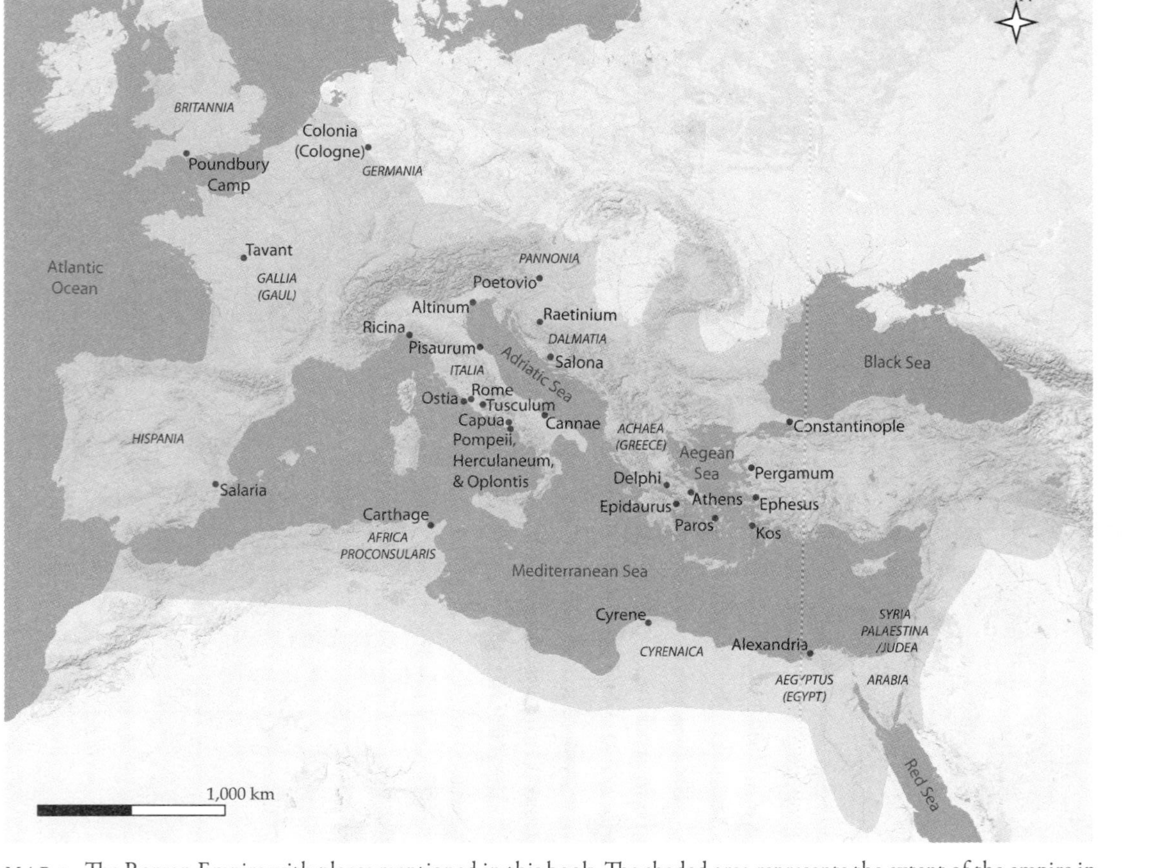

MAP 1. The Roman Empire with places mentioned in this book. The shaded area represents the extent of the empire in the 2nd century CE. Map by Stephen Bartlett.

Introduction

THIS BOOK IS A BIRTH STORY. It takes place in the Roman Empire—a vast territory that encompassed the Mediterranean Sea, extending from present-day Algeria, up to Great Britain, over to Azerbaijan, and down to Egypt. Ancient Rome, as well as the many societies that lie between it and us in time, was incredibly hostile to birthing people. None of their histories have survived fully, so this is not an ordinary birth story. It is a mosaic crafted from the experiences of many women who lived during the first few centuries of the Common Era. These women exist today in fragments—from letters, medical case histories, legal documents, poems, myths, funerary inscriptions, bones, medical instruments, magical amulets, artwork, and anecdotes. Those texts that we today consider "histories"—full of detailed descriptions of war and death—tend to be least informative on the topic.

This book is also a feminist history of the cultural forces that shaped the experience of giving birth in the ancient Roman world. Under the aegis of the Roman Empire, male doctors claimed expertise and authority for themselves with treatises on midwifery and obstetrics, new gynecological instruments, and an emphasis on anatomical and theoretical—rather than practical—training. There was tension in this emerging medicalization of childbirth. Male medical writers represented pregnancy and birth as a conflict between mother and fetus, undermining women's experiences and bodily knowledge. At the same time, they recognized the real—if threatening to them—value of women's expertise and their communities of care around birth. Midwives attended women in labor and held medical and legal authority despite unflattering portraits of them in male-authored texts. These nascent tensions anticipated great conflicts in the centuries to come: the encroachment of male doctors into birth, the criminalization of midwives, and the cloaking of childbirth in secrecy and shame. From the Middle Ages to the 20th century, the takeover of childbirth by male doctors and man-midwives grew ever more extreme, culminating in the near eradication of midwifery in the 20th-century United States. This book is the story of where that conflict began. The very forces that make this history hard to write—patriarchy, misogyny, and the suppression of women's voices—attest to the challenging circumstances in which birth happened.

NATALITY

Why write a history that is so hard to write? Because a radical corrective is needed to the story of the Roman Empire. As Jennifer Banks argues in *Natality: Toward a Philosophy of Birth,* birth has long played second fiddle to death. "Death," she writes, "has been humanity's central defining experience, its deepest existential theme, more authoritative somehow than birth, and certainly more final."[1] Nowhere is this elevation of death—and its companion, war—more apparent than in the Roman Empire.

Recently, a viral social media trend asked, "How often do you think about the Roman Empire?" This question was directed primarily at young men, who, we all learned, think about it quite frequently—upward of once a day. But what Roman Empire are they thinking about? They mean the one of Brutus and Cassius and the tyrant Julius Caesar, of the emperors Augustus and Marcus Aurelius, Trajan's Column, Caligula's orgies, and the gladiators in the Colosseum. Theirs is a Roman Empire obsessed with war, death, sex, and aggressive masculinity. It is a culture full of stories about the exploits of war, including the rape and violation of women's bodies, but few about birth. It has left behind many visual depictions of sex—in statues, wall paintings, oil lamps, and graffiti—and only a few images of birth. A society that tells war and sex stories but not birth stories is out of balance. This essential part of the Roman experience has been denied, first by its own culture and second by the historians who study and write about it. More insidiously, the dearth of natality in both Rome's narrative of itself and in our historical narrative of Rome makes this narrative attractive to the most destructive aspects of masculinity within our own culture.

Part of my contention in this book is that telling birth stories matters—even birth stories that are two thousand years old and fragmented. We cannot understand ancient Rome without its birth stories, and we do not have a full picture of birth without birth stories from ancient Rome. As challenging and imperfect as this history is, it must be told.

BIRTH STORIES

In her 1998 essay in *American Baby* magazine, writer and educator Laura Stavoe wrote two sentences that have taken on a life of their own: "There's a secret in our culture, and it's not that birth is painful. It's that women are strong."[2] These lines appear on T-shirts, bumper stickers, Instagram accounts, and inspirational birth websites. Some people have lifted these words up as a testament to the idea that birth isn't really that painful (or even painful at all) and women are strong enough to withstand physiological birth without medical interventions; others have critiqued them as wildly irresponsible on the same grounds. But in June 2011, Stavoe wrote to a blog called *Birth Trauma Truths* to set the record straight. Her words, she explains, were not a judgment on the type of birth a woman should have or the amount of pain involved in birth, but a response to "the rather old-fashioned idea (popular in my mother's generation) that we should not talk about birth stories because it would scare women about the pain." Stavoe's intention was to propose "that in sharing our [birth] stories we would learn what so many women have been able to bear over the centuries in its myriad forms."[3] The secret that women were attempting to keep from each other was that birth was painful. But, Stavoe argued, in the poor attempt to keep this fact hidden, a more important fact was lost: women are strong. By suppressing birth stories, we suppress stories of women's strength and glory.

Others have recognized the importance of telling birth stories. In *Pregnancy, Delivery, Childbirth: A Gender and Cultural History from Antiquity to the Test Tube in Europe,* Nadia Filippini writes about the shame and secrecy surrounding pregnancy in 20th-century Italy and the suppression of birth stories. "Childbirth," she writes, "was a taboo subject, erased from language and storytelling: children were taught that babies were brought by storks or that they were born under cabbage leaves."[4] In *Sumud: Birth, Oral History, and Persistence in Palestine,* Livia Wick explores how humans make sense and meaning of their lives through storytelling by recounting the stories of Palestinian women giving birth under Israeli occupation. Birth stories, she explains, involve "the selective refashioning of experiences to make ourselves alive and part of the world."[5] Birth stories for Palestinian women in particular are stories about beginnings that lead to isolation and reduction—after giving birth, they are confined to their homes by curfews, separated from natal families by checkpoints, and deprived of husbands due to detainments and arrests. Telling their birth stories is a way for them to assert their participation in the human community.[6]

Even or perhaps especially when birth is very hard and very painful, it's important to tell these stories. In *Invisible Labor: The Untold Story of the Cesarean Section,* Rachel Somerstein chronicles her efforts to make sense of her birth—an emergency c-section in which her anesthesia failed. What became important for Somerstein was to tell her birth story, and to contextualize her story within the long (hi)story of cesarean section. She writes about the intense need for "emplotment" people experience after giving birth—"putting nonfiction events into a storyline, so that they form a complete narrative."[7] Telling birth stories helps us make sense of our experience within an established framework. It can also help other birthing people to hear these birth stories.

The power of the birth story is something I know well. As the daughter of a certified professional midwife, I grew up listening to birth stories told by circles of midwives around bonfires, on the chilly shores of Lake Michigan, in hotel conference rooms, and in the bedrooms, living rooms, and kitchens of laboring people. For my whole life I have witnessed a particular phenomenon: whenever someone learns that my mother is a midwife, their birth story comes rushing out. Birth stories beget more birth stories. They are offered up in awe, for catharsis, as a warning, as a celebration. Midwives are the collectors of birth stories. Midwife Geradine Simkins writes, "As midwives, we have stories to tell," stories full of "hard-earned wisdom."[8]

When I was preparing to give birth to my child in the spring of 2023, I reflected on the many births that I had seen—the first when I was four years old and watched my mother birth my sister on my parents' bed in our rented townhouse in Baltimore, Maryland. The midwife helped me cut the umbilical cord and I cried when blood squirted onto my pajamas. I thought about the women I saw give birth in a geodesic dome tent in Jacmel, Haiti, during the summer of 2011. When the temperature got to be over 100 degrees in the tent, we would set up makeshift spaces for the women outdoors, on a wooden platform, with sheets hung for privacy. Many of them arrived at the clinic on foot, alone, in hard labor. Some of them had malaria. I learned enough Haitian so that I could hold their hands and tell them that everything was going to be okay.

In the weeks leading up to my child's birth, I talked with friends who had given birth, listened to birth story podcasts, and read collections of birth stories. But I didn't know just how important those stories would be until I was in my own labor. It turns out, birth stories are what get us through the births.

The birth of my son was difficult. Labor was long and painful. He had an asynclitic (tilted) head, making it hard for him to descend down into my pelvis. I had to *work* to get him out—squatting, lunging, walking up and down stairs, doing supported head stands off the couch—and so did my birth team. I needed a lot of hands-on support, especially hard hip squeezes and pulls. When my son's head finally emerged, the reason for the head tilt became clear—his short umbilical cord was wrapped around his neck.

Many of the methods and tools I used to bring him into the world would not have been out of place at an ancient Roman birth. To ease my pain, I put hot water bottles on my back and inhaled the fragrance of lavender. I submerged my body in warm water and relaxed into massages provided by loving hands. Early in labor, when I needed some rest, I drank a glass of wine, which allowed me to sleep. Later, when contractions seemed to be stalling, I drank castor oil to intensify them. My mom and partner helped me change positions and physically supported me through contractions. Their words of praise and encouragement sustained me. When I was at the most intense point of labor, transitioning to full dilation, subconsciously, in a trance-like state, I whispered over and over again, "Please god I need a break"—an involuntary prayer and incantation. As night fell and I began pushing, the only light in my living room came from one beeswax candle.

Throughout my labor, my birth necklace lay in my sight. While I do not hold any particularly powerful beliefs in divinities or magic, the beads and charms on the necklace, gifted to me by my friends and family members, prompted me to focus on all the women throughout history who had done exactly what I was doing in that moment—my mother, my aunts, my grandmothers, my great-grandmothers, and all my relatives going back to the wattle-and-daub huts of ancient Europe.

Although I have witnessed many unmedicated births at homes and birth centers, labor was more intense than I imagined. At a few points I wept and wanted to give up. As I neared the point of pushing, with the contractions lasting up to three minutes and little break in between, I remembered a birth story I had read the night before. Mariahna Nelson-Schafer had written about her long, painful labor with her daughter, Ajahna.[9] As Mariahna got close to pushing, a lip of cervix was preventing her from being fully dilated. She wrote, "I decided right then, I was going to have to just let it hurt more." I thought of Mariahna and I repeated her words to myself: "You're just going to have to let it hurt more." This mantra gave me the strength to birth my baby. As he emerged from body, my mother somersaulted him out from the cord wrapped around his neck and passed him through my legs. I reached down, bringing him out of the water and up onto my chest. I leaned back into my partner in euphoria and relief.

It was my choice to give birth at home without pain medication. I was grateful to be able to mix the traditional practices of physiological birth with modern innovation. When my placenta took a while to emerge, my midwives, Kerry and Katrina, were able to give me a shot of synthetic oxytocin in the thigh to stimulate expulsive contractions. And I appreciated their administration of a local anesthetic while they stitched up my second-degree tear. In ancient Rome, birthing women would not have had these choices. For them, birth attendants would have been critical to successful birth outcomes. And so they were for me. What sustained me through my labor was the attention and stamina of a loving birth partner, the encouragement and wisdom of an experienced midwife, and the birth stories.

A WOMB OF ONE'S OWN

This book begins at preconception and goes through the early postpartum period. Each stage is anchored by one woman's story and supported by pieces from many other women's stories. Birth was so tied into womanhood in ancient Rome that the two were nearly inseparable. Not only were women expected to give birth, but by giving birth they reinforced their womanhood. In our own culture today, birth and womanhood are not so entwined. Trans men and nonbinary people give birth. Chestfeeding complements breastfeeding. My language in the book acknowledges these ancient and modern realities. When talking about pregnant and birthing people in ancient Rome, I use "women," but when talking about them today, I generally use "people."

Some of the stories that follow are more detailed than others. Where specifics are lacking, I sometimes fill them in through informed speculation. I don't know if ancient Roman women told each other birth stories.

I like to think that they did. I like to think that they told each other birth stories to help each other through births. Given the saturation of their lives in patriarchy and misogyny, they would have dearly needed them. This book is my attempt to reinstate their stories of pregnancy and birth, to give back to each ancient Roman woman a womb of her own.

ONE

Cyrilla Faints in the Bath

ON JULY 28, 162 CE, in the city of Rome, a woman named Cyrilla fainted in the bath.[1] She had been suffering from copious vaginal discharge for weeks. A sense of embarrassment or modesty had kept her from consulting a male doctor about the condition, but she had been under the care of her "usual midwives."[2] They were using the traditional remedies for this type of ailment: astringent (drying) herbs, taken orally and applied in ointments to her vulva. The thinking was that her flux, as it was called, was caused by excessive fluidity not only in her uterus, but throughout her whole body. But the treatments were not working, and her condition was only getting worse.

At the same time, her belly was starting to swell. One of the women taking care of her began to suspect that she was pregnant and started the normal prenatal care, which included a daily bath.[3] Although the baths did not seem to be helping much, they didn't seem to be doing any harm either—until she fainted.

Cyrilla was carried from the bathing room to a couch while her attendants shrieked. A physician named Galen, who had recently been invited into the home by Cyrilla's husband, Boethus, heard the cries of the attendants and came running into the room. Grabbing a nard oil ointment, he began to rub her lower belly, which he found to be the consistency of soft, curdled cheese. He directed the panicking women who were gathered around—likely enslaved women in Cyrilla's household—to rub her hands and feet and to apply smelling salts under her nose. Cyrilla quickly regained consciousness. No labor ensued and nothing solid came out of her vagina.

Galen, who had been adamant that it was a false pregnancy all along, felt that he had been proven right. But he was still perplexed about the cause of Cyrilla's continuous discharge. Consulting together, Cyrilla's midwives, Galen, and her other caretakers, who included additional male doctors, decided to keep drying out the excess moisture in her body with astringent and styptic (blood-stanching) substances, but also with heat therapies, such as having her lie in a bed of warm sand. Finally, Galen asked Boethus to give him full control over Cyrilla's case, taking her out of the care of the midwives and other doctors. Pausing the ineffective astringent remedies, Galen made a decoction of wild spikenard and celery to evacuate her bowls and bladder. He administered daily massages and body rubs with honey, alternating soft and rough cloths, and he fed her a mild diet of wild poultry and fish. He was thus able, in his understanding, to disperse the excess moisture from her uterus thorough the rest of her body and purge it through her bladder, bowels, and pores. By mid-October, Cyrilla had improved dramatically. There was minimal sign of flux. By the end of the month, she had recovered a healthy color in her face and the flux was completely gone. Boethus sent Galen 400 gold pieces as a gift for curing his wife.

What was wrong with Cyrilla? Why did she get sick? How and why did she get better? What were Galen's aims in writing this narrative of her illness? What was Cyrilla herself experiencing? If we can answer some of these questions about Cyrilla, we can start to get at the experience of being a person who could get pregnant and give birth in ancient Rome. We will see that Cyrilla—an upper-class woman married to a highly placed Roman politician—was hardly a typical Roman woman. But in many ways her experience *was* typical. What happened to her that day in the bath, and everything that occurred afterward, was part of a standard script for women of reproductive age in ancient Rome.

We will look at Cyrilla's story in this chapter and the next, first putting her in her social context in ancient Rome and looking at the various pressures on her to reproduce. Then in chapter 2 we will turn to the beliefs and practices that informed the way medical professionals, and Cyrilla herself, understood her body and what was happening to it.

BOETHUS'S WIFE

Let's start with what we know and what we don't know. We don't actually know that this woman's name was Cyrilla. We do know that her husband was Titus Flavius Boethus and that he was a Roman senator during the reign of the emperor Marcus Aurelius (161–180 CE). Boethus's family originally came from the Roman province of Syria-Palaestina (formerly Judaea).[4] After living at Rome for many years, he was sent to be governor of Syria-Palaestina around 166 CE, and he died of an illness a few years later. We know that he was close with the physician Galen, who moved to Rome from Pergamum (in modern-day Türkiye [Turkey]) in 162. Galen only tells us that he treated Boethus's wife in the summer; it could have been any of the five summers from 162 to 166.[5]

Otherwise, all the details about the progression of Boethus's wife's illness, including her treatment by the midwives and nurses, fainting in the bath, and the useless shrieking of her attendants, come from a case history in Galen's book *Prognosis*.[6] Throughout his account, Galen refers to her only as "Boethus's wife." By giving her the name Cyrilla, I aim to reclaim and recenter her as a historical figure in her own right. She was not just the wife of Boethus or a patient of Galen, but a real Roman woman with her own hopes, fears, and desires. We have to rely on the writing of Galen to find her, but we don't have to tell her story in precisely the way he did.

Often, specific women have been lost to history because their names have been overshadowed by their connections to their fathers, husbands, and sons. In ancient Rome, a man had at least three names, while a woman generally had only one—a feminized form of one of her father's names. There were so many Julias and Tullias that to distinguish them, we reduce them to "Caesar's daughter" or "Boethus's wife." We don't know the name of Cyrilla's father, but as a nod to Roman naming conventions and their emphasis on connection to a male relative, I've given her a name based on that of her son, Cyrillus. We know his name because he features in another of Galen's case histories, in which he is treated for a stubborn fever.[7]

In writing down Cyrilla's dramatic scene, Galen had his own aims: to show the inadequacy of the medical theories and practices that the midwives and other consulting physicians were using, to display his own superior skills of diagnosis and treatment, and to advertise his relationship with the highly placed Boethus. Galen was a prolific and self-aggrandizing practitioner. He left us the single largest surviving body of texts written in Ancient Greek, and much of his writing is devoted to showcasing himself as the best medical practitioner in a medical marketplace saturated by doctors from competing philosophical schools, midwives, root cutters, priests, magicians, and even Roman estate owners, who treated their own family members and slaves with a variety of herbal-based home remedies.[8]

With this context in mind, we may rightly question whether it was truly "embarrassment" and "modesty" (as Galen says) that caused Cyrilla to consult midwives instead of a male doctor, or whether she was just accustomed to consulting the midwives. Galen adds the detail that these are her "usual midwives" and "the best in the city." The fact that he calls them "the best" only makes his own improvements to their treatments all the more impressive.[9] We should also be suspicious of the misogyny inherent in Galen's characterization of the attendants as shrieking and useless. But as to the other particulars of the case, we have to take him at his word. His account is all we have. There is nothing particularly fantastical or out of the ordinary in his description of Boethus's wife, her ailment, the assumptions made by the attending midwives and consulting physicians, or the treatments administered to her, even Galen's treatments. The only aspect that is remarkable is that Boethus gave Galen 400 gold coins after she recovered—a truly staggering amount of money. At the time, one gold coin (an *aureus*) was the monthly wage of a Roman infantry soldier.[10]

What we can see from this account is that Cyrilla was a woman of reproductive age. She had already had at least one son that we know of, and her husband was a wealthy, well-connected man who had served for part of a year as a consul, the highest office at Rome under the emperor. He would soon be appointed governor of a province. He may have been in his thirties or forties, and she would likely have been at least ten years younger than him, if not more.[11] She was probably between twenty and thirty years old.[12]

We can make an educated guess that Cyrilla was in the middle of her reproductive years. She was a mother and a *potential* mother. On a basic level, a potential mother was someone who was expected and likely to get pregnant at some point in the near future. But potential mothers in ancient Rome were also people who were subject to various social, legal, and medical controls that aimed to increase their reproductivity while consequently limiting their freedoms. We'll never know for sure how Cyrilla felt about her own fertility, but it's safe to assume that Cyrilla experienced intense pressure to have children from her family and her wider community. Understanding these pressures of potential motherhood is the key to understanding her condition and how it was treated.

PRONATALISM AND CLASS IN ROME

The Rome that Cyrilla inhabited was an intensely pronatalist society.[13] Childbearing was valued and promoted in both formal and informal ways, and this was true for women of all social and economic classes. As we have already seen from Cyrilla's story, Rome was populated with women who were free, enslaved, and freed (formerly enslaved).[14] Wealth disparities could be extreme, with elite women living in abundant luxury and poor women often destitute. Much of the evidence we have pertains to free, wealthy, politically connected women like Cyrilla. But with a critical eye, we can see the other women too. Look, for instance, at the (almost certainly) enslaved women tending to Cyrilla in her household and the working women she hired as her midwives. While these women appear as accessories to Cyrilla's story, if we center them in their own lives, we see that they too experienced great pressure to have children.

During his reign, Augustus, the first emperor of Rome, created laws specifically related to reproduction. Known as the Julian Laws, they dictated who could legally marry (Roman citizens) and who could not (enslaved persons, sex workers, and those serving in the military) and gave tangible rewards to wealthy citizens who bore large numbers of children within legitimate marriages. They imposed penalties on those citizens among this same rank who failed to have children. The rewards included the right to inherit from a deceased spouse (otherwise the inheritance usually went to the spouse's family of birth). The amount of spouse-to-spouse inheritance that was allowed increased with the birth of each additional child.[15]

The "Law of Children," as this second part of the Julian Laws was called, conferred even more benefits on especially productive parents: citizen men who fathered at least three children within a legitimate marriage earned career advancements and reprieve from civil obligations, specifically the requirement for wealthy Romans to provide public works and games. Citizen women who had three children (for free-born women) or four children (for freed, formerly enslaved women) earned the right to no longer have a male guardian.[16]

Ironically, Augustus himself only had one child, a daughter named Julia (from his full name, Gaius Julius Caesar Augustus). All of his sons, including the second emperor, his successor Tiberius, he adopted from other members of his family. It's also not clear how much of an effect this legislation actually had on the birth rate in the Roman Empire. It doesn't seem that it was a particularly effective way of increasing the birth rate of legally recognized children, let alone the overall population, since it only applied to a small group of very wealthy citizens and would not have affected most of the inhabitants of the Roman Empire.[17] However, the Julian Laws did signal clearly that Rome was interested in prolific reproduction. In fact, there is evidence that some male heads of households instituted their own informal versions of the Law of Children. In a book on Roman agriculture written in the 1st century CE, a Roman military veteran and farmer explained his own system of rewards for enslaved women on his plantation: "An enslaved mother of three sons gets exemption from work; a mother of more gets her freedom."[18] Three or more sons, however, was a tall order. It's unlikely that many, if any, enslaved women got to take advantage of this policy.

As the Law of Children was expanded by later emperors, its explicit aim of encouraging reproduction became clearer. In the early 2nd century, the emperor Hadrian made it possible for married citizen women who had the requisite number of children to inherit from their own deceased children, even without an explicit will. Later, the Roman jurists, the men in charge of interpreting the law and passing judgment on legal cases, expanded Hadrian's provision to include mothers with children born outside of legal marriage, as well as to mothers who were sex workers.[19] The property and income requirements to be eligible for the Law of Children also dissolved over time.

Beyond the legal system of rewards and punishments for childbearing, there were strong cultural and social incentives to have children. Free women of all economic classes stood to benefit socially from having children. Giving birth within a legally recognized marriage initiated the transition from girl to woman. Women who had successfully given birth to thriving children were able to remarry if their husbands died or divorced them.[20] The pressures on enslaved and non-citizen women were different. Enslaved women were expected to have children for their enslavers' use.[21] In chapter 11 we will look at how they were incentivized to do so with promises of freedom. Non-citizen women were counted on to provide the next generation of non-citizen laborers for the empire, including fresh soldiers for the ever-expanding Roman military.[22] Thus, the majority of women in the Roman Empire, with the exception of a small few who were religiously and legally obligated to remain virgins—such as the Vestal Virgins who tended the sacred flame of Rome to protect the Roman state—were expected to have children.[23]

For freed (formerly enslaved) women, children were especially important for intergenerational family-building and continuity. Anyone who was enslaved either lost all legal family ties or never had them in the first place. Even if and when they got their freedom, they did not regain their ancestors. As historian Angela Hug has pointed out, with "no family lineage from which to draw their descent, they had no choice but to look forward."[24]

POTENTIAL MOTHERS

Before they became mothers, Roman women were potential mothers—young women of reproductive age whose fertility could be harnessed for social, cultural, political, or economic benefit. Even once they had given birth to one or more children, Roman women continued to exist in a state of potential future motherhood. This constant potentiality had an impact on what they could do with their bodies and how they were allowed to exist in the world.

The pressures of potential motherhood are perhaps best seen in the conflict between the medical recommendations for the age at which girls should marry and get pregnant for the first time and the age at which Roman girls actually married and started having babies. Physicians at the time were aware of the risks that sexual intercourse, pregnancy, and birth posed to women, especially to teenage girls. But their words of caution often went unheeded by elite householders, who wanted their daughters and wives to marry young and get pregnant fast.

Rufus, a Greek physician who studied at Alexandria and practiced medicine at Ephesus, on the western coast of modern-day Türkiye (Turkey), during the reign of the emperor Trajan (98–117 CE), was emphatic that young women should delay marriage and sexual intercourse until the fifth year after the start of menstruation, or about age eighteen.[25] He viewed these years as important for the growth and development of the adolescent body. Girls who gave birth before this age tended to produce weak babies and could damage their uteruses.[26] He may have been following the example of Aristotle (4th century BCE), who cautioned that although girls could get pregnant earlier, pregnancy was quite risky, since their bodies were not ready for childbearing until age twenty-one.[27]

Soranus, a Greek physician who practiced at Rome and was a later contemporary of Rufus, advised that girls were in good shape to get pregnant starting at age fifteen, provided that their bodies were in a moderate, healthy state: not manly, compact, and solidly built, nor excessively fat, loose, or moist.[28] Though, really, his perspective was that permanent virginity was actually the healthiest choice of all, since a woman who stayed a virgin did not take on any of the risks of intercourse, pregnancy, and birth.[29] But Soranus conceded that the point of marriage was for producing children, and he realized that his treatise had to be aimed more at mitigating rather than eliminating the risks that childbearing posed to young women.[30] One of his goals seems to have been to convince male heads of household that girls should not be subjected to sexual intercourse *until* they had menstruated for the first time. In his understanding, it was possible for girls to get pregnant prior to first menstruation—a pregnancy that would be very dangerous, since the young girl's body was not big enough and her vagina not opened up enough to allow the safe passage of an infant. In addition, her small uterus likely would not allow enough room for a fetus to grow properly.[31]

Soranus's advice to wait at least until the onset of menstruation for first intercourse is sobering when we consider the age at which girls were being married off. In the Roman Empire, legally, girls could be married starting at age twelve. This age was set based on an upsetting standard known as *viripotens,* "capable of sustaining a man"—that is, in vaginal intercourse.[32] These girls were almost certainly not yet menstruating, and pregnancy and birth would have been quite dangerous for them. On this point we only have access to the experiences of wealthy, socially elite girls—those whose families had enough money to be the subject of literary texts or who could afford to set up tombstones in their honor.

Herennia Cervilla, a woman from Ricina in northwestern Italy, died in the 3rd century at the age of eighteen. She had three children. Her tombstone, set up by her husband, Caius Carrenas Verecundus, tells us that she died "in pain" (*dolens*), which may indicate that she died in childbirth.[33] Herennia would have had to start getting pregnant quite young in order to have three children by the time she was eighteen. She may have been married before puberty. Similarly, Quintilian, a Roman writer from the 1st century, writes about his wife, who died at age nineteen. She had given birth to two sons, the younger of whom died at the age of five, a few months after his mother.[34] There are many more such examples from tombstone and literary evidence: Marcella, who died on her wedding night at age twelve or thirteen; Julia, daughter of the emperor Augustus, who was married when she was fourteen; Agrippina the Younger, wife of the emperor Claudius and mother of the emperor Nero, who was married to her first husband, Gnaeus Domitius Ahenobarbus, at age eleven or twelve.[35]

It's likely that poorer women were not subjected to marriage at such a young age. Wealthy women were frequently used as pawns to keep power within families or to establish alliances with other wealthy families.[36] They were often married off before puberty. Less wealthy and less socially elite women would likely have gotten married a few years after puberty and would have started having babies then.[37]

Given the wealth and high status of her husband, it's likely that Cyrilla was a young bride. If she was thirteen or fourteen at her wedding, her husband would have been well into his twenties, if not his thirties. She may have had a child when she was a teenager. We only know of one living son, but it is possible that she had other children who do not appear in Galen's accounts. Perhaps she had miscarriages or stillbirths, or maybe her children died when they were young from the many dangers that abounded for young infants and children.[38] The fact that Galen refers to the midwives on the case as "her usual midwives" suggests other pregnancies.[39] These were clearly women Cyrilla was in the habit of employing.

Galen's imperfect record here is frustrating. We wouldn't even know that Cyrilla had the one child if he hadn't been the subject of another case history. What Galen chose to share about a particular case was generally what he thought was pertinent or what illustrated a larger point about his own expertise. He did not deem Cyrilla's history of childbearing to be relevant. The fact that she was a potential mother was assumed. His job was to get her healthy again so she could have future children. Regardless of how many living children they had, married Roman women probably spent most of their reproductive years dealing with pregnancy in one way or another: being pregnant, trying to get pregnant, or trying to prevent pregnancy.

The marriages and pregnancies of these very young women show how important the status of potential mothers was. The medical writers were in a delicate conflict with potential fathers and grandfathers over the bodies of young (elite) Roman women. Although they knew, medically speaking, that it was safer, and ultimately more productive in the long run, if the girls waited a few years after first menstruation for their bodies to develop before having sex and getting pregnant, male heads of household seem to have been eager for the girls to be married and impregnated as soon as possible.

Although doctors and husbands might have disagreed about *when* women should start having babies, it's clear that they had a shared understanding of women as potential mothers. But there were a number of things that could go wrong with women's bodies on the road to motherhood. As Cyrilla's story continues in the next chapter, we will see how medical writers from the 5th century BCE onward presented medical intervention as the solution to these problems.

TWO

Cyrilla's Flux and Other Fluids

HOW DOES CYRILLA'S STORY prompt us to think about women's bodies in ancient Rome? What does it say about how their bodies appeared in medicine and science? Does it tell us anything about how they experienced their own bodies?

Once they began menstruating and having sex, Roman women were engaged in a constant struggle with their leaky, changeable, unreliable bodies—or at least this is what the ancient medical texts would have had them believe.[1] Medicine at the time operated on the theory of humors, or fluids. There were different permutations of this theory, but one model (which would go on to prominence in the Middle Ages) held that the body was made up of four basic humors: black bile, yellow bile, phlegm, and blood.[2] Black bile—"melancholy," from *melan*, "black," + *chole*, "bile"—was tied to the spleen and associated with the cold and dry of autumn. Yellow bile from the gallbladder was hot and dry, like summer, and would cause people to be hot headed and temperamental. Blood—hot and wet—was associated with spring. Finally, cold and wet phlegm was associated with winter and was the term for any white milky or viscous substance produced in the body. Phlegmatic individuals were sluggish and reserved. Health and disease in the body were understood as a balance or imbalance among these humors.[3]

This principle of balance was also applied more generally. Medicine was often a process of bringing balance to the body, from tight to loose, hot to cold, dry to wet, and vice versa. These differences were also associated with a person's sex. Men were seen as hot, dry, and tight/compact;

women as cold, wet, and loose.[4] In one medical text long in circulation by Cyrilla's time, sexual difference existed at the level of the flesh.[5] Male flesh, it contended, was firm and compact, female flesh porous and spongy. A metaphor illustrated the difference: male flesh was like woven cloth; female flesh was like raw wool. If you left a scrap of each suspended over a vessel of water overnight, in the morning the wool would have soaked up more liquid than the woven cloth. So it was with the flesh. Women's flesh was thought to soak up more fluid, especially blood—understood as the digested form of food in the body—than men's flesh.[6] These distinctions were not value-neutral. The underdeveloped rawness and excessive fluidity of the female body made women unstable—physically and psychologically. And so, enter gynecology.

From at least the time of the Hippocratic doctors, who emerged in the 5th century BCE in Ionia (around Ephesus on the western coast of modern-day Türkiye [Turkey]), gynecology was a distinct part of medical practice.[7] The Greeks and Romans didn't have obstetricians in our modern sense of the word, since women's reproductive care was overseen by midwives. But there were medical writers starting to produce texts devoted to the pathology and treatment of female bodies. Medicine in the ancient Mediterranean was an unlicensed, unregulated, competitive endeavor. In this environment, women's bodies—the interpretation of them and the treatment of their particular ailments—were a lucrative area of practice. We see this medical competition at work in the story of Cyrilla. The physician Galen is at first in conversation and then in competition with the midwives treating Cyrilla, as well as the other, unspecified physicians consulting on the case. The story is ultimately about his triumph. Along with the 400 gold pieces, he also gains the respect of Boethus, one of the most powerful men in Rome and a direct conduit to the emperor, Marcus Aurelius.[8]

The degree to which different physicians separated the treatment of women from the treatment of men (and from other branches of medical practice) varied depending on the theories of each. Some of the big questions of the time included whether women were made of the same physical substance as men and whether they had conditions that were unique to them. For the Hippocratics, whose theories were popular at Rome in the 2nd century CE, the answers were "no" and "yes": women were not made of the same substance as men, and they had conditions that were uniquely female. They thought that women's bodies were fundamentally different from men's bodies. Thus, women had their own physiology and their own unique diseases.[9]

Much of Hippocratic gynecology dealt with the "economy of fluids" in female bodies, that is, their humors, but also just their general *wetness*.[10] This wetness was understood to be necessary for reproduction; it was this excess fluid that formed and fed the developing fetus.[11] During pregnancy, this fluid would heat up in the uterus, evaporate, and solidify into a fetus—like bread baking in an oven, or milk solidifying into cheese.[12] But the rest of the time the woman had to go around with all that extra fluid in her body. The consequence was that she was generally too wet. The body's self-regulating mechanism for this fluid was menstruation. If the body did not become pregnant, it purged the excess fluidity in a more or less regular evacuation.

Menstruation signaled that the body was in a healthy state—not pathologically holding onto excess moisture—*and* that it was ready to take in the male semen and generate a fetus. Further, it indicated that the channels within a woman's body were open.[13] These channels were the veins and arteries that were conduits for transporting excess moisture from the woman's body, either to be purged or to support the growth of the developing fetus. They also included the passage from the uterus to the outside of the female body—what we call the vagina or birth canal, and what the ancient Greek and Roman physicians called the neck of the uterus. They labeled the parts of the female reproductive system from the point of view of the doctor—the outer part of the genitals were the lips (*labia*), then there was the mouth (*os*) and neck (*cervix*), then the body of the uterus, which terminated at its bottom (*fundus*).[14]

In contrast, male bodies were thought to produce little in the way of excess fluids. What they did produce could be evacuated through their pores as sweat. In extreme cases they might evacuate excess fluids from the anus in the form of burst hemorrhoids or other versions of "male menstruation," but this was much rarer than the monthly period experienced by female bodies.[15] Due to its reputation for being hotter, drier, and more tightly and compactly constructed, the male body was seen as fundamentally healthier than the female body. The colder, wetter, more loosely formed female body was, on the one hand, necessary for human reproduction, but on the other was considered inherently less healthy, on a day-to-day basis, than the male body. Its excessive moistness was thought to be the origin for all kinds of ailments, from headaches to cancers. Thus, there were medical texts devoted specifically to the management and care of the female body.

Galen, taking a different approach than the Hippocratic doctors, did not think that women were fundamentally different from men, nor that they needed their own type of medicine. He treated all patients—men, women, and children—using the same medical theories and principles.[16] The majority of his case histories involve male patients.[17] He did not produce much theoretical or anatomical writing devoted specifically to female patients.[18] However, when he did treat female patients for female complaints—issues having to do with their breasts, uteruses, or genitals—he showed that he knew how to apply the basic principles of therapeutic fluid regulation to their treatment.[19] In the case of Cyrilla in chapter 1, we saw him applying drying and dispersing remedies and redirecting her excess fluids to evacuate out of her urethra and bowels.

According to the way that Galen and his contemporaries conceptualized the body, excess fluids could be purged out of any orifice. Menstrual blood did not necessarily need to come from the uterus and out the vaginal canal. It could also come out in the urine or stool. In the medical writings of Celsus, a wealthy Roman man with wide-ranging academic interests who lived during the early 1st century CE, many types of bleeding could be related to menstrual purgation, including nosebleeds, bleeding from the gums, and blood erupting from abscesses.[20] If the extra fluid failed to emerge from the body on its own, the doctors could cut open a vein, usually at the elbow or ankle, to let it out.[21]

Medical writers thought that amenorrhea (lack of menstruation) indicated a number of potential issues: that the woman's body was still immature, was not producing excess fluids, and had small, constricted passageways; that something was blocking and narrowing the pathways of the body, causing fluids to build up, stagnate, and putrefy; or that the woman had overexerted herself in exercise, changing the nature of her flesh to such an extent that she had become in some sense masculine and thus did not have excess moisture to purge.[22] Of course, the lack of menstruation may also have indicated pregnancy and the growth of a fetus.

Excessive menstruation, as well as other sorts of vaginal discharges or "fluxes," indicated other types of bodily dysregulation. The fluxes could be bloody, phlegmy, or choleric (having too much black bile), aligning with a humoral theory of the body. They might signify that the body was too wet and loose, with a great deal of fluid to evacuate. According to the doctor Soranus, this excessive fluidity could be caused by overeating, lack of exercise, and a generally sedentary lifestyle.[23] The discharges could also indicate that there was something faulty with the closing mechanism of the womb. In the ancient world the uterus was sometimes imagined as an upside-down jar with a mouth that could open and close.[24] Proper functioning of the uterus depended on the jar opening regularly to admit male semen or allow for the outflow of excess fluid during menstruation, and then closing and locking in order to hold in the semen and the developing fetus. It would need to open again to allow for the exit of the fetus during childbirth. Female bodies in flux were not in good shape to become pregnant. Excess fluids, continually dripping or gushing from the neck of the womb, would likely drown out or wash away any male semen ejaculated into it.

Overall, in these texts women's medical issues are reproductive issues. Women's bodies were moist and unstable for the sake of reproduction. At the same time, this inherent moistness and instability could make it hard for them to reproduce. Gynecological texts from the 5th century BCE onward present medical expertise as the answer to this problem.[25]

THE WANDERING AND SUFFOCATING WOMB

Beyond the issues caused by fluid dysregulation, there were other troubles that could afflict reproductive-age women in ancient Rome. While these conditions came from and were centered around the uterus, their effects could be felt throughout the entire body. They had to do with the nature of the uterus and its unique place and function within the body. For Cyrilla's case, understanding the nature of the uterus and what could go wrong with it from the ancient Roman perspective will help us see how she and the other women around her may have understood her condition.

The nature of the uterus, according to some people in the ancient Mediterranean, was that it was able to move around the interior of the body—up and down, side to side. This phenomenon has been dubbed the "wandering womb" by modern scholars.[26] The ancient medical writers called the main condition caused by the mobile uterus "hysterical *pnix*," which means "uterine suffocation." Through its movements, they explained, the uterus could overwhelm, envelope, and suffocate other organs, or even the woman herself, cutting off the respiratory passageways within the body.[27] In the Hippocratic treatise *Diseases of Women* 2 (5th century BCE), the author describes the uterus as being able to move from the lower abdomen up to the head, cutting off airflow through a woman's neck.[28] It could "fall upon" or "attack" the liver, heart, ribs, bladder, or hips, and it was able to move downward as well, extruding out of the vagina such that it could be seen or felt via a manual examination of the external genitalia.[29] Perhaps this language was meant to instill in women an idea of their own bodies as attacking them. The solution offered by the doctors was defense through intercourse, pregnancy, and childbirth.

The litany of ailments that the wandering womb could cause was expansive: a sensation of strangulation, body shivers, fever, pain in the groin, thick urine, a large and hardened abdomen, teeth grinding, loss of appetite, difficulty sleeping, fretfulness, jerky movements, vomiting of phlegm, extreme thirst, pain on touch, fainting, loss of voice, irregular breathing, biting sensations in the uterus or stomach, inflammation of the womb or stomach, and swelling in the legs and feet.[30]

Clearly these ideas about how the uterus could move and the damage its movements could do to the body come out of an understanding of the body that was very different from our own. We have already seen that the uterus was sometimes interpreted as an upside-down jar. Specifically, it was imagined as a cupping vessel, a medical instrument used by doctors in the ancient world to draw excess or diseased fluids and pollutions from the body ("cupping" is still performed by many paramedical practitioners today).[31]

But the idea that the uterus could move and strangle comes from another metaphorical image common in the ancient Mediterranean: the uterus as octopus. This comparison probably arose from observed similarities between the octopus and animal uteruses, which the Greeks and Romans had access to through animal dissections.[32] In particular, the uterus of the cow was comparable to the octopus: it had a similar rubbery texture, pale pinkish color, and curling tentacles/horns with caruncles that could look like suckers. The attributes of the octopus were well known to the ancient Greeks. They observed its intelligence and changeability and ascribed to it a wily, crafty nature. They then projected these same features and characterizations onto the uterus.[33] In his *Timaeus,* a philosophical text from the 5th century BCE, Plato describes the uterus as "a living creature who longs for child-making."[34] Whenever it has gone too long without a child, it becomes "irritable" and "wanders" through the body, cutting off respiration and causing all manner of illness.

In this same part of the treatise, Plato also describes the penis as an independent, animal-like entity with raging desires. But while the desires of the uterus were reproductive, those of the penis were imagined as sexual. The penis sought orgasm, while the uterus sought to house and grow a fetus. And while both organs moved, it was only the womb's movements that were seen as pathological.[35]

Descriptions of the wandering womb portray a uterus that is unmoored in the body. It's possible that for some people in the ancient Mediterranean, the uterus did not have a designated place because it was the only organ that was unique to the female body—the male body being seen as the standard.[36] The ancient medical writers recognized that at least theoretically, the uterus could be removed without harming the rest of the body. Soranus writes about such operations being performed on pigs.[37] But there is no evidence that a hysterectomy was ever performed on a living woman in ancient Greece or Rome.

The idea of a wandering womb isn't completely bizarre. Uterine prolapse was a known condition in antiquity and one that may have occurred frequently given the number of times women gave birth.[38] If the womb could move down out of the vagina, surely it could also move side to side or up toward the diaphragm. And when the uterus prolapsed, it was described as feeling "like the head of an octopus."[39]

KNOWLEDGE OF THE BODY

The fact that the image of a cupping-vessel-like uterus—solid and rigid, with a fixed opening and closing mechanism—appears to be entirely at odds with the image of an octopus-like uterus—soft-bodied, flexible, and constantly in motion—doesn't seem to have bothered people in the ancient world. Conceptually, the uterus was a vessel for collecting fluids, *and also* an octopus that could crawl around the interior of the body, wrapping its tentacles around other organs and suffocating them, as an octopus envelops and consumes its prey. Perhaps different metaphorical images of the uterus made sense in different contexts, or from different perspectives. The one (the cupping vessel) is notably passive, while the other (the octopus) is active. The image of the uterus as cupping vessel works for thinking about the process of fluid regulation in the female body: opening, closing, holding, leaking. It also makes sense for pregnancy, if we think about the fetus growing in the uterus as a cucumber growing in a clay pot, as one of the Hippocratic writers does in a text called *Generation:* "It's like if someone were to put a growing cucumber . . . into a cup: it will grow like the cup in size and shape . . . so it is with an infant."[40] In this analogy, the uterus is a firm-sided vessel whose size and shape determines the size and shape of the growing fetus. A small cup-like uterus will result in a small, weak fetus, while a larger vessel allows the fetus space to achieve its full size.

The octopus-like uterus, then, could represent a more sensorial, embodied experience of the uterus. What does it *feel* like to have a uterus? Maybe it feels like an octopus crawling around inside you and attacking your other organs. Maybe the sensations of contractions in labor feel like octopus tentacles reaching out and squeezing your insides.

How did the ancient Greeks and Romans reconcile these metaphors of the uterus with actual human uteruses? They rarely, if ever, had access to uteruses outside the human body. For the most part, with one notable exception, the Greek and Romans did not practice human dissection. During a brief period in the 4th and 3rd centuries BCE, two physicians named Herophilus and Erasistratus practiced human dissection in Alexandria, Egypt.[41] Herophilus wrote anatomical treatises, including one about the uterus, that do not survive today but that were used and referred to by the medical writers who came after him. Otherwise, there were religious and cultural taboos against human dissection. Doctors had to rely on animal dissection—of dogs, pigs, monkeys, sheep, and cows—as well as on the writings that Herophilus left behind.[42]

From references in later sources, it is evident that the anatomical knowledge that Herophilus gained from performing human dissections circulated throughout the Mediterranean.[43] In his treatise on the anatomy of the uterus, Herophilus described the ligaments and tendons that attach the uterus to the interior of the body. Later anatomies of the uterus incorporated these tendons and ligaments into their understanding of the interior of the body. In a medical treatise from the 2nd century CE, the physician Aretaeus explained that there are ligaments at both the fundus (the top of the uterus) and the cervix; the ones at the fundus are narrow, allowing for less movement, while the ones at the cervix are broad, like the sails of a ship.[44] Soranus, too, described the thin membranes that connect the uterus to the bladder, rectum, hips, and sacrum.[45]

We might think that widespread knowledge of these anchoring ligaments and tendons would have dispelled the idea of the wandering womb. There was certainly some hostility to the idea of a wandering and strangling uterus starting to crop up in the 2nd century, but not nearly as much as we might expect. In his *Gynecology*, Soranus posts a single challenge to the idea of an animal-like uterus: "The uterus does not rush forth like a wild animal from its lair."[46] This admonishment fits into a larger dismissal of "superstition" that is a theme in Soranus.[47] But overall, belief in the wandering womb and uterine suffocation persisted.

Aretaeus, with his careful description of the sail-like uterine ligaments, actually provided one of the most vivid descriptions of the mobile, animal-like womb. He did not ignore the anatomical discoveries of Herophilus but incorporated them into his image of a malevolent, sentient uterus. Despite the fact that the uterus was attached to the body via ligaments, these ligaments, he explained, could expand and contract, giving the uterus full range of motion throughout the interior of the abdomen.[48]

DOCTORS' TREATMENTS

The thread running through all of the gynecological writings, from the Hippocratics to Soranus and Galen, was the message that there was *a lot* that could go seriously wrong with the uterus. Even as anatomical knowledge grew and the theories underlying uterine ailments changed, one theme stayed constant: the (alleged) need for medical intervention. Doctors presented regular gynecological care as essential, both for the health of the woman herself and for her ability to make babies. They positioned themselves as the caretakers and facilitators of potential mothers.

What we see in Soranus's gynecological treatise is that doctors in the Roman Empire made it their business to get female patients in the best state to conceive. His reasoning went something like this: because of the inherent tendency of the female body toward ill health, caused by its excessive moistness, particular regimens of diet and exercise were key to keeping it healthy. When something went wrong with the flow of fluids, the doctors might prescribe herbal remedies in the form of drinks, douches, ointments, plasters, pessaries, and fumigations. They would also employ manual therapies: massage, scrubs, and bloodletting. The remedies followed well-established principles of herbal medicine that are still used today. Astringent substances were used to dry up excess fluids, while loosening herbs like diuretics (for urine), emmenagogues (for menstruation), emetics (for vomit), and laxatives (for feces) were used to break up and purge blockages and swellings in the body.

To deal with the threat posed by the mobile womb and uterine suffocation, the Hippocratic gynecological texts recommended a combination of odor therapy and uterine fumigation.[49] The idea was that the animal-like uterus was able to sense and respond to strong odors. It could be enticed and attracted by sweet-smelling substances such as frankincense, myrrh, and rose; and contrastingly, it could be repelled by foul-smelling substances such as burning hair or pitch, bitumen, and turpentine. These principles of attraction and repulsion were used to compel the uterus's movements. If the uterus had charged up toward the upper abdomen or into the neck, then foul smelling substances would be held up to the woman's nose to repel it downward, while at the same time a sweet-smelling fumigation (vapors from a steam bath or smoke from incense) would be directed up her vagina to entice it in the same direction. If the uterus had moved down, the opposite arrangement would be used, with pleasant incense at the nose and foul-smelling smoke in the vagina.

The writer of the Hippocratic text *Diseases of Women* 2 described the elaborate process of fumigating the uterus.[50] He instructed the practitioner to make a hole in the lid of an earthenware pot, into which a slim metal pipe could be inserted, making sure to fit the pipe precisely so that no vapor could escape out the sides of the hole. The pot contained the fumigating substance—in this case, foul-smelling garlic and seal oil. The pot was set into a depression in the ground with a fire built underneath it. The patient was to sit over the pot, inserting the metal pipe into her vagina, so that the steam went directly up to her uterus.

It's clear that these same remedies were still being used in the 2nd century CE, although in some cases with different theoretical underpinnings. Soranus's uterine therapies included odor therapy and fumigation, but his explanations for why they worked were different.[51] Fumigation and odor therapies didn't "attract" or "repel" a sentient animal-womb, he said, but sweet smells and caustic pessaries mechanically manipulated the inflamed or loosened uterine membranes. These remedies worked due to principles of constriction and relaxation, tightening and loosening.[52] For him, uterine concerns could be divided into retained fluids and hard growths (things were too tight), excessive fluids and lax membranes (things were too loose), and inflammation. His treatments were the same as those in earlier texts. There were still uterine movements, but they were confined to the "neck" and "mouth" (the area around the cervix).

Soranus wrote, "The orifice of the uterus and its neck suffer bending, flexation, sometimes laterally, forward, or backward and sometimes upward or downward, and sometimes becoming entirely dislocated."[53] These ligament-anchored bendings and flexings of the cervix and vagina could give the feeling of a moving uterus. Therapies acted mechanically on the flesh; they didn't depend on a sentient uterus. The upshot was that although Soranus argued against the idea of a mobile, animal-like uterus, his remedies for uterine issues remained largely unchanged from those of earlier medical texts. Even if he did not believe in the idea of a wandering womb, his patients probably did. The consistent remedies were likely intended to appeal to patients' beliefs about their own bodies.[54]

Galen, too, ridiculed the notion of a wandering and animalistic womb. He scoffed that it was "totally absurd" that anyone would think that a "dried-up womb would turn toward other organs looking for moisture."[55] "It is completely senseless," he went on, "to consider the uterus an animal." Nonetheless, Galen was finely attuned to women's beliefs about their own bodies, writing, "I have seen many 'hysterical' women, as they call themselves and as the older female physicians call them, from whom it is likely they heard the term."[56]

In the "hysterical" condition Galen describes, those afflicted are in a catatonic state: they have low to no pulse and minimal respiration and are weak and non-responsive. Some appear to be dead. The female doctors, practicing the same type of Hippocratic medicine as Cyrilla's midwives, attribute this affliction, what they call the "uterine condition," to the mobile womb. Galen has an alternative theory. The cause, he explains, is retained menstrual fluid or female semen. This female semen was analogous to male semen, and Galen thought that it was produced in the uterus and contributed to reproduction. When not evacuated regularly in the monthly period, it could putrefy, causing a number of pathological symptoms and even eventually killing the woman. The disease particularly afflicted women who had previously been sexually active, especially "those who had been pregnant and were eager to have intercourse but were now deprived of all this."[57] The deprivation of intercourse could cause a back-up of the female semen, even in a woman who was menstruating regularly.

Despite his novel theoretical explanation, Galen employed the same remedies as those who were treating the wandering womb.[58] In the same treatise, he recounts a story he has heard of a woman who was a widow for a long time.[59] Beset by various disturbances and tensions, she turned to a midwife for help.[60] The midwife diagnosed her as having a "pulled-up womb"—that is, a wandering womb. The widow used the remedies that were typical in this situation: a heating medicament applied manually to the genitals, meant to coax the womb back down to its appropriate position in the body. The remedy worked. The woman experienced contractions of pain and pleasure like those "experienced during sexual intercourse" and "emitted a large quantity of heavy semen." In the midwife's estimation, the widow had reset her wandering womb. But according to Galen, she had released retained seed, blocked up in her uterus from long widowhood and lack of intercourse. Even though the explanations were different, the remedy was the same. As for the widow, she probably didn't care what Galen thought. The midwife's remedy was effective and she was cured.

Other texts by Galen show him giving credence to the idea of the mobile uterus. In a letter to a friend, he advises using odor therapy to deal with a "rising uterus," and in a book of herbal remedies, he suggests that a woman inhale foul-smelling substances for the same condition.[61]

The need to appeal to patient beliefs arose from the nature of the medical marketplace of ancient Rome. Along with the services of medical doctors like Soranus and Galen, women had access to other forms of therapy. They could engage the services of midwives (as Cyrilla did), root cutters (herbal medicine suppliers), temple priests, or fortune tellers.[62] While we might think that there is a divide today between rational medicine and magic or superstition, patients in the ancient world did not feel the same.[63] Despite the rhetoric of doctors suggesting otherwise, from a patient's point of view, medicine, religion, and magic were not in competition, but instead were complementary.

As much as ancient doctors might have wanted to set themselves apart from other medical practitioners by championing "rational" medicine and eschewing superstition, such distinctions would have made little sense to their patients. People seeking treatment in the ancient world likely used multiple therapies at the same time. In Cyrilla's case, her first course of action was to seek out her usual midwives. Even once Galen was brought on the case, he was still coordinating her care with these midwives as well as with Cyrilla's other attendants. But Cyrilla had other therapies available to her as well, therapies that we might today call religious or magical. For Cyrilla and women like her, these therapies gave them agency in their own care that increasingly powerful, male-dominated "gynecology" did not.

OTHER THERAPIES

Doctors weren't the only game in town in the 160s. Cyrilla probably sought out other therapies as well. Perhaps she commissioned or purchased a prefabricated uterine amulet—a small oval gemstone inscribed with religious/magical formulas and figures and gynecological iconography (see fig. 1). Of all the objects that remain from the ancient Greco-Roman world, these amulets are some of the most tantalizing.

A few hundred of these uterine amulets from around the Mediterranean have been found and catalogued.[64] They date to the first centuries CE. They are very small—only a centimeter or two across—and would likely have been mass-produced by amulet carvers who were perhaps stationed close to healing temples and sanctuaries. Women purchased them directly from the carvers or indirectly from priests or midwives.[65] They carried them in pockets and pouches, or wore them tied around the body on strings, or set into rings, brooches, and necklaces.

The amulets are important because they reveal a type of gynecological therapy distinct from the medical texts.

When amulets come up in the medical texts, they are tolerated. Soranus tells us that amulets are ineffectual but largely harmless.[66] Galen actually sees some use in them. He famously tests a green jade amulet, tied around the neck, for digestive issues that he is experiencing. He finds it effective, largely, he suspects, based on the mineral properties of the jade rather than anything in particular that is inscribed on the amulet.[67]

What do these amulets show and how do they match up with the gynecological texts? Many of these tiny amulets are inscribed with uteruses in the shape of an upside-down cupping vessel (see fig. 1).[68] These cupping-vessel-like uteruses have large keys at their mouths, signifying the opening and closing of the cervix.[69] A few of the amulets also feature, on the back side, a uterus in the form of an octopus—a circular body with squiggly legs radiating outwards from one half.[70] The amulets contain inscribed magical formulas in Greek lettering, as well as Egyptian gods such as Isis, Bes, baby Horus, Khnoum, Anubis, and Cnoubis.

The cupping-vessel-like uterus represents the holding function of the uterus—for fluids and fetuses. The key signifies a uterus that is working properly—opening to let out menstrual fluid and take in semen and closing to hold in the fetus—and that it is locked in place, not wandering throughout the body. The octopus-like uterus represents the uterus's capacity to cause significant harm in the body by moving, smothering, and suffocating, as well as its ability to grasp onto semen and contract during childbirth. The magical formulas appealed to a protective deity of the uterus (Ororiouth) and worked to bind the uterus in place.[71] And the deities were traditional protectors of women (Isis, Bes), children (Horus, Khnoum), and interior functions of the body (Chnoubis).[72] Their presence on the amulets signaled that they were being invoked to guard potential mothers, as well as prenatal and birthing women.

In nearly every amulet, the figures (uteruses and deities) are surrounded by an ouroboros, the snake that eats its own tail, signifying a

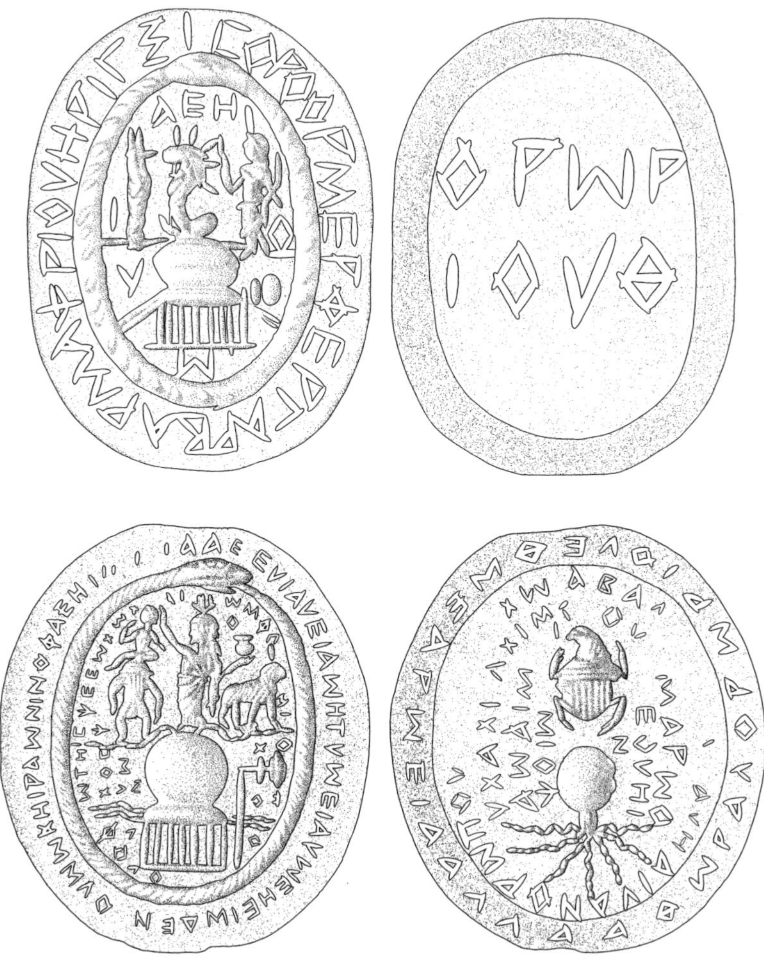

FIGURE 1. Front and back of two uterine amulets made from hematite with cupping-vessel-style uteruses, octopus-style uteruses, ouroboros snakes, figures, magical symbols, and formulas; such amulets were worn on the body for a variety of gynecological and obstetrical purposes. Top: CBd 176, 20 × 15 × 3 mm. Bottom: CBd 747, 23 × 20 × 3 mm. 1st–4th century CE. British Museum. Drawings by Hayley Monroe.

binding, protective action taken against a sentient, malevolent entity.[73] The Egyptian deities stand on top of the uterus, weighing it down so that it can't charge up to the neck and strangle the woman. Some of the amulets are inscribed with an explicit command directed at a misbehaving uterus: "Womb, retract!" Another proclaims simply, "Therapy for the womb." Yet another gets personal: "Restrain the womb of Maxeima."[74] Amulet carvers could add names to concentrate and intensify the power of the amulet, ensuring that its effects were felt by the right person.

Unfortunately, we cannot know the extent to which medical texts were influencing the images on these amulets. Nor can we know the extent to which the women purchasing these amulets were making choices based on how they envisioned their uteruses. The mass-produced nature of these amulets implies that there was standard iconography that was expected to appear on them. Nonetheless, it is interesting that at least some of these amulets show two radically different ideas of the uterus on the same gem—the cupping vessel and the octopus. It also matters that the use of and market in amulets was driven by women—likely women of all social and economic classes.[75] The amulets that survive are made of semi-precious gemstones—hematite, carnelian, jasper—but there were thousands more amulets made of cheaper, perishable materials—wood, leather—that do not survive.[76] These would have been less expensive and more widely available.

Another issue with the amulets is that we don't know where individual ones come from. When amateur archaeologists first started digging them up in the 19th century, they would pocket these small finds. The gems ended up in private antiquities collections—where many remain today—and only some made their way into museums. It would be great to be able to look for geographical patterns in the iconography of the gems. Maybe those with octopus-wombs came from places on the sea, from people who were familiar with octopuses and their ways.

The best that we can say is that there were similar metaphorical images of the uterus used by different types of medical practitioners, and that women had their own ways of treating their uterine ailments, separate from the medical doctors. Even women who were illiterate and never had access to the theory-dense medical writings of Aretaeus, Soranus, and Galen could see the pictographs on the amulets. They may not have understood the lettering or the particular resonances of the different Egyptian gods if they were not themselves Egyptian, but that didn't matter. The important thing was that the amulets were produced (supposedly) by people who did.

As much as it's tempting to trace the history of medicine through the medical texts alone, the amulets show us that what was going on was richer and more complex than that story suggests. Medicine wasn't neatly divided between the "rational" therapies of men like Soranus and Galen and the medical-magical treatments of priests and amulet carvers. The history of reproduction is not a simple line of progress from superstition to reason. Even today there are people with valid concerns about the overmedicalization of childbirth. In the ancient world too, especially from the perspective of patients, Galen may not have seemed like the best option. He may have acted like his expertise is what saved Cyrilla. But what would that same episode have been like from Cyrilla's perspective?

THE TROUBLE WITH CYRILLA

From what Galen tells us, Cyrilla was suffering from excess fluid in her body.[77] Galen did not say why, but it's clear from his description that he thought that the excess fluid was not only causing her to have continuous vaginal discharge—the "female flux"—but that it had also built up inside her uterus, solidifying and putrefying into a semi-solid mass. This mass was the source of her abdominal swelling, which her female attendants mistook for pregnancy.

In order to treat her, the midwives followed herbal principles. They administered astringent, drying herbs, probably in the form of teas, as well as vaginal douches and pessaries.[78] Their aim was to dry up the excess fluids throughout her whole body. But the treatments were not working. When she started to develop a hard mass in her abdomen, they thought she was pregnant, and they began giving her daily baths. It seems like it was these daily baths that caused Cyrilla to faint, as she simultaneously expelled a large amount of liquid from her vagina.

What Galen realized is that the drying herbs alone were not helping Cyrilla. The midwives, expert as they were, had been treating the symptoms (vaginal discharges) but not the root cause of the disease. Although he does not spell it out for us, it's likely that what Galen saw as bringing about Cyrilla's massive, watery purge was the whole-body warming effect of the bath. He recognized that in addition to trying to stem the flow of fluids from Cyrilla's vagina, he also needed to break up and disperse the putrefying mass in her abdomen. That's why he started massaging her upper stomach with nard oil, and why he got her attendants to start rubbing her hands and feet, bringing blood and sensation back to her extremities. For twenty days following the critical moment in the bath, Galen concentrated on dispersing the abdominal mass, warming Cyrilla's body with beach sand and giving her daily massages with alternating soft and rough cloths. Rather than using only astringent, drying remedies as the midwives had, he started using purgatives—emmenagogues, diuretics, and laxatives—in order to expel the excess fluids from her body.

As Galen tells it, Cyrilla got better because he was a more astute observer of her illness than her midwives and other doctors. His remedies themselves weren't unique, but he applied them in just the right way at just the right moment. For him, this episode displayed his superior medical prowess. Having recently moved to Rome from Pergamum, he used this episode and the others in the collection to advertise his medical skills and to make a name for himself among Rome's elite.

From Cyrilla's point of view, she must have realized that something was wrong with her when she had the continuous vaginal flux instead of her menstrual period. In addition to consulting her usual midwives, it's possible she also purchased an amulet to correct and protect her malfunctioning uterus. Maybe she imagined her uterus as a leaky clay vessel. Perhaps she experienced the sensation of an octopus crawling around in her abdomen.

When the abdominal mass started developing and the midwives told her that she was pregnant, she may have felt relief that the remedies, medical and magical, had worked. Instead of expelling her husband's semen, her uterus had held onto it, closing and locking up properly to hold her growing baby. Perhaps she thought the amulet had been effective at stopping the destructive movements of her octopus-like womb.

Or maybe the news that she was pregnant was frightening or emotionally fraught. As the mother of a young son, Cyrilla had prior experience with pregnancy and childbirth. Depending on how that birth had gone, she might have been concerned about having to go through the process again. Given the fact that her son was seven or eight years old, it's likely that she had had other pregnancies as well. Perhaps she had other children that we don't know about because Galen didn't care to mention them. Or maybe she had a history of miscarriages and stillbirths.

Galen attributes Cyrilla's reluctance to involve him to "embarrassment" and "modesty." But maybe Cyrilla was content with the healthcare that she had previously received from her midwives. It's not surprising that up to this time, her medical care did not involve a male doctor. Recall that it was her husband, Boethus, who got Galen involved. Perhaps he was trying out the new fad in his social network.

From our vantage point in the 21st century, there seems to be a kind of inevitability to the encroachment of medicine and medicalization upon childbirth. But in Cyrilla's time, in the 2nd century, we can see how Galen's foray into gynecology and reproductive health was as much a matter of jockeying for power, money, clientele and prestige as it was about providing superior medical care. Cyrilla's potential motherhood and her female troubles, combined with her high social and economic status, made her a perfect candidate for medical intervention and manipulation.

What would we say was wrong with Cyrilla today? Maybe she had ovarian cancer, or a benign cyst or tumor. Perhaps she experienced uterine fibroids or an ectopic pregnancy. It could have been any of these things, but crucially, from Cyrilla's point of view, it was none of them. We are all limited to experiencing things that have been named and defined by the culture in which we live. It's not that ovarian cancer did not exist in ancient Rome; it almost certainly did. But what we experience, what we call it, and how we define that experience are determined by the cultural narratives and the language available to us. Retrospective diagnosis—trying to understand the illnesses of the past through categories of the present—can be interesting and useful, but it has limitations.[79] We are missing crucial pieces of information from Cyrilla's case history that would let us know whether what happened to her was malignant or benign. Galen was not always interested in the same information that we are, and what functioned as crucial signs to him do not always translate to pieces of information salient to us. Even more frustratingly, Galen does not give us access to what Cyrilla was thinking and feeling about what was going on in her body.

All we know is that Boethus's wife was a woman of reproductive age. She had a serious problem with her vagina or her uterus that was likely interfering with her ability to get pregnant. In fact, we are told, there were a lot of uterine problems that could affect the reproductive function of women who were similar to Boethus's wife in age and life stage. The impression that the medical and literary texts from the Roman Empire give is that the most important role these young women served was as mothers and potential mothers. In order for them to carry out their duties, their moist, leaky, fleshy bodies needed to be carefully monitored, controlled, and remedied—by doctors and husbands. Potential mothers were under threat from their very own bodies. They could produce excess fluids—more than their bodies could purge during their menstrual periods. Their wombs could malfunction or even rebel, crawling and rushing around inside their bodies, suffocating organs, expelling semen.

Generally, women were under the care of midwives, female relatives, or other attendants. We don't know exactly why Galen took on this case, though we do know that Boethus asked him to and that he rewarded his efforts with an enormous sum of money. What this episode demonstrates is that there was room—lucrative room—for Galen, and presumably for other elite, overwhelmingly male medical practitioners, in gynecology. The message from doctors like Aretaeus, Soranus, and Galen was that, going forward, their services would be necessary to prepare and maintain women for the all-important task of human reproduction.

THREE

The Self-Observant Women Get Pregnant

Kos, 410 BCE

Demetria adjusts her chiton, draping the fabric evenly over both shoulders, and gargles with salt water to clear her throat. She trills up and down a scale, warming up her voice. She's been hired to sing at a banquet. But she won't get paid for the gig; the money will go to her enslaver, a wealthy woman named Basilia. She feels an uncharacteristic twinge in her belly. Nerves? Indigestion?

By the end of her set, Demetria knows that whatever is ailing her is not typical. She goes to Basilia and explains her symptoms. After asking a few more questions, Basilia recognizes the signs. Demetria is pregnant. Thinking only of diminished profits if her best singer is out of commission, Basilia consults with her relative, who is a doctor. She explains the situation and the doctor—a man named Hippocrates—advises Basilia to have her singing girl jump up and down, vigorously kicking her buttocks in a move called the "Lacedemonian Leap." Demetria does as she's told and performs several leaps and kicks, wearing only her chiton and no undergarment. A white viscous mass falls out of her vagina and onto the floor. Hippocrates will later say that this mass is a six-day-old fetus.

Rome, 172 CE

Flavia, Helena, and Claudia stand in the marketplace talking. Flavia runs a vegetable stand with produce from her garden on the outskirts of the city. Today, she's selling some leeks to Helena, who is enslaved and does the market shopping for her household. Claudia is a midwife who assisted at the birth of Flavia's children as well as the births of many children in Helena's household. They're all in their forties and have known each other for many years. They've each given birth to several children. Flavia's daughter Cornelia, who is helping her mother at the market, is six months pregnant with her first baby. They're chatting about mutual friends and acquaintances, exclaiming over Cornelia's pregnancy, and bemoaning the price of grain.

Suddenly, a pompous man comes up to them, flanked by an entourage of followers and onlookers. Claudia recognizes him and greets him by name. He's a Greek doctor who has been in and out of the city for the past decade. He and Claudia have worked together on some cases involving female patients. She sighs inwardly and makes a subtle gesture toward the other two women to indicate that she is annoyed. The doctor asks if he can have a word with the women. He has a few questions of a delicate nature that he would like to ask them. They have just the sort of expertise he's looking for.

The women agree to a chat. Flavia hands the vegetable stand over to Cornelia and they move to the edge of the market where the crowd is thinner and less chaotic. The doctor's eager hangers-on follow. With very little preamble, he launches in, explaining that he has been conducting some experiments to determine when and how pregnancy occurs. He's been observing female animals during and after mating, noting which animals discharge semen and which ones hold on to it. Matching that up with those animals who subsequently get pregnant, he's been noticing a pattern. The female animals that discharge semen after mating do not become pregnant, while those that hold onto it do. He asks the women if they have noticed something similar in themselves after having sex. He explains that he trusts their judgment because he knows that they are rather self-observant. In his work with Claudia, he has been impressed with the midwife's knowledge and expertise.

The women laugh. Yes, they say, when the semen stays inside them after having sex, they become pregnant. Flavia makes a crude joke accompanied by hand gestures and there are fresh peals of laughter. But, Claudia says, you want to know something else? The doctor leans in eagerly. The women describe what conception feels like. They tell him that when they conceive, they can feel their uteruses moving—crawling—and grasping onto the semen. The doctor's eyes light up. As he takes his leave, the women shake their heads in amusement.

These two episodes are partly fictitious, extrapolated from skeletal passages in ancient medical texts. The first appears in a Hippocratic text called *Nature of the Child*, which is one of the earliest embryological texts in the

Western world.[1] We don't know exactly when it was written or when the events it describes took place, but it was sometime in the late 400s or early 300s BCE. It's a treatise concerned with how the fetus forms and develops in the uterus. Its writer—Hippocrates or one of his followers—does not name the singing girl or her enslaver, nor do we hear about the girl's feelings or perspective.[2] But we are told that the leaping and buttock-kicking did cause an abortion and that a small mass of congealed sperm, looking like a partially formed fetus, fell out of the girl's vagina.

The second story comes from Galen, the 2nd-century doctor we encountered in the previous two chapters.[3] He's the pompous man in the marketplace. In a text called *Semen*, he writes of his quest to understand conception using three different methods: observing farm animals during and after mating; consulting earlier medical writings, primarily by Hippocrates and Aristotle; and speaking with women who are "rather self-observant."[4] Again, we don't know exactly when the events described took place, but it was likely sometime in the late 160s or early 170s CE.

These two stories are significant because they provide evidence for the same hypothesis: pregnancy happens when semen stays in the vagina after sex. Although the first story was written in the 5th or 4th century BCE, it, along with the other Hippocratic gynecological writings, was in wide circulation in the 2nd century CE and hugely influential on Galen. It showed, according to Galen, that male semen congeals to form the physical body of the fetus.[5] The Hippocratic text goes on to describe the appearance of the aborted embryo:

> It was as if someone had removed the shell of a raw egg, and the fluid part inside could be seen through the internal membrane.... It was red and roundish; broad, white strands were visible inside the membrane, pressed together with thick, red serum, and around the membrane on the outside there was bloody material.[6]

The Hippocratic writer, and Galen after him, explained that the red, bloody parts starting to form the embryonic body were from the red, bloody menstrual fluid, retained inside the womb at the time of conception. The white strands and the viscous membrane were evidence that the white, viscous male semen had stayed inside the uterus after intercourse and was also forming part of the developing embryo. Why is that important? There was a debate going on at the time as to whether the male semen contributed to the physical makeup of the fetal body or merely ignited a spark of life in the inert menstrual fluid. Some of Galen's rival physicians at Rome, the self-identified Aristotelians and the Peripatetics, thought that semen was more like the carpenter that fashions wood into a couch—the creator of life, but not a physical part of the finished product.[7] For Galen, the semen was more like rennet in milk, causing it to solidify into cheese, *and also* remaining as part of the final product.[8] It was important for him that the male semen did both—it contained the spark of life *and* it contributed to the material makeup of the fetal body. According to Galen, the semen turned into veins, arteries, and nerves—the strong, stretchy conduits of blood, feelings, and intelligence running through the body.[9]

This debate over the role of the semen in generation paralleled a similar debate about female contribution to generation. Physicians and theorists in the 2nd century CE debated whether women had a "seed" like men that was emitted during sexual intercourse (and orgasm), or whether their contribution to generation was only the blood of the menstrual fluid, which collected in the uterus for the purpose of forming the fetal body.[10] Beyond archaic debates about the powers of sperm, what's interesting about the passages is how women's knowledge functions in these male-authored medical texts.

How real were Galen's self-observant women? How many were there? How old were they? By what criteria were they deemed self-observant? Did Galen actually talk to them, or does he just say that he did, to add authenticity to his investigation? These are unanswerable questions. Galen inserts the testimony of the women—whom I'm calling Flavia, Helena, and Claudia, but whom Galen leaves unnamed—between his own observations of mating farm animals and the medical and scientific writings of earlier men. The lived experiences of these women, he asserts, are more reliable than the writings of long-dead scientists and physicians. But they are less reliable than his own observations.

The hierarchical nature of Galen's three-step approach is evident. He states that he started with the "clearest" means of investigation: he observed female animals—horses, dogs, asses, cattle, goats, and sheep—during and after mating.[11] Only once he had made these observations did he ask the women what they experienced. Then, to bolster his conclusions, he turned to the writings of other scientists and physicians. One of these writings was the Hippocratic *Nature of the Child*, and specifically the story about the enslaved singing girl and her self-induced abortion. Finally, intrigued by the women's claims that they could feel the uterus grasping the semen at the moment of conception, he returned once again to the female animals. He dissected a large number of pregnant animals, noting that every time, he could see the uterus wrapped around the embryo.[12] To his satisfaction, this wrapping and clinging of the uterus to the embryo proved the claims of the self-observant women. So his investigation begins and ends with his own observations of female animals. Galen acknowledges that the women's contributions are significant, but they are less important than his own experiments on animals.

Galen's story also reveals popular ideas about the nature of the uterus. In the act of conception, Galen writes that the uterus was "like a physician's cupping vessel."[13] The sucking action pulled the semen up through the vaginal canal and the bulbous, cup-like quality of the uterus made it a good home for a fetus. But the description given by the women themselves sounds like nothing so much as that octopus-like uterus that we saw in chapter 2. Just as the octopus grasped and enveloped its prey with its suckered tentacles, the uterus grasped and enveloped the sperm. Galen seems to adopt the women's language when, later in the treatise, he writes, "The whole uterus wants to wrap itself around the semen . . . it seizes the . . . [semen], just like an octopus seizes what it touches with its suckers."[14] This uterus in the process of conception "wants," "wraps," and "seizes"; it's like an octopus grasping with its suckers. Together, these metaphors of the physician's cupping vessel and the octopus reveal beliefs about the mechanism of conception.

In this chapter and the next we will examine ancient medical understandings of conception and explore how a Roman woman would have dealt with the problem of infertility. We will consider medical theories of and recommendations for infertility, as well as other avenues of aid she would have had available to her. As we will see, according to medical theory, it was women who were largely responsible for reproductive failures, but medical men who held the solution.

PLEASURE AND CONCEPTION

As is evident in the story of the midwife Claudia and her friends, in the 2nd century it was understood that conception occurred through sexual intercourse and the mingling of male semen with menstrual fluid in the uterus. Although they didn't know about the ovum, medical writers of the time argued for the existence of female semen that was analogous to male semen. Expanding on a principle from Aristotle (4th century BCE), Galen described the female body as a comparable but lesser version of the male body.[15] For him, the male body was the physiological standard. Since he saw the female body as a second-rate male body, any physiological processes that took place in the male body were also thought to occur in the female body, but in an altered or less effective way.

If male and female bodies came from the same mold, why were female bodies seen as second-rate? The short answer is patriarchy. Men held power; therefore, they had to be better in every way, including in the makeup and functioning of their bodies. But male physicians also sought to give a *rational* explanation for women's comprehensive subordination; they located female inferiority in the processes of conception and fetal development. Here's how it worked in Galen: He imagined the male and female genitals as analogues of one another. The male genitals ejected or popped out from the body during fetal development, he thought, due to a hot and dry uterine environment. The hot, dry environment allowed the embryo to fully develop and "set"—just like that bread in the oven or cheese in the pot—into the completed male form.[16] The female genitals, though, remained internal and underdeveloped due to a cold, wet uterine environment.[17] So male and female started from the same stuff but were differentiated due to the condition of the womb during development. The female, Galen was careful to explain, is a necessary but incomplete outcome of reproduction.

In a treatise called *The Function of the Parts of the Human Body*, Galen provides a memorable image: the male and female genitals are inverses of each other. If you were to turn the penis up into the body, you would get the vagina and uterus.[18] This image endured for centuries in Western medical and scientific thought. A drawing from the famous 16th-century Italian anatomist Andreas Vesalius's *On the Makeup of the Human Body* shows the tenacity of Galen's analogy. Despite Vesalius's extensive dissection of actual human bodies, he included a drawing of the vagina and uterus based on Galen's 2nd-century description (see fig. 2).[19] What appears to be the head and glans of a penis is actually the vulva and labia. The shaft is the vagina, and the bulbous part at the top is the uterus, which has been opened to show the hollow interior.[20]

Of course, Galen is roughly correct in his description of what we now call genital homology; male and female reproductive organs develop from the same parts in utero, and for every structure in the male there is a corresponding altered structure in the female; for example, the glans of the penis is the same as the glans of the clitoris.[21] But while today fetal sex differentiation is largely attributed to chromosomes, for Galen and his contemporaries, the female was a necessary, but, in a sense, *failed* outcome of reproduction.

The ancient physicians also took genital homology in a much more sinister direction. Given the supposed similarities between the male and female sexual organs, Galen thought that, like the male, the female ejaculated semen during sex.[22] The complete development of the male (due to the hot, dry circumstances of his development) explained why the penis, an external organ, had the power to ejaculate sperm outwards and into other bodies, while the underdevelopment of the female explained why her ejaculation remained internal and invisible.[23] The evidence for internal ejaculation was the white substance that flowed out of some women—such as the widow discussed in chapter 2—when aroused.[24] But even when this semen could not be seen, it was thought

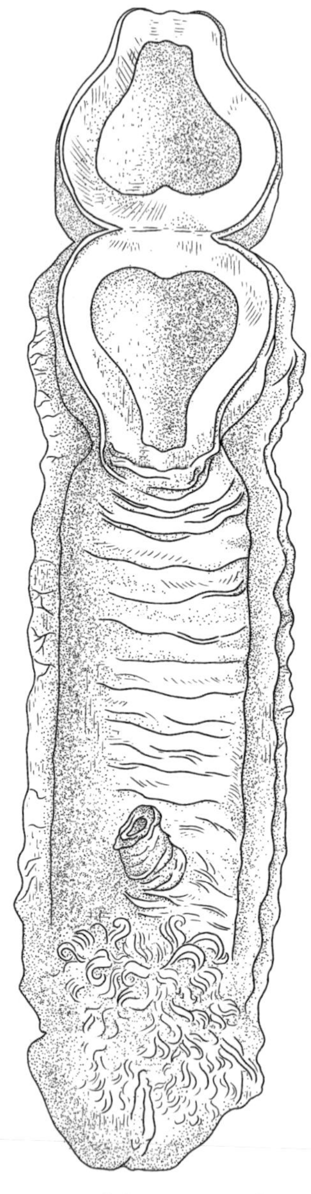

FIGURE 2. Illustration of the uterus and vagina from Andreas Vesalius's *On the Fabric of the Human Body,* 1543. Drawing by Hayley Monroe.

to be a necessary ingredient for conception. Pregnancy was always a sure proof that the female seed had been ejaculated.

It was also evident that ejaculation was generally pleasurable for men. Soranus took the genital analogue to its logical conclusion: since ejaculation felt good to men and since the female body was an inverted version of the male body, then ejaculation must feel good to women too. And since ejaculation was necessary for pregnancy, then women had to experience sexual pleasure to get pregnant.

But let's not think for a second that Soranus was an advocate for female sexual pleasure. The connection between pleasure and conception was applied retroactively. If a woman got pregnant, that was proof that she had ejaculated and felt pleasure. Even if a woman was raped, a subsequent pregnancy *proved* that she—or at least her body—had "enjoyed" the encounter.[25]

In his *Gynecology,* Soranus writes:

> Just as males can't ejaculate sperm without desire, in the same way females can't conceive without desire. Just like when food that is eaten without desire . . . isn't ingested and digested well, so too the sperm can't be taken up and, if taken up, can't lead to pregnancy without an urge and desire for intercourse. This can even be said about women who get pregnant after being raped: for these women desire was present, but the judgment of the psyche overshadowed it.[26]

Conception, Soranus says, is similar to digestion. To be digested well, food must be eaten with desire, otherwise there is indigestion or even vomiting. Similarly, to "conceive"—to grasp, take in, and hold on to the semen—the female body must engage in intercourse with desire. This desire of the body can act independently of the woman's psyche. Indeed, the psyche can even overshadow and *deceive* the desire of the body. A woman can think in her mind that she does not want to have sex, while her own body betrays her.

This supposed connection between pregnancy and pleasure has never been fully excised from popular understandings of the female body. In 2012, Missouri senatorial candidate Todd Akin espoused a similar view, explaining, "If it's a legitimate rape, the female body has ways to try to shut the whole thing down"—the idea being that in a body experiencing rape, physiological processes that lead to pregnancy just stop.[27] If the woman gets pregnant, then it wasn't a legitimate rape—she actually wanted it all along. We know that the people of Missouri were not impressed by Akin, who failed to oust his political rival, Claire McCaskill. But how would such an idea have impacted women in 2nd-century Rome?

This notion reinforced a principle from Greek philosophy that was central to Greco-Roman gynecology: men were governed by the soul and the principle of reason, while women were governed by the body and the principle of passion ("sensation" or "suffering"). Even if a woman might try to control her body by means of her psyche—by preventing conception from taking place after non-consensual, unwanted intercourse—her body, governed by its own desires, could betray her. The woman who could not control her body (every woman) needed outside intervention.

But notice that female sexual pleasure was not part of the description of conception given by Flavia, Helena, and Claudia, Galen's self-observant women. They mention a "grasping" sensation, but not one of ejaculation or pleasure. This is not to say that they didn't feel pleasure during sex, but that it was not a part of their description of conception. Rather, it was an idea that came from medical theory by way of analogy to the male body.

TURIA'S INFERTILITY

Flavia, Helena, and Claudia spoke as women who could conceive easily. But what about women for whom this was not the case? As we saw in chapter 1, fertility was very important. Naturally, then, infertility was an easy inroad to medical control of women's bodies and the reproductive process.

In 10 BCE, an upper-class Roman woman named Turia died and was commemorated by her husband in a eulogy that he had carved into stone.[28] The eulogy is unique for its length and its content. Turia's husband commends her many actions—private and public—to preserve him and their property through the tumultuous and deadly years of civil war when the first emperor, Augustus, was coming to power. Most notably, we learn that she died childless, having been married to her husband for forty years.

The lack of children was a source of great sadness for Turia and a circumstance for which she took full responsibility. Her husband writes, "You were despairing of your fertility and pained over my childlessness."[29] The childlessness was his, but the infertility belonged to her. In her affection for her husband, Turia even went so far as to suggest divorce. He could marry someone else who was able to give him children. Or, if he was not amenable to divorce, given their unusual level of marital harmony, then she would at least find a fertile woman to produce children for him. Turia herself would take on the role of a sister or mother-in-law to the new woman. Turia's husband refused both options.

But what would forty years as an infertile woman have been like? A few lines in the eulogy hint at Turia's experience. Her husband laments that, despite all of Turia's efforts, Fortuna—the Roman goddess of chance and fortune—put an end to their hopes for children: "What you planned and what you attempted! Perhaps in some other woman this would be remarkable and worth commemorating, but in you it is nothing at all to marvel at, compared to the rest of your virtues, and I pass over it."

What is it that Turia's husband "passes over"? What did Turia "plan and attempt"? I think he must be referring to her efforts—religious, magical, and medical—to counter her infertility.

MEDICAL THEORIES OF INFERTILITY

The general medical truism was that infertility could be the fault of the man, the woman, or both.[30] But as historian Rebecca Flemming has pointed out, while infertility was *in theory* a problem that could afflict either partner, in practice fertility treatments were applied to female, not male, bodies.[31] There are a few medical suggestions for treating male infertility: men are advised to do hardening and drying things such as drinking red wine, eating fortifying foods, and avoiding warm baths.[32] But on the whole, it was women who were infertile and women's bodies at which the doctors directed their medical treatments.[33]

Hippocratic medical writers explained female infertility as a temporary state that could be remedied with appropriate medical intervention.[34] In *Diseases of Women* 1 and *Barrenness* (5th century BCE), infertility is essentially an inability of either the semen to reach the uterus or of the uterus to grasp onto and retain that semen. These problems and their proposed remedies lay with the uterus. The writers of these medical manuals provide general principles for understanding the causes of infertility, diagnostic processes, and a series of mechanical, herbal, and dietary remedies.[35]

Fundamentally, not having sex would cause infertility—not just, as you would think, because sex is necessary for getting pregnant. Long abstinence—such as in unmarried women and widows—could cause diseases and malfunctions of the uterus that could lead to long-term infertility.[36] Penile penetration during sex served to expand the passageways of the female body.[37] Mechanically, it opened and widened the birth canal. It also stimulated sexual desire in the rest of the female body, causing blood to flow to the uterus and opening the passageways throughout the whole body. These passageways conveyed nutriments to the uterus for a (potential) developing fetus, and for facilitating the monthly purge of built-up bodily fluid via menstruation. So the absence of penetration could cause a number of problems. The birth canal, including the vagina and cervix, could close up, trapping menstrual fluid inside the uterus, leading to uterine ulcers and, ultimately, permanent infertility.[38] Or the lack of penetration could cause the vagina and cervix to bend and kink, not being routinely kept straight by the insertion of a penis. This bending and kinking could prevent the man's semen from entering the uterus when sexual intercourse finally did occur.[39]

Regular pregnancies, too, were key to the continued ability to become pregnant. In one sense, pregnancy, according to the Hippocratic writers, fulfilled the uterus's function. Holding a developing embryo and bringing it to term "satisfied" the uterus and ensured that it would not go wandering around the body looking for an infant and causing physical distress and malfunction. In a more mechanical interpretation, pregnancy weighed the uterus down, preventing it from floating or bending freely inside the abdomen. Uteruses that were not weighed down by a fetus, such as those in very young women who had never had sex or in older, post-menopausal women, were uteruses in danger of moving and suffocating other parts of the internal body.[40] In the Hippocratic gynecological texts, pregnancy itself was a remedy for female afflictions. At the most extreme end, a text called *Girls* advised pregnancy as a cure for a psychological disease that afflicted young women, causing them to want to hang themselves.[41]

The Hippocratic writer of *Diseases of Women* 1 identified the cause of infertility according to the point in the process at which reproduction failed—for example, when semen ran out of the vagina immediately after intercourse, the problem was that the cervix was closed, obstructed, bent, or kinked.[42] Remedies were herbal or mechanical. To clear an obstruction, the physician could prescribe pessaries, poultices, fumigations, or sexual intercourse.[43] To straighten a bent cervix, the writer advised the insertion of lead probes or sounds; and to widen a too-small vagina or cervix, a woman might use graduated dilators made out of pine wood (see fig. 3).[44] If semen ran out of the vagina in the days following intercourse, then the uterus was too moist; the uterine walls did not grasp onto the seed and it washed away.[45] Drying remedies were recommended for the entire body. The uterus might also require a cleaning.[46]

These were principles that could be used to diagnose and treat infertility. Not only was medical intervention helpful, it was necessary to prevent catastrophe. The writer emphasizes repeatedly that if the woman is diagnosed and treated quickly with the appropriate remedy, then she will likely recover and conceive. If her condition is left to fester, though, she could experience permanent infertility. He writes, "If the patient is treated, she will recover, but if she is not treated, after a while she will suffer everything I've described and it will be more severe."[47] And then again, "If the patient

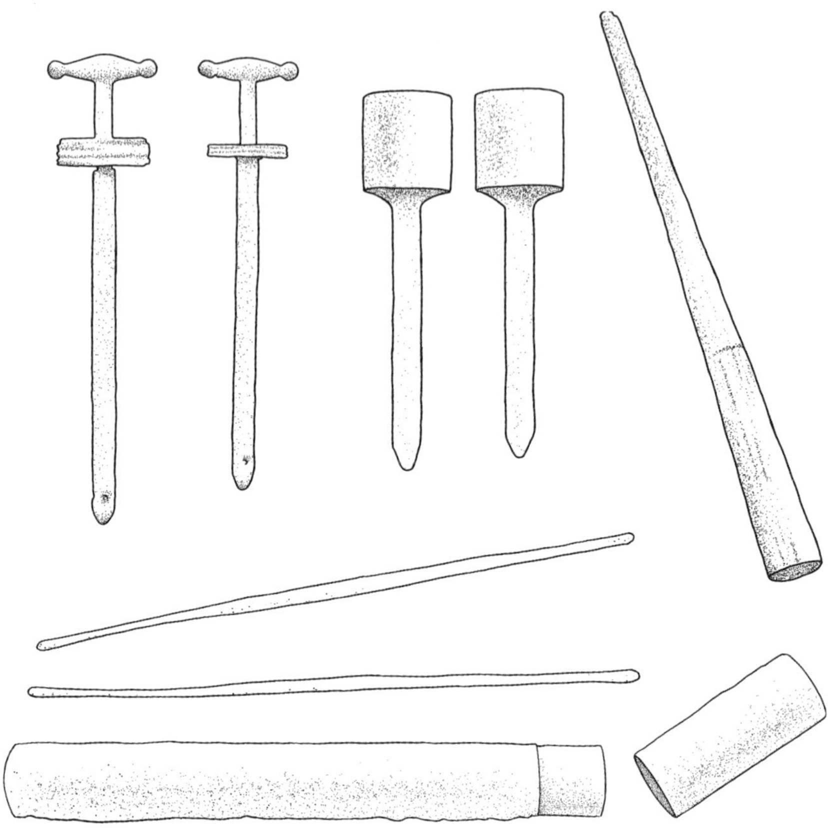

FIGURE 3. Roman medical instruments, clockwise from upper left: two clyster plungers with handles and two clyster tubes, which were operated like modern vaginal cream applicators and could be used to inject medicinal creams into the vagina or anus; a hollow lead graduated dilator, which could be used to widen the vagina or cervix and to insert medicaments; two lead probes with a lead carrying case—among a range of uses, these could be inserted into the vagina and cervix in an attempt to straighten the pathway to the uterus. Pompeii, 1st century CE. Located in the Health Sciences Library, University of Virginia. Drawings by Hayley Monroe.

is treated, she will recover even if the disease is far advanced and she will usually live; but she won't be able to have children."[48] The message was clear: medical expertise, provided here by Hippocratic doctors, was essential to female fertility and successful reproduction.[49]

Other Hippocratic treatises expanded on these principles. In *Barrenness,* as a remedy for uteruses that could not retain semen, the writer recommended, "Grind up lead and the stone that attracts iron, tie them up in a cloth, and after dipping the bundle in breast milk, insert it into the vagina."[50] For a uterus that was determined to be too small, or which had had several consecutive miscarriages, the remedy was to inflate the uterus using a bellows (like the one used for a fire) and then fill it with expanding substances, such as gourd flesh or squirting cucumber, and to have the woman eat bloating, gas-producing foods such as garlic. Diets were coordinated to match the issue with the womb. Women whose uteruses were hard and closed off were given foods and drinks that were thought to have softening effects on the whole body, such as puppy meat, octopus, and boiled vegetables.[51] They might be given warm baths to soften and loosen the entire body.[52]

These remedies were medical, mechanical, and magical. We can see the medical principles at work in the herbal remedies and diets that were intended to correct the imbalances of the body. The mechanical interventions included the probes, dilators, and bellows to pump air into the uterus, along with the organic substances—gourd flesh and squirting cucumber—used to fill and stretch the too-small uterus. A "magical" treatment can be seen in the "stone that attracts iron," which was meant to be shaved and formed into a vaginal pessary. It was its property of "attraction" that was important. Just as the stone attracted iron, it would also, it was thought, attract bodily fluids—semen, menstrual blood—or even the uterus itself.[53]

This power of attraction can be understood through the principle of sympathy. In a general sense, "sympathy" referred to the actions and interactions of all things in the universe. Together with its opposite, "antipathy," it formed a kind of push and pull, action and reaction principle.[54] Sympathy was important to philosophical, medical, and magical understandings of the body, sickness, and remedy. Some philosophical schools, such as Stoicism, recognized sympathetic connections throughout the whole universe, while some medical writers, such as Soranus, limited their understanding of sympathy to interactions that took place within the body—for example, pain that was referred from one part of the body to another. Magic was often understood as the practice of manipulating the invisible, sympathetic connections that existed *between* objects.[55] In the manipulation of sympathy, whether medical or magical, particular objects or substances could be used for the properties they exhibited: attracting, repelling, growing, decaying.[56]

Let's consider an example that shows how remedies we might call "medical" and "magical" diverge and overlap: the use of products from the olive tree to treat a fever. "Medicine" involved applying olive oil to the body to bring down the fever, while "magic" called upon the user to write a special character on either side of an olive leaf and wear it around the neck as an amulet.[57] But sometimes the distinction between medical and magical manipulation was not completely clear.[58] Another magical treatment for a fever instructed the user to "take [olive] oil in your hands and say seven times, 'SABAOTH,'" before spreading the oil "from the sacrum to the feet."[59] The oil is rubbed on the body like a medical treatment, but this remedy also enlists the aid of Sabaoth—a manifestation of the Hebrew god—and the repetition of his name seven times, an important magical number.

The objects or substances used in the manipulation of sympathetic connection had the properties of or symbolically represented the outcome that was being sought.[60] The amulet made of "the stone that attracts iron" was supposed to be dipped in breast milk. This breast milk was thought to contain the power of a successful pregnancy, which would transfer to the infertile woman undergoing the treatment.[61] Similarly, the squirting cucumber plant mimicked the action of the ejaculating penis, spewing out seeds when touched. The use of this plant as a uterine expander was probably intended to impart a kind of fertilizing action to the uterus.[62]

Similarly, a whole category of remedies involved the use of feces and other filthy ingredients to treat infertility.[63] One recipe for a closed cervix called for the woman to mix hawk excrement with sweet wine and drink it while fasting. Another instructed her to mash up goose feces with rose perfume and apply it to her vagina.[64] Immediately afterward, she was to have sex with her husband. These ingredients were likely meant to act as fertilizer.[65] Just as manure was used to fertilize a field, these animal feces would work to fertilize a barren woman. The treatment was medical and magical. The distinctions drawn between medical, magical, and mechanical treatments are largely a product of the modern world.

As much as the Hippocratic writers claimed to be innovating—in their systemization of symptoms, diagnoses, and cures—the methods and components of their practice had been around for a long time. The Hippocratic medical writers likely appropriated orally transmitted knowledge of herbal medicine from female midwives and healers.[66]

Their writings oscillate between tradition and innovation, between at-home therapies and physician-directed treatments. On the one hand, the writer of *Barrenness* appealed to popular understandings of sympathetic magic with his prescriptions of magnetite, breast milk, and squirting cucumber. At certain points in the treatise, he directs women to administer the medications and therapies to themselves, suggesting that women had some prior knowledge of and facility with these practices.[67] On the other hand, the writer repeatedly emphasizes the importance of correct diagnosis and swift treatment for long-term relief. He positions himself as the one able to provide the diagnosis and to prescribe the correct remedies. We see here the beginning of the long, fraught history of the medicalization of reproduction. At this point it does not seem to be a hostile takeover, but one that integrates multiple forms of knowledge. There seems to be room here for women's understanding of their own bodies as well as for traditional remedies.

This coordination of tradition and innovation can be seen in the stories of Demetria and of Flavia, Helena, and Claudia. Galen recognizes the value of women's knowledge both for his own investigations and to his potential readers. Women know things about their bodies that Galen can only externally observe. Women like Claudia and her friends—

women who are midwives and healers, or who have given birth themselves—are self-observant and can be trusted. Demetria's story also involves experienced women: an enslaved professional, who by definition was perpetually sexually available, and her enslaver, a woman responsible for managing the reproductive lives of other women. But the existence of "rather self-observant women" implies the existence of rather less self-observant women. For the few women—midwives, grandmothers, and sex workers—who had knowledge, there were many, many more, Galen would have us believe, who knew nothing.[68]

TURIA'S TRIALS

What is it that Turia "planned and attempted" in her decades-long struggle with infertility? Although this chapter has largely focused on medical theories and treatments, Turia's first recourse was probably religious. As her husband's reference to the goddess Fortuna shows, fertility and infertility were thought to be granted by the gods. Although there were certain obvious deities who were associated with reproduction, such as Juno Lucina—Juno in her capacity as Lucina, goddess of childbirth—almost any deity could be petitioned for help with fertility.[69] The important thing was to get a powerful god or goddess on your side who would work on your behalf to persuade other deities and to manipulate the sympathetic threads holding the universe together. Turia probably appealed to many of them.

Let's say that she paid a visit to the temple of Juno Lucina on the Esqualine Hill in the eastern part of the city of Rome. She may have brought garlands of flowers and incense as gifts for the goddess. As she entered, she would have been surrounded by votive dedications, made by those whose prayers had been answered. Perhaps, in particular, her eyes were drawn to a collection of terracotta wombs—objects given in thanks for fertility and a successful pregnancy (see fig. 4).

Roman women throughout the western Italian peninsula would go to a temple or sanctuary and make a vow to a deity: answer my prayer—

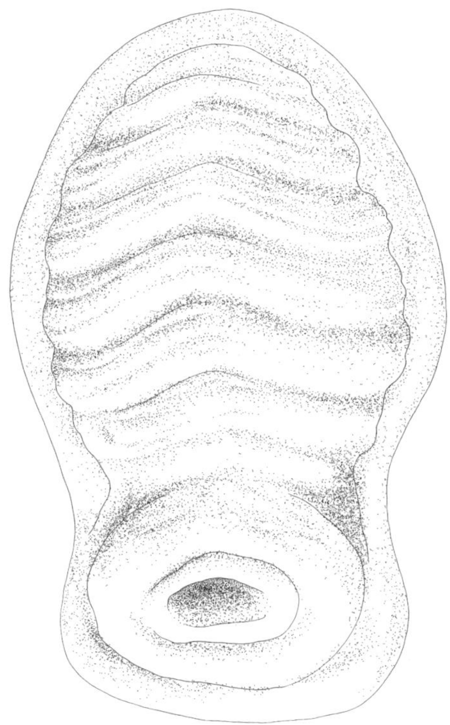

FIGURE 4. Roman terracotta votive womb. 4th–1st century BCE. Wellcome Collection A636076. Drawing by Hayley Monroe.

for fertility, a healthy pregnancy, a successful birth—and I will dedicate an object in thanks. The terracotta wombs were the fulfillment of the vow. There are hundreds of them. Many have narrow or wide ridges or waves. These could represent the powerful contractions of the uterus during birth. Women would have been thanking the goddess for a healthy uterus and a strong, swift birth.[70]

Other womb votives have small clay balls inside that rattle around freely and can be seen via X-ray. The balls could represent the male and female seed contributed by each partner, or they could represent developing embryos. They may be thanks for conception or for the healthy and safe development of the fetus.[71] Turia, of course, would never have had the chance to dedicate her own terracotta womb.

A root cutter—a procurer and provider of plants and herbal medicines—may have supplied her with darnel (a wheat-like grass) to burn with frankincense or saffron as a vaginal fumigation, or wild carrot to make an aphrodisiac drink.[72] Perhaps she consumed particular foods to promote conception: cow's milk, snails cooked in saffron, anise, stinging nettle seeds in grape syrup, or root of the man orchid.[73]

As her repeated prayers to the gods and herbal remedies proved unsuccessful, Turia probably visited soothsayers and fortune tellers, hoping to gain a glimpse into her future and perhaps discover the cause of her infertility. There were many types: knucklebone throwers, animal entrail readers, dream interpreters, and more.[74] But their proclamations could be confusing. When a woman dreamed that her womb had been sealed, one interpreter told her that she was barren—her womb was sealed off to the sperm. But when she sought a second opinion, another told her that she was pregnant, since "it's not customary to seal up something that's empty."[75]

Perhaps—secretly and in desperation—Turia sought out more illicit magical cures. Amulets, spells, or potions could work as aphrodisiacs to promote sexual desire, fertility, and conception, such as a fertility remedy that entailed eating hyena's eye with licorice root and anise.[76] Many of the remedies involved reciting or writing magical spells and formulas to make the ingredients effective.[77] Magic was not just sneered at by doctors, it was actively distrusted and, eventually, outlawed. Aphrodisiac potions—with the power to promote conception, not just arouse desire—were particularly suspect. They were banned under the Cornelian Law Against Murderers and Poisoners.[78]

Whereas religion was an *appeal* to the gods, magic was an attempt to *force* them to do your bidding (for example, by using their secret names) or to circumvent their authority altogether. But here too the line was blurred. Two thin lead tablets dated to the 1st or 2nd century CE were found folded seven times, rolled up, and fastened together with a nail in the sanctuary of the goddesses Demeter and Kore (Persephone) in Corinth.[79] The tablets are engraved with a curse against a woman named Karpimē Babbia and an appeal on behalf of the writer: "Bring a monthly destruction upon Karpimē Babbia, subdue and destroy her soul, heart, mind, and wits! Make me fertile!"[80] The bid for fertility includes a string of indecipherable magical letters, appeals to Hermes of the Underworld, and invokes Eupher—a powerful name invoked for opening a mouth (here, the mouth of the womb).[81] The writer's bid for her own fertility is paired with a request for destruction of another woman's fertility—an interference with her menstrual period.[82] The tablets are located in a religious space—the sanctuary of Demeter and Kore—but involve a kind of religion-adjacent, magical activity. Perhaps Turia was desperate enough to resort to such measures.[83]

Finally, to what lengths did Turia allow doctors to go? When drinks, vapor baths and fumigations failed, perhaps she was subjected to bloodletting from her arm or the application of the physician's cupping vessel to her inner thighs.[84] Maybe she endured vaginal clysters with medicaments or painful cervical expansion with lead dilators (see fig. 3).[85] The writer of the Hippocratic *Barrenness* advises:

> Dilate the uterus with five eight-inch hammered lead dilators: the first dilator should be thin, the second one thicker, and the ones after that successively thicker still. Dilate for five days. The woman should always have a bath before she makes the insertion, and she should tie bandages around her loins so that it [the dilator] does not fall out . . . she should push the dilators progressively higher such that the last one will be as high as possible.[86]

This treatment involved inserting progressively thicker eight-inch-long lead dilators up through the cervix in order to open and expand it. The doctor prescribed the treatment and provided the tools, but the patient was responsible for administering this painful procedure to herself.

Turia never got the child she desired. But she was alive at a time—the late 1st century BCE—when the fertility treatments of Greek doctors were increasingly spreading around the Mediterranean. Doing everything that she could to remedy her infertility would have involved subjecting herself to many lengthy, laborious, and painful medical procedures. More than one hundred years later, as Cyrilla was fainting in the bath and Galen was consulting with Flavia, Helena, and Claudia in the marketplace, medicine made an even larger incursion on women's reproductive bodies. In the next chapter, we will see how, in the 2nd century CE, one doctor in particular was making the business of being born *his* business.

FOUR

Controlling Conception

IN THE EARLY 2ND CENTURY, the physician Soranus did something unprecedented. He wrote a gynecological treatise in which he argued unequivocally for medical intervention in the process of human reproduction. He also showed elite Roman men how to be knowledgeable readers and controllers of women's bodies. His claim was that by following his prescriptions, these elite Roman men would be able to mold their wives into optimal makers of optimal babies.[1]

Why does this matter? Soranus made the first significant step in a fundamental shift—fully realized in the 20th century—wherein pregnancy and childbirth came to be seen as pathological rather than physiological processes.[2] We cannot know how much of an impact his writings had on the women of his time, but in the long trajectory of childbirth, the ideological shift to which he contributed has been the most consequential change in birth in the Western world. He created a model for male medical control of reproduction.

Soranus, like Galen, was a Greek doctor who came from the region of Ionia around Ephesus on the western coast of modern-day Türkiye (Turkey). While biographical details are sparse, it's clear that he made his way to Rome sometime during the reign of the emperors Trajan (ruled 98–117) or Hadrian (ruled 117–138).[3] There, he made a name for himself caring for wealthy patients and publishing treatises on a wide variety of medical topics, including fevers, drugs, ophthalmology, and surgery. But his most enduring work was his *Gynecology*.[4] It circulated in the western part of the Roman Empire and was translated into Latin. Parts of it survived in later compilations until at least the 12th century.[5] The *Gynecology* has already had a large presence in this story, and it will continue to do so. It is the earliest comprehensive medical text in the Western tradition dealing with menstruation, conception, prenatal care, childbirth, postpartum care, breastfeeding, and child-rearing.

SORANUS'S *GYNECOLOGY*

Soranus flipped the main tenet of Hippocratic gynecology on its head. For the Hippocratics, pregnancy was inherently healthful and therapeutic.[6] It could relieve menstrual difficulties, wandering womb, uterine suffocation, and more. For Soranus, on the contrary, pregnancy was pathological. He said that it "causes physical degeneration, muscular weakness, and premature old age," and that permanent virginity was healthier for women.[7] But this was no proto-feminist manifesto about the dangers of repeated and closely spaced pregnancies for women's bodies. Pregnancy, he said, despite being pathological, was necessary for producing children.[8] Or as historian Anna Bonnell Freidin has put it, according to Soranus, reproduction was not "healthful," but it was "natural."[9] The role of the doctor—and the husband—then, was to get women in the best possible shape to conceive and to shepherd them through the risky processes of pregnancy, childbirth, and the postpartum period. Because pregnancy was dangerous, medical intervention was necessary. Because conception was difficult, the woman who wanted to become pregnant—or the man who wanted her to become pregnant—had to follow the advice of the doctor.[10] Soranus also aimed to show men how to take control of the reproductive process, from choosing an appropriate woman with whom to procreate to choosing the best midwives and wet nurses.

Hippocratic gynecology used tests for determining a woman's ability to conceive. One involved putting a strong-smelling substance such as bitter almond or garlic in the vagina overnight.[11] If the garlic or bitter almond could be smelled on the woman's breath in the morning, then her internal passageways were open and she was fertile. Another involved rubbing her eyes with a red stone. If the red color could be seen in her saliva, she was fertile, if not she was not.[12]

Soranus, on the contrary, told Roman men that they could follow his directions and assess a woman's fertility based on her age, physicality, and temperament. That is, he established principles by which a good, fertile woman could be recognized and chosen from the outside—cutting out the middleman, who was probably a midwife. Soranus encouraged Roman men to select a woman in generally good health, between fifteen and forty years old, with a moderate physique—not mannish, compact, and overly sturdy, nor too flabby and moist.[13] His argument was that her uterus matched the condition of the rest of her body: if a woman was hard-bodied and mannish, her hard uterus would repel the sperm; if she was too fat, fleshy, and moist, her lax, untoned uterus could not grip the sperm and would quickly flush it out. He also seemingly encouraged men to assess or even track the menstruation of prospective partners. Another way to tell if a woman had a fertile body, he explained, was if she had a regular menstrual period made up of blood (not water) in which she bled a moderate amount.[14]

Soranus advised manual evaluation of a woman's cervix—likely performed by a midwife—in order to assess her fertility. He explained that a woman was fertile if her cervix "lies relatively far forward [in her body] and in a straight line."[15] A cervix that was deviated or that lay further back would have a harder time taking up the sperm.[16] Finally, a suitably fertile mate could be judged by her temperament. Those women were likely to be fertile who were "calm and cheerful" since, as Soranus explained, a "sorrowful" or "passionate" temperament "expels the fetus due to heavy breathing."[17] That is, sad and emotionally volatile women eject the sperm with their dramatic crying and sighing.

Soranus empowered Roman men to take control of the reproductive process through their assessment of potential mates. But if a suitable mate was not chosen, the doctor could help. In addition to pathologizing pregnancy, Soranus also individualized it. He explained that rather than follow general principles—such as the belief that the menstrual cycle followed the moon, or that there were fertile and infertile times of year—each woman's body held particular signs about her fertility.[18] The job of the Roman man—in consultation with the doctor—was twofold: to recognize the particular signs of fertility in a particular woman's body *and* to do some general things to get her body in the best state to conceive.

Soranus explained that a woman's body gave off signs that it was fertile and ready to be impregnated. A man could read these signs and time sex appropriately. Intercourse, Soranus wrote, should happen as the woman's menstrual period was ending, when she was sexually aroused, when she was not hungry or too full or intoxicated, and after she had eaten a small meal and been given a massage.[19] Each of these elements was key to conception. When the menstrual period had ended the uterus was at its driest point, when it was least likely to flush out the semen. Arousal would likely lead to orgasm and ejaculation of the female semen.[20] If she was hungry, her body and her uterus would be too weak to receive and retain the semen. If she was too full of food or intoxicated, her body and uterus would be disturbed and would reject the semen.[21] The small meal gave her strength for intercourse and conception and the massage dispersed any congestions and "superfluities" in the body so that it was ready to receive the seed.[22]

Perhaps these prescriptions don't sound too bad—a light meal, a massage, and even an orgasm. But they were more about the control that a Roman man could exert over the reproductive process than about making it a pleasant experience for women. It's clear that Soranus was talking to Roman men, not to the women themselves. He uses passive and impersonal grammatical constructions to talk about female bodies: "The best time [for intercourse] is after a massage has been given and a little food eaten."[23] He compares the Roman man to a farmer preparing his fields for planting: "Just as the farmer sows only after he has sifted the soil and removed any foreign objects, in the same way we advise that intercourse for the purpose of reproduction should happen after the body has been given a massage."[24] The female body was a commodity that had to be cared for and prepared in the appropriate way in order to produce the greatest yield.

The stakes of this reproductive control were high. The aim was to prevent dangerous conception—that is, conception that resulted in a child with a damaged body or soul. This kind of conception could come from a woman who was not being properly managed. Any fault, though, did not lie with the man doing the managing, but the woman herself. The man could do things to mitigate a woman's corrupting influence on the sperm, but the woman had to comply. In Soranus's reckoning, men could take control of reproduction, but women could be blamed if something went wrong.

Dangerous conception, Soranus argued, could come from overindulging in food and wine. Such overindulgence could damage the sperm. If a woman who had indigestion or was intoxicated managed to conceive, the corrupted state of her bodily fluids—the blood and *pneuma* (breath) that she supplied to the freshly conceived sperm would harm it. He wrote, "There is a risk that because of bad material [menstrual fluid and female semen], the seed [male sperm] will change for the worse."[25] *Pneuma* translates to "breath," but for the ancient physicians and philosophers it was much more than that. Significantly, it was *vital* breath, a concentrated, refined form of blood, responsible for all the functions that we associate with the nervous system. It was responsible for perception and thought *and* it was a material substance that was one of the important building blocks of the fetus.[26] Intoxication affected perception and thought and therefore affected the actual substance of the *pneuma*. Bad *pneuma* would make bad babies. Thus, Soranus cautioned women against overeating or drinking wine when they were trying to conceive.

The effects of intoxication could be quite sinister. Soranus cautioned that an intoxicated woman could be a "victim of strange phantasies," which would harm the fetus right at the moment of conception.[27] He was referring to something called "maternal impressions"—the notion that whatever a woman saw with her eyes or her mind's eye during conception would affect the body and soul of the fetus.[28] For example, he said that women who happened to see monkeys while having sex gave birth to children that looked like monkeys. This effect could also be manipulated toward positive ends. Soranus wrote that the ugly tyrant of the Cyprians had his wife look at beautiful statues while they were having sex so that she would give birth to beautiful children. Similarly, horse breeders placed "noble horses" in front of the mares while they were breeding to make them conceive the best horses. Soranus did not invent the idea of maternal impressions; it crops up in Roman texts as early as the 1st century CE.[29] But his is the first surviving work that incorporates maternal impressions into a cohesive regimen for conception.

Soranus does not specify what he means when he writes about fetuses that have been harmed in body or soul. But he is also the only ancient physician to recommend that midwives assess newborn babies to determine whether they are "worth rearing."[30] The alternative would have been exposure and abandonment—more on this in chapter 11. Importantly, these eugenicist concerns about bodily and psychic perfection were aimed at wealthy men—those who would have hired Soranus to treat infertility or to enhance their reproductive success.

What should we make of these elaborate conception regimens? What would it have been like to be a woman whose husband was following Soranus's advice? Certainly, by offering Roman men a prescription for conception, Soranus was bringing some order to a chaotic and confusing time. It must have been inscrutable why some acts of intercourse led to pregnancy and others didn't. It's possible that his advice, much of which involved providing attentive care, soothing baths and massages, and a mild diet, would have led to better outcomes. But his motives were hardly feminist. It's clear from his explanations that he thought women were largely to blame if anything went wrong. His recommendations for diet, exercise, and entertainment presuppose that anything and everything the woman did could potentially harm the fetus. He made it the role of the (potential) father to make sure that his wife was doing everything possible to get pregnant and to produce the best possible child.

Soranus's wasn't the only word on conception. Pregnancy, and particularly fetal development, had long been a topic of debate among philosophers. They were not interested in providing prescriptions and regimens to promote conception. Rather, they were making technical, theoretical arguments about the nature of the soul. In essence, they were trying to answer some of the big universal questions: where do we come from and how did we get here? In the process, some of them provided a not-quite-feminist but certainly more woman-positive take on conception, maternal impressions, and the relationship between pregnant woman and fetus.

Porphyry, a 3rd-century Neo-Platonic philosopher—an intellectual follower of Plato—imagined the woman as the "captain" of fetal development—a relatively positive and active metaphor.[31] According to Porphyry, both the male and female partners had generative, life-giving powers that they imparted to the embryo. It was only because she had sustained contact with the developing fetus that the woman's mind, body, and soul affected the fetus more than the man's.

These views make sense when we consider that Porphyry did not think there was a difference between men and women at the level of the *psyche* or the soul.[32] Unlike earlier philosophers—including Plato himself—and medical writers who dabbled in philosophy, he thought that men and women were equal in this regard. It therefore makes sense that he would have assigned women the powerful role of captain, not as an indication of their culpability, but as an expression of their power over the inferior, developing soul of the fetus. This idea of equality seems to have played out in his life as well. One of Porphyry's main intellectual correspondents was his wife, Marcella.[33]

READING THE SIGNS OF CONCEPTION

At the start of chapter 3 we met Flavia, Helena, and Claudia, three self-observant women who helped the physician Galen understand the mechanism of human conception—how the uterus takes up the male sperm following intercourse. They gave voice to a common understanding at the time that women could feel conception taking place in their own bodies. They said that they could feel the uterus crawling and grasping as it took up the sperm from the man's penis. Soranus wrote that women were conscious of a "shivering sensation" at the end of intercourse, which meant that they had conceived.[34] Other early signs of conception may have been apparent to women themselves, but not necessarily to outsiders: headaches, nausea, dimmed sight, food aversions, and vomiting.[35] Women might feel heavy in their loins and experience swelling in their breasts.[36] For some women, it might have taken an experienced woman—a midwife, an older relative, or a women who had been pregnant several times—to explain these signs. It wasn't until later in the pregnancy that the signs of conception were apparent to outside observers, including husbands. Menstruation stopped and signs could finally be read on the flesh of the body. The blood vessels in breasts appeared prominent and livid, and the under-eye area grew dark and greenish. Something like pregnancy melasma could appear. The abdomen grew.[37]

Soranus systematized these signs of conception, arguing for an almost forensic analysis of potentially pregnant women: "Evidence of conception must be worked out from many signs lumped together and by their differentiation."[38] Soranus explained that an outside observer could know that conception had happened if, after intercourse, the cervix was closed, but soft and responsive to the touch, and if the vagina was dry or only slightly moist.[39] This description implies an invasive manual procedure shortly after intercourse. We are meant to imagine, I think, that a Roman man would hire a midwife or a female doctor to conduct the procedure while he acted as overseer (though perhaps some intrepid Roman men attempted their own examinations).

Knowing the signs of conception, according to Soranus, was not just a matter of interest. It was a matter of safety. Remember, as far as he was concerned, pregnancy was a pathology—bad for the woman, but good for producing babies. Furthermore, there were conditions that could mimic the signs of pregnancy. These conditions could be dangerous. They might threaten the woman's life or her future fertility.

The most serious kind of false pregnancy was called a *mole*, from the ancient Greek word meaning "millstone."[40] Just as an ancient millstones was a heavy, hard-to-move rock, the uterine *mole* was a heavy, hard-to-move mass. One 1st-century-CE description of the *mole* called it "a shapeless and inanimate mass of flesh that resists cutting."[41] It could form because of a problem with a woman's monthly period. The menstrual fluid could get backed up, congealing into this impenetrable, lifeless lump. The *mole* was especially dangerous because it gave off the same signs as pregnancy: both caused the belly to swell and both stopped menstruation.

But the *mole* could be differentiated by its lack of movement.[42] And the medical practitioner could identify a *mole* through palpation and tapping on the abdomen.[43] Soranus brags that while other physicians refuse to treat the *mole*—on the assumption that it is incurable—or only treat it when it is first beginning, he will treat it "even when it is chronic."[44]

It's hard to imagine that some or even many women, especially those who had been pregnant before, would not have been able to tell the difference between a pregnancy and a *mole*. Just as Galen's self-observant women could describe in detail the sensation of conception, it's likely that women would have had a strong, embodied sense of pregnancy. What we see in Soranus, then, is an attempt to establish criteria for the *external* observation and confirmation of pregnancy—confirmations that could be made by the father or his agent.

Controlling conception also meant controlling the metaphorical landscape of conception. Which metaphors were favored by women and which ones were emphasized by the male medical writers? How might these metaphors have affected the embodied experience of conception?

In chapter 2 we saw two contradictory metaphors for the uterus: the octopus and the cupping vessel. I speculated that these metaphors were meant to represent different aspects of the organ: the cupping-vessel-style uterus, signifying the uterus's capacity to hold fluids and fetuses, and the octopus-style uterus, representing the embodied experience of having a uterus that could crawl, grasp, suffocate, and contract. The words of Flavia, Helena, and Claudia (Galen's self-observant women from the start of chapter 3) corroborate this picture. They told him that when they conceived, they could "feel the uterus moving, sort of crawling and slowly contracting into itself, when it grasps the semen."[45] This description sounds a lot like an octopus. It also sounds like the crawling and squeezing sensations that accompanied the wandering womb and uterine suffocation. But here the actions of the octopus-style uterus are productive, not destructive. Without the crawling, grasping action of the uterus, the semen slips back out and conception fails. What we see in the women's report is the *utility* of the octopus-like womb. It is not merely a destructive force; its octopus-like qualities have a purpose. The women endure the negative aspects of the crawling, strangling, suffocating, and sentient octopus-like uterus because, as they tell Galen, those same properties are necessary for conception. The image of the octopus-like uterus, in fact, was uniquely related to childbirth.[46]

This connection between octopus-like uterus and birth can be seen on the amulets that women used to manage their gynecological health, which we saw in chapter 2.[47] Those amulets with an octopus-like uterus feature other symbols of birth—a laboring woman, the Egyptian god Khnoum (the ram-headed fashioner of children), or the infant Horus.[48] Some of these octopus-style uterine amulets also have a cupping-vessel-style uterus, implying a coordination in these two metaphorical aspects of the uterus to promote conception, pregnancy, and birth—the octopus-like uterus to grasp the semen and to initiate the birth contractions and the cupping vessel-like uterus to hold onto the fetus and the fluids necessary for its nourishment.[49] The metaphor of uterus as octopus also seems to have originated with women, or at least to have been approved by women. Tellingly, as we have seen, Soranus ridiculed the idea of an animalistic womb, scoffing that "the uterus does not rush forth like a wild animal from its lair."[50] Rather, he compared the uterus—and, in fact, the whole body of the woman—to something more easily controlled and managed: a field.[51]

In the analogy of woman to field, the man, as farmer, is in control of the reproductive process. Soranus used the metaphor of farmland to describe women's bodies, cautioning that just as poor soil destroys seeds and plants, so too female bodies in an "abnormal state" do not "grasp the semen injected into them" but weaken or kill it.[52] He advised the man/farmer, "Just as every season is not right for sowing seeds to grow fruit, so too in humans not every time is right for conception."[53] In this analogy, the man took on the roles of assessor, planter, and cultivator. He first determined the suitability of a particular womb/field for impregnating/planting, assessing the woman/womb/field that lay before him. He then took the active role in impregnating/planting. In seeing to the diet and regimen of his wife/field, the elite Roman man/farmer cultivated his semen/seed as it matured into the fetus/plant. The uterine *mole*—the hard growth in the uterus that mimicked pregnancy—functioned metaphorically as a rock in the field/womb. Its presence signaled barrenness/infertility, and it was the responsibility of the husband or doctor to remove it, just as a farmer removed rocks from his field before planting.

The role of the woman/womb/field, however, was not entirely passive. Just like the octopus-like womb, the field-like womb had to "grasp the semen."[54] When women were compared to fields, they also took on this active, desiring part of the metaphor. Indeed, we have already seen in chapter 3 how female desire was a key component in human generation. The man/farmer might oversee the process, but the woman had ultimate responsibility for the generative power and fruits of her womb.

Galen took an interesting middle line between the octopus-like uterus and the field-like womb, perhaps due to his conversations with the self-observant women. In *On the Dissection of the Uterus,* a text he wrote early in his career and gave to a midwife, he described the uterus as having "tentacles."[55] But in the majority of his writings, including *The Shaping of the Embryo,* he imagined the fetus as a plant, with the uterus acting as the supplier of nutritive matter, like a field.[56] In *Semen,* he wrote, "What the earth is to plants, the mother is to [the fetus], irrigating [it] with nutriment."[57]

In one final metaphor that we have seen in this chapter, the Neo-Platonic philosophers viewed the woman as the captain of the developing fetus. As captain she had creative agency over the body and soul of the embryo. Philosopher James Wilberding has argued that this attribution of creative agency to the mother is "proto-feminist,"[58] though that may be going a bit far. Due to her extended contact with the fetus, the mother had an enormous responsibility. What started off as creative agency could easily have degenerated into culpability. The mother, as captain, had to make sure to regulate her psychological state and internal imaginings at the time of conception.[59] Otherwise, she was not acting as appropriate manager of the fetal soul.

The metaphors of conception adopted by male writers presented a double bind for women in the ancient world. Either they were unruly, desiring fields that needed a farmer/husband/doctor to assess their fecundity and see to their proper clearing, plowing, and planting; or they were captains, controlling the construction of the fetal body and soul. Either way, they were ultimately responsible for the reproductive outcome. The state of their own bodies, minds, and souls determined whether conception would occur and, if it did, how the fetus would develop.

Galen's self-observant women likely didn't know it, but from the vantage point of the 21st century we can see that they were living through a major shift in the understanding and representation of pregnancy. Galen was speaking to these women at a moment when reproduction was being increasingly medicalized. He, and likely the women themselves, drew heavily on Hippocratic medicine, in which the gradual medicalization of reproduction had started as early as the 5th century BCE. As we saw in chapter 3, these first several hundred years of medicalization were marked by integration rather than conflict. Traditional remedies had a place alongside medical interventions. Physicians seemed to be making choices particularly to appeal to their female patients. However, they were also positioning themselves as experts in the field of women's medicine. The Hippocratic writers published manuals and treatments for infertility, systematizing it as a diagnosable and curable disease—provided that there was timely intervention by a doctor.

Soranus, in a significant departure from Hippocratic tradition, presented pregnancy as pathological rather than a healthful or therapeutic state. He made medicine and the doctor indispensable to the tricky—and potentially dangerous—process of conception. He involved the father, empowering him to monitor and control his woman. Soranus's writings would have a long afterlife in the Latin-speaking North African parts of the Roman Empire—the home of early Christin church fathers such as Saint Augustine, Tertullian, and Cyprian, all of whom mention or refer to the works of Soranus.[60] They were likely drawn as much to the patriarchal nature of his work as to the useful medical content.

Male physicians also colonized the metaphorical space of conception. While the self-observant women described their uteruses using animalistic language, the male medical writers preferred the analogy of a field. In this metaphorical landscape, the doctor and husband acted as farmers, judging the fertility of the field/body/womb. The man had to recognize and facilitate the right conditions for sowing/impregnating and then monitor the diet and regimen of his wife in order to bring about optimum conception and fetal development. He was like a farmer, readying his soil and planting the seeds. The doctor might have to be called in to remove a rock/*mole* from the field/womb. In the Neo-Platonic tradition, the woman was viewed as the captain of the fetal soul and the active builder of the fetal body. But in this role, she was responsible for the quality of the materials that went into sparking the fetus into life and molding it—materials of both the body and the soul. Since the fetus was effectively part of her body, she was responsible if anything went wrong in its physical or psychic development.

It's probable that women like Flavia, Helena, and Claudia monitored their menstrual cycles and paid attention to when they got pregnant. Whether they wanted to get pregnant and have children, as most women likely did, or whether they wanted to prevent pregnancy, as some women did because of their jobs, their own health conditions, or some other personal or economic reason, knowledge of their own bodies was key. We hear from Galen that they envisioned the moment of conception as an animated event—the animal-like womb crawling and grasping the semen. How might they have been affected by Soranus's and Galen's descriptions of the field-womb? Perhaps rather than as unruly fields needing to be tended by a male farmer, they imagined *themselves* as attendants and cultivators of that fetus/plant. Maybe the description of the Neo-Platonists resonated with them and they imagined themselves as builders or craftspeople.

In the next chapter we will consider the experiences of women in ancient Rome who got pregnant and didn't want to be, or whose pregnancies were dangerous, unviable, or inconvenient for (illicit) lovers or enslavers. We will see that women who wanted or needed to terminate their pregnancies not only had to contend with the dangers of risky abortifacients, but also had to face a storm of misogyny in the form of antiabortion screeds and laws.

FIVE

Corinna Has an Abortion

IN THE 1ST CENTURY BCE, Corinna lay exhausted and near death.[1] She had gotten an abortion after having an affair. She was the mistress of a famous writer, Publius Ovidius Naso ("Ovid"), who documented his reaction to her abortion in a pair of poems. In the first he describes the mixture of anger and fear that he feels as he prays to Greek and Egyptian gods to spare her life. In the second he pans outward, chastising all women who have abortions. Across the two poems he touches on many antiabortion classics: he suggests that Corinna is promiscuous—"She's pregnant by me—or so I think"; he calls the abortion a "great risk"; he accuses women of having abortions out of vanity over their physical beauty—"No doubt you'd take your chances . . . just to keep your bellies free of wrinkles with your crime?"; he fearmongers about population decline—"If mothers in antiquity had behaved this way, the human race would have perished from this crime"; and he asserts that women often get a swift comeuppance, since they usually die as a result of the abortion. He uses the words "destruction," "crime," "violation," "murder," and "desecration" to describe the act. Those who perform abortions are "unsure" and inexperienced—they don't really know what they are doing. And when a woman dies after a botched abortion, everyone says, "She deserved it!"[2]

What should we make of this vitriolic screed? It doesn't sound far off from the rantings of antiabortion zealots today. So, was abortion as contentious an issue in ancient Rome as it is in the modern United States? Were the ancient Romans as strongly opposed to abortion as these poems seem to imply? What did Corinna do to have an abortion? Were there reliable and effective methods for terminating pregnancies?

We will see that Ovid was not alone. Ancient Roman men left an extensive record of their misogynistic outrage. Women, they complained, practiced abortion widely, depriving them of heirs and slaves. Roman law displayed concern for the rights of fathers and enslavers and discomfort with various types of women's knowledge that could be used to concoct body-altering potions, especially abortifacients and aphrodisiacs. At the same time, many forms of contraception and abortion were available to women, recorded in herbals and medical treatises. With these methods, women had to balance efficacy and risk. Ultimately, we should not take the record we have at face value. Despite their bluster, many men were probably supportive of abortion. And, in many cases, what may seem to us to have been abortions were actually important methods of fertility treatment.

VIEWS ON ABORTION

When Corinna was having her abortion, in the late 1st century BCE, antiabortion sentiment was increasing in both pagan and Christian literature, all of it written by elite men. Later, in the 2nd to 4th centuries CE, Christians attempted to distinguish themselves from pagans through their condemnation of abortion. But the reality is that both groups published dramatic, moralizing tirades against abortion and the women who (allegedly) had them. Roman law was also hostile to abortion, but ostensibly for different reasons. It was concerned with how abortion—carried out by a woman without the knowledge of the father—could deprive (elite) men of heirs and deprive the Roman state of citizens. Finally, the medical texts display a contradiction, especially from the 2nd century CE onward. They offer mild to severe criticism of abortion, but nonetheless lay out extensive procedures for how to abort, including specific recipes for abortifacient drinks and vaginal suppositories. The sheer amount of medical information on abortion suggests that they were happening with some regularity. Not only were abortions a standard feature of healthcare, they were also a standard part of *fertility* care. That is, abortion—or what we would consider to be abortion today—was often a precursor to pregnancy. It was an important treatment for infertility.

A typical pagan attitude toward abortion can be seen in a poem by the 1st- to 2nd-century satirical writer Juvenal. He paints a lurid picture of women using abortion to hide affairs and worrying over their youthful good looks. His criticism is aimed particularly at upper-class women:

> But at least [poor] women endure the dangers of childbirth and put up
> with all the work of breastfeeding that their position in life forces on them.
> By contrast, scarcely any laboring woman lies in a gilded bed.
> So powerful are the skills and drugs of the woman
> who makes [rich women] barren and hires herself out to kill humans in the belly.
> Be happy, you unfortunate man. Offer your wife whatever [potion] she
> has to drink yourself. After all, if she wanted to stretch and
> torture her womb with jumping baby boys, you might
> turn out to be father of an Ethiopian. Soon you would have a discolored heir in
> your will—one that you'd never want to see in the morning light.[3]

Juvenal contrasts wealthy women with poor women. In the lines just before these, he chastises rich and poor women alike for seeking out the services of fortune tellers. Wealthy women pay expensive foreign soothsayers, while poor women seek out cheap prophesies in the marketplace. But at least poor women, he writes, go through the danger of pregnancy and childbirth. They don't have another option. Rich women, though, can procure the "skills and drugs" that cause abortions. He calls this murder. Here the rich pregnant woman hires an assassin to "kill humans in the belly." But Juvenal advises his male readers to accept these abortions gratefully—his wife might be concealing an affair that she had with an Ethiopian man. In the Roman world, paternity was granted to the birthing woman's husband, regardless of her sexual history. So the hypothetical cuckold in this poem might be forced to bequeath his property to a "discolored heir." The child's dark skin color reveals the infidelity. The authorial voice is sardonic. Abortion is murder, but having another man's child for an heir is worse.

These accusations of adultery and abortion were common. The 1st-to-2nd-century writer Tacitus accused Octavia, sister of the emperor Augustus, of having an abortion to conceal an affair.[4] Like Juvenal, he drew an unflattering contrast between elite Roman women and non-elite women. In this case, he praised barbarian German women, living on and outside the borders of the Roman Empire, for not using birth control or having abortions in an attempt to limit the number of their children, like spoiled Roman women did.[5]

Monotheistic attitudes were similar, but with the added threat of eternal damnation. The *Sibylline Oracles*—a collection of anonymous prophesies that was first composed by Jews and then revised by Christians, perhaps as early 30 BCE—provides a startling vision of the punishments awaiting women who committed the sin of abortion or infanticide:

> Those who defiled their flesh with vicious acts,
> And who undid the belt of maidenhood
> In secret union; who their unborn load
> Aborted, or cast out the child, once born,
> Unlawfully; witches and poisoners
> Them too the wrath of the heavenly, deathless God
> Shall fasten to the pillar, where a stream
> Of quenchless fire flows round.[6]

Here, women who procure abortions are unmarried virgins who have had secret affairs. To hide their sexual transgressions, they either abort the fetus or leave the child outside to die after it is born. Their punishment is to be tied to a pillar in hell while "a stream of quenchless fire flows round." The witches and poisoners who provide abortions are subject to the same fate.

As Christianity developed its theology over the first several centuries CE, condemnation of abortion became a mainstay of its moral philosophy. A late-1st- or early-2nd-century Christian manual called the *Didache* (literally "teaching") defined abortion as murder: "You will not murder offspring by means of abortion."[7] Tertullian, a Christian writer living in Carthage (modern-day Tunisia), explained how opposition to abortion was an objection to murder more generally: "Since murder is altogether forbidden to us, it is not permissible even to destroy what has been conceived in the womb, while blood is still being gathered into a human."[8] In his estimation, abortion is murder because "what has been conceived in the womb" is equivalent to a child that has already been born. The Christian antiabortion rhetoric is similar to the pagan antiabortion rhetoric, but the Christians have the additional threat of divine punishment.

ABORTION IN THE LAW

In the 3rd century, abortion came under the Cornelian Law Against Murderers and Poisoners. The law read, "If it is proved that a woman has done violence to her womb to bring about an abortion, the provincial governor shall send her into exile."[9] Romans—and Roman law in particular—were suspicious of potion and poison dealers. Those who supplied the abortifacient drinks were also subject to punishment. Lower-status providers were sentenced to hard labor in the mines, while those of higher status were sentenced to exile and partial forfeiture of their property.[10] That the law was primarily concerned with the distribution of body-altering potions more than abortion specifically is shown by the fact that aphrodisiac and fertility potions were similarly punished.[11]

A Roman jurist explained the law against abortion with reference to a courtroom speech from 69 BCE in which the lawyer Marcus Tullius Cicero described a Milesian woman who was bribed by rival heirs to get an abortion.[12] She was convicted of a capital offense. This woman, Cicero explained, "had destroyed the hope of the father, the continuity of his name, the support of the family line, the heir of the household, a citizen marked out for the republic."[13]

This line displays typical Ciceronian bombast. He was a self-aggrandizing lawyer and politician known for his rhetorical flourishes. If it had gone no further than his published speech, we might not make much of it. But the fact that this passage from 69 BCE provided the precedent and justification for a law written hundreds of years later suggests that there was a widespread belief in the Roman Empire that abortion was a threat to paternal and civic interests. The fear was that due to the choices of a woman, a man might not be able to secure his legacy. Further, there was the idea that the unborn infant belonged to the state. The unborn fetus was the future heir of its father and future citizen of Rome.[14]

Although the fetus did not have a fixed status in the law, the principles of paternal and civic interest repeatedly crop up. At times the fetus was described as "part of the woman or her insides."[15] At other times it was considered a full human being in its own right.[16] But when it was considered a full human being, this was primarily in relation to inheritance and property rights. According to one judicial decision, the fetus was considered to be "in the category of human" (*in rebus humanis*) when it stood to gain some material advantage upon birth.[17] If there was the possibility that it might inherit money, property, or a title, then it had a claim on humanness. In the law, the fetus was presumed to be male for the purposes of its potential future rights. However, both male and female children could inherit from their fathers, and daughters were valued as heirs along with sons.

Another legal decision was primarily concerned with who had control over the fetus.[18] It stated that a man did not have to acknowledge his unborn child if his wife (or ex-wife) pretended that she was not pregnant—or even flat out denied it. A man was not responsible for supporting a doubtful or concealed pregnancy. But even in such a situation, once the baby was born, the man could take it and make it his heir. His claim to custody trumped the mother's.

Both of these scenarios deal with a particular kind of fetus—one whose father had enough property to be concerned with having an heir. The law did not protect the fetus as a human being per se. It protected the potential future heir of a man with property. Other Roman legal decisions reinforced this principle. A fetus could be appointed its father's potential heir, with the understanding that it would assume the full status of heir upon its birth.[19]

If a free, pregnant woman was condemned to death, Roman law stipulated that she give birth before she was executed.[20] Her fetus had the potential to be born a free Roman citizen and so was not subject to the punishment meted out to its mother. If this fetus was the product of a free, Roman marriage, then it was under the power of its father—a legal condition that gave Roman fathers the right of life or death over their children, even grown children.[21] In this way, a Roman woman was a temporary holder and caregiver to a fetus who was ultimately going to be under its father's control.

These laws and principles did not apply to the many enslaved pregnant women in the Roman Empire. In the eyes of the law, such women were not potential or expectant mothers, but producers of a commodity. Their children were the potential future property of enslavers.[22] Legally, the relationship between an enslaved woman and her fetus was often depicted as being like the relationship between fruit trees in an orchard and the fruit they produced.[23] Her children were considered to be an addition to the property and estate of the enslaver, just as the fruit from the fruit tree was an addition to the property of the tree's owner. Enslavers could sell or send away the offspring of enslaved women.[24] Enslaved pregnant women were subject to men and to the law but in a quite different way from free women.

In terms of the Roman state's interest in unborn children, we can imagine that it had the same sort of interest that any monarchical, militaristic state has in its citizens: it wanted to reproduce its pool of available laborers and soldiers. Certainly, much of this work was done by enslaved people, but in order for the Roman state to continue being a giant, powerful empire, it needed to constantly reproduce its free population.[25]

In the literature of the Roman Empire, abortion is presented as murder. Women who have abortions are vain, adulterous, wicked, and—in the Christian literature—going to hell. The legal texts come up short of calling abortion murder but nonetheless offer paternal and civic concerns as reasons to prohibit it. If we return to the Juvenal passage, though, we can see how morality and the law were often intertwined. Despite rhetorical flourishes about the murder of fetuses and the culpability of pregnant women, Juvenal is ultimately concerned about paternal and civic interest. His graphic description of abortion-seeking women starts with drugs and murder ("So powerful are the skills and drugs of the woman who makes [rich women] barren and hires herself out to kill humans in the belly"), but ends with inheritance concerns and racism ("Soon you would have a discolored heir in your will"). The alleged issue is the destruction of a human being, but the actual issue is the usurpation of the father's will by an unacceptable heir.

ABORTION IN MEDICINE

The medical texts of the empire, particularly those of the 2nd century and later, exhibit a tension around abortion. They generally contain a broad declarative statement about the immorality or danger of abortion, while at the same time giving extensive instruction in how to abort.

A 4th-century medical text from Constantinople is on the more extreme end. It states, "It is never right to provide an abortion to anyone" but then goes on to give nine abortifacient recipes—to be used when the life or health of the mother was in jeopardy.[26] Two centuries earlier, the physician Soranus was milder in his critique. He explained that there was a controversy among contemporary physicians, with some physicians prohibiting abortifacients altogether and others prescribing them "with discrimination," refusing to provide abortions "because of adultery" or "out of consideration for youthful beauty."[27] These physicians only prescribe abortion when pregnancy and birth would be dangerous to the mother because the uterus is too small or due to some other physical difficulty. Soranus puts himself in this second category, adding that "it is safer to prevent conception than to destroy the fetus." Nonetheless, in addition to several contraceptive methods, he gives a detailed procedure for how to induce an abortion, including two recipes for abortifacient vaginal suppositories and one abortifacient drink.[28] The phrases "because of adultery" and "out of consideration for youthful beauty" are clearly echoes of the antiabortion screeds that were popular among the upper-class men of the Roman Empire. Soranus is paying lip service to the concerns of his clientele. But both contraceptives and abortifacients are key parts of his gynecological manual.

PREVENTING PREGNANCY

As an upper-class woman involved in a long-term affair, Corinna was probably well versed in contraceptive measures. She may have followed something like a fertility awareness method, tracking her menstrual cycles and avoiding intercourse during her most fertile period. Today we know that the most fertile period is during ovulation, which is generally midway through the approximately twenty-eight-day menstrual cycle, or about fourteen days before the start of menstruation (but there is quite a bit of variation from person to person and from cycle to cycle). However, the general wisdom at the time was that the most fertile period was right as menstruation was ending.[29] As we saw in chapter 3, there was no awareness of ovulation. Rather, people believed that female "seed" was released during orgasm, just like the male semen. The time right as menstruation was ending was seen as the most fertile because the uterus was freshly cleansed and not overloaded with menstrual fluid.

Perhaps Corinna practiced a version of the pull-out method. Today, coitus interruptus involves removing the penis from the vagina right before ejaculation. But in the ancient world, it was the woman, not the man, who was supposed to act at the critical moment, holding her breath and drawing back as the man ejaculated inside her. That way she could prevent the semen from being propelled too far up into her vagina. After sex she was advised to squat down, sneeze, and wipe all around her vulva and vagina to expel and clear out the seed. She was supposed to drink something cold (to counter the heat that made conception happen).[30] Another mechanical method involved inserting a tuft of wool into the vagina prior to intercourse, either alone or dipped in a medicinal preparation.[31] This method was akin to the modern-day sponge or even diaphragm.

Maybe Corinna relied on herbal contraceptives. These took two main forms—those inserted vaginally and those taken by mouth. She could have smeared her vagina and cervix with old olive oil, honey, cedar resin, balsam tree juice, or myrtle oil (alone or mixed with white lead) prior to intercourse. There's no exact explanation for how they worked, but it seems likely that these viscous or sticky substances were meant to trap and hold the semen, preventing it from entering the uterus. Or she could have used a vaginal suppository made of astringent, clogging, and cooling herbs that were meant to close the cervix. Soranus provides recipes for several contraceptive pessaries; ingredients that feature prominently include pomegranate peel and oak gall, both highly astringent. He advises against a monthly contraceptive drink, arguing that it skirts the line between contraceptives—of which he generally approved—and abortifacients—of which he approved only in certain circumstances. However, it seems that these monthly contraceptive teas and pills were popular, since he mentions that some people think them advisable, and he himself gives recipes for four.[32]

If she was truly anxious about getting pregnant, Corinna may have used a combination of methods. She probably also wore a contraceptive amulet.[33] Magical handbooks contained recipes for these, such as one that advised the user to "take a pierced bean and attach it as an amulet after tying it up in a piece of mule hide."[34] Mule body parts were popular ingredients in contraceptive amulets.[35] They, like the amulets described in chapter 3, worked via the principle of sympathy. The sterility of the mule—a cross between a horse and a donkey—was supposed to rub off onto the person wearing the amulet.

But despite her best efforts, Corinna found herself pregnant. We know what she did next and what the consequences were. She got an abortion and nearly died in the process. But what did her abortion actually look like? Was it mechanical, herbal, or instrumental? How did it go wrong? These details we do not get from Ovid. But many of the abortifacient methods that were available to Corinna would have been risky, especially if her abortion was successful.

HOW TO HAVE AN ABORTION IN ANCIENT ROME

A pregnancy could be terminated through physical and herbal means.[36] Physical methods included taking hot baths, bloodletting, and moving the body vigorously, such as by riding or jumping and leaping about, like Demetria and her Lacedemonian Leap. Herbs could be administered orally or vaginally. Although abortifacient remedies and methods have been preserved in the writings of men, it was likely women who were preparing and performing them, either on each other or themselves.[37] When they record their sources, the male writers tell us that they have learned about abortifacients from women—primarily sex workers and midwives.[38]

Dioscorides, a military doctor who traveled around the Mediterranean with the Roman army in the 1st century CE, recorded the medicinal uses of the plants, resins, and minerals he came across. Many of these were abortifacients. He listed herbs and spices such as white and black hellebore, scammony, cardamom, garden cress, shepherd's purse, and soapwort as having the power to "destroy the fetus" when inserted as a vaginal suppository or applied via uterine fumigation.[39] As he himself was not an expert in all the places and plants he encountered, he likely got this knowledge from local healers, many of whom would have been midwives and other female practitioners.

In his *Gynecology,* Soranus gave detailed instructions on how to have an abortion.[40] In the first thirty days after conception, the aim was to separate the embryo from the wall of the uterus. He advised the pregnant woman to walk about energetically, be shaken by draft animals, leap forcefully, and carry things that were too heavy for her. She was to be given vigorous massages on her lower abdomen, mons pubis, and inner thighs, take long daily baths, and consume wine and pungent foods. In short, she was to do the opposite of what was recommended for someone trying to get pregnant. Soranus also advised the use of diuretic concoctions (for inducing urination), pungent suppositories and vaginal clysters, herbal sitz baths, poultices, and plasters.

He provided a specific treatment plan: for two or three days, have the woman take long baths, use softening vaginal suppositories, and largely abstain from food and wine. Then administer bloodletting, taking away a large quantity of blood. The idea was to disturb the uterus, making it loose so that the embryo would fall out. If the bloodletting did not work, then an abortive vaginal suppository should be used as a last resort. Recommended ingredients included myrtle, wallflower seed, lupine, rue, sweet bay, cardamom, sulfur, wormwood, and myrrh. Because these recipes were dangerous for the woman, they were only to be used if the physical and mechanical methods did not work. He cautioned against abortifacients that were too powerful and also against using anything sharp-edged to try to separate the embryo from the uterus. His concern was that other parts of the body might be injured.

Soranus's step-by-step process focused on harm mitigation. His main concern was not the morality of abortion, but the safety. He emphasized the importance of trying to induce an abortion within the first thirty days after conception, which would have been the safest for the woman. Throughout his descriptions of abortive methods, his focus was on relaxing the pregnant woman and her body. The idea was that if the uterus could be made loose, it would gently release the embryo. He advocated for the use of gentle herbal abortive remedies. Finally, his caution against using sharp objects implied that there was a more dangerous method that was not part of his medical practice. This sort of mechanical abortion would have involved massive risks for the woman, including laceration and infection. Overall, his abortive methods progressed from least to most risky: from vigorous exercise, to hot baths and softening vaginal suppositories, to bloodletting, and finally to abortive suppositories and drinks with caustic herbs such as rue and wormwood, which had to be administered in the right dose so as to not poison the patient.

SILPHIUM

The most widely discussed and mythologized contraceptive and abortifacient herb from the ancient world is a plant called silphium. Today, popular articles on ancient birth control and abortion will tell you that silphium—a member of the giant fennel family found in the North African region of Cyrenaica (modern-day eastern Libya)—was so highly prized for its abortifacient properties that Greek and Roman colonizers of Cyrenaica harvested it to extinction.[41] Indeed, there does seem to have been an ancient plant called silphium that was literally worth its weight in silver. It grew only in Cyrenaica and was likely extinct by the end of the 1st century CE due to overharvesting and to desertification—a process of human-induced climate change—caused by deforestation, cropland expansion, and overgrazing of livestock by Greek and Roman colonists.[42]

But the claim that silphium was driven to extinction due to its widely appreciated contraceptive and abortifacient properties is likely false. Silphium was, in the first place, a culinary delight.[43] The Cyrenaic variety seems to have been the most delicious, with a pleasant-smelling resinous stalk, though other types of silphium grew in in the eastern parts of the empire and in Persia (modern-day Iran). It was also a panacea. Dioscorides described it as being therapeutic for tumors, anal swellings, cataracts, toothaches, warts, calluses, chronic cough, spasms, epilepsy, and more.[44] This sort of multipurpose utility was not unusual. Herbal preparations worked off of general principles, rather than being specific to a certain body part or ailment. Silphium reduced swelling and encouraged the elimination of excess or putrid fluids from the body. Dioscorides mentioned that when "drunk with pepper and myrrh," it could "bring on the menstrual period." This remedy sounds like an abortifacient, especially since Dioscorides did not give any further explanation.

But if we look at the Hippocratic gynecological texts, we see that silphium was actually a key ingredient in fertility treatments. It was used for cleansing the uterus—inducing the outflow of menstrual blood and other fluids—in order to prepare it for conception and pregnancy. If a woman habitually miscarried at two months, the Hippocratic writer of *Superfetation* recommended silphium as part of a treatment to "wash out" the uterus.[45] He advised mixing strained gourd pulp with boiled honey and a little silphium. The woman was supposed to spread this mixture on a spatula and insert it into her vagina. At the same time, she was to "eat a large amount of garlic . . . a stalk of silphium, and whatever else will produce gas to inflate her uterus."[46] The patient did this treatment for many days until her menses appeared. Once she had stopped menstruating—at what was believed to be her most fertile time of the month—she was to have intercourse. In this treatment silphium, taken vaginally and orally, inflated and cleansed the uterus, preparing it for pregnancy. Even though it induced menstruation, it was not meant as an abortifacient.

"ABORTION" AS FERTILITY TREATMENT

There was a difference between remedies to induce menstruation and abortifacients. In fact, the Greeks and Romans drew several distinctions in their methods of fertility management. Contraceptives prevented pregnancy, abortifacients ended it, and a third group called emmenagogues (literally "things that draw down the menses") cleared the uterus out, preparing it for pregnancy. They recognized the connection between menstruation and pregnancy. So, if a woman wasn't menstruating and she also wasn't pregnant—as far as they could tell—then she needed an emmenagogue to get her period going. Emmenagogues could be but were not necessarily also abortifacients.

One of the most serious conditions that required treatment with emmenagogues was the uterine *mole,* discussed in chapter 4. As a false pregnancy, not only did it cause problems for the pregnant woman's health, but it also monopolized the space that should be available for a real pregnancy. If a midwife or doctor determined that a woman had a *mole,* they would prescribe purgative remedies: suppositories, sitz baths, cupping, bloodletting, and emmenagogues. Their purpose was to cleanse or purge the uterus and to restart menstruation.

There was a great variety of herbs available and accessible to women at all economic levels that could be used to cleanse the uterus and induce menstruation. Dioscorides lists over a hundred cultivated and wild herbs, plants, and animal parts that can be used as emmenagogues. Wild herbs such as rue, pennyroyal, marjoram, Cretan spikenard, Cretan thyme, catmint, stinging nettle, squirting cucumber, lovage, common centaury, and hazelwort were ubiquitous around the Mediterranean.[47] Cultivated plants, too, such as leek, onion, garlic, garden cress, radish, cabbage, and fig could have been found in home gardens.[48] Lanolin and soapwort (see fig. 5), which was used to clean wool, could both be used for drawing down the menses.[49] Anyone who processed wool would have had ready access to these materials. Expensive imported resins, such as myrrh and storax, were likely harder to come by, but given the number of alternatives available, lack of financial means would not have prevented anyone from accessing this treatment.[50]

Since many of these herbs were also used to terminate pregnancies, however, (and since pregnancy termination was essentially a purging of the uterus), what was the difference between emmenagogues and abortifacients? Were emmenagogues just a euphemistic or secretive way of prescribing abortifacients?

It's true that the herbs that were used as emmenagogues and abortifacients overlapped. For instance, Dioscorides records that soapwort "brings on the menstrual period" and "destroys fetuses."[51] And in his *Gynecology,* Soranus lists rue and wormwood as powerful abortifacient herbs *and* prescribes them as treatment for a condition called "air in the uterus," which caused infertility by destroying the sperm during intercourse.[52]

But just because an herb or mineral could be used as an emmenagogue and an abortifacient or as a contraceptive and an abortifacient doesn't mean that every time it was used it was actually secretly an abortifacient. Part of the issue is that the Romans didn't have birth control methods that prevented ovulation from taking place like we do today with the pill and the IUD. So contraceptives, abortifacients, and emmenagogues were *functionally* the same in that they broke up and expelled intrauterine

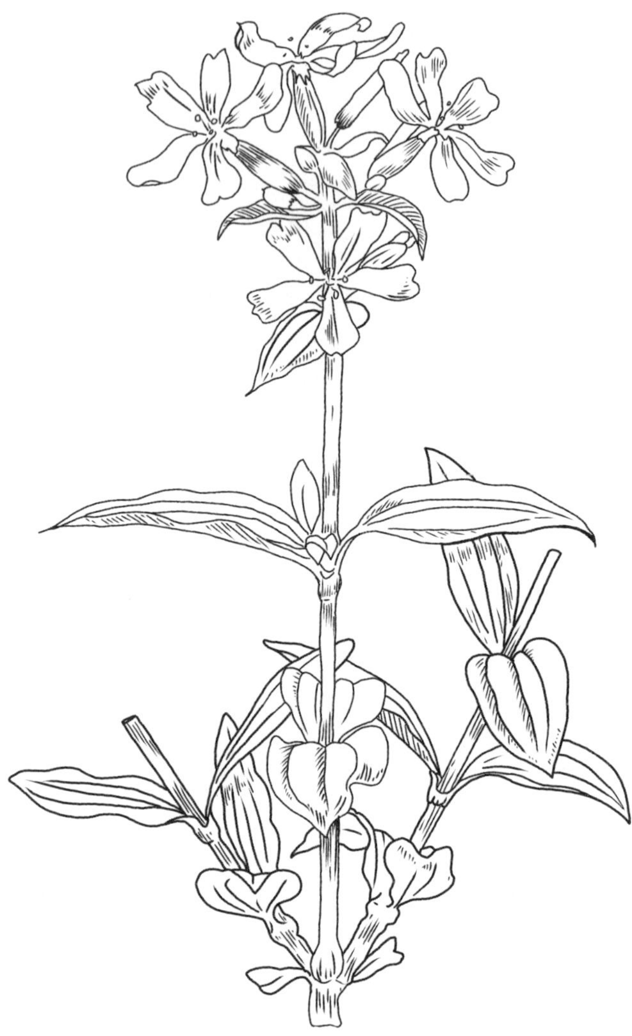

FIGURE 5. Soapwort, *Saponaria officinalis* L. A common plant in the ancient Mediterranean that was used for cleaning raw wool. It could be used in a vaginal suppository to bring on menstruation or cause an abortion. Drawing by Hayley Monroe.

material. But the conceptual differences were important. Unlike abortifacients (and contraceptives), which were fundamentally anti-pregnancy, the purpose of emmenagogues was to prepare the uterus for conception. They were an important part of reproductive health as treatments for infertility.

Occasionally—and this may be the cause of some confusion in modern interpretations—Dioscorides will categorize an herb as good for starting menstruation and for "drawing down" or "expelling" fetuses. Such is the case, for instance, for wild olive, wine flavored with allheal, cinnamon, myrrh, and iris.[53] These certainly sound like abortifacients. But what Dioscorides is identifying in these instances is that these substances could be used to remove a dead fetus. The entry for dittany of Crete explains that it "expels deceased fetuses" when drunk, applied topically, or used in a vaginal fumigation.[54] Similarly, the entry for Mecca balsam shows that stillborn, not living, fetuses are the targets of such herbs—its juice "draws down both the afterbirth and fetuses."[55] The context is clearly one of birth, not abortion. The phrases Dioscorides uses consistently for abortifacients are "destroys fetuses" or "kills fetuses," not "draws down fetuses." In the Hippocratic *Diseases of Women* 1, a woman is given a drink of clover and white wine if she "is not cleaned after birth" (that is, if her placenta or lochia does not come); similarly, a clover suppository "causes menstruation and expels a fetus."[56] This remedy is for clearing out matter, not destroying it.[57]

It's also possible that an expulsive was used in coordination with an abortifacient. Once the abortifacient "destroyed" the embryo, the expulsive would then be used to remove it from the uterus. There is no direct evidence that this is what happened, but Dioscorides is clearly recording two different types of action when he says that some herbs "draw down" or "expel" fetuses and others "destroy" them.

Conceptually speaking, emmenagogues, expulsives, contraceptives, and abortifacients were different. The purpose of emmenagogues would have been to instigate or assist menstruation, clearing out and purging the uterus to prepare it for intercourse and conception. Women taking emmenagogues likely would have been looking for the early signs of conception so as to avoid foods and herbs that might interfere with pregnancy. Similarly, expulsives would have been used in the case of a stillbirth, to clear out the impacted fetus. Contraceptives, conversely, would have been used deliberately and consistently to prevent conception from taking place. And abortifacients were for the express purpose of destroying a fetus.

Throughout the medical and non-medical texts, while abortions are dangerous, purging supports fertility. In his 1st-century-CE encyclopedia, Pliny the Elder, using an analogy to lead mines, explains, "It is a remarkable fact in the case of [lead] mines that only when they have been abandoned do they replenish themselves and become more productive . . . just as a miscarriage seems to make some women more prolific."[58] According to Pliny, women's bodies, like mines in the earth, sometimes become more productive when they have been cleared out and left to sit fallow for a while.[59] Or, as one of the Hippocratic writers put it, "To get a woman pregnant, first clear her and her uterus out" (that is, with an emmenagogue).[60]

This relationship between purging and conception can be seen in the herb called birthwort, *aristolochia,* which literally means "best birth." Dioscorides writes that it gets its name "from the belief that it is very helpful to women in childbirth." It was able to "draw out all birth matter compacted in the uterus, the menses, and embryos/fetuses" when drunk or used in a vaginal suppository.[61] Birthwort could be used for speeding up a birth, expelling the placenta or lochia, or removing a stillborn fetus. In a gynecological text from the 5th to 6th century CE, the author includes it in a pessary, along with Mecca balsam, myrrh, rose oil, and other ingredients, to promote conception. The physician writes, "Have her keep it in [her vagina] for two hours and then take it away and have sex [with her husband] and conception will occur immediately."[62] Birthwort was an herb intended to promote childbirth, not prevent it.[63]

Certainly, a woman could have used emmenagogues and expulsives as contraceptives and abortifacients. To this point, Soranus discourages the use of emmenagogic drinks for the purpose of contraception (that is, drinks taken monthly "to induce menstruation") on the grounds that not only do they "prevent conception, but also destroy anything already conceived."[64] And he explains, "Some say that an expulsive is the same as an abortifacient, while others say that it is different."[65] So there was some recognition that emmenagogues, expulsives, and abortifacients could be the same in effect if not necessarily in intent. Soranus was writing some fifty or so years after Dioscorides, and it's possible that attitudes on this front were changing. As antiabortion sentiment ramped up among both pagans and Christians, women's practices might have come under more scrutiny. Many centuries later, in the mid-19th century, when abortion was criminalized in the United States, the ability to hide abortions under the guise of emmenagogues became very important. Abortifacient pills were advertised in newspapers as therapeutic remedies for "drawing down the menses." But it is impossible to say to what extent this kind of subterfuge was being practiced in ancient Rome. For the most part, it seems that there would have been deliberate reasons for using emmenagogues *or* abortifacients without pretense.[66]

EFFICACY

How effective were abortifacient methods? Certainly a sharp object would have worked, but at what cost? The consequences in the pre-germ-theory world would have been dire. The work of historian John Riddle in the 1980s and 1990s, using modern scientific studies to assess the efficacy of ancient abortifacient herbs, suggests that that the Romans did have some abortifacients that worked. Riddle's work has been controversial because, as some scholars have pointed out, we often do not know the dosage or potency of the abortive herbs and recipes that are mentioned in the ancient texts.[67] It's hard to know whether the ancient Romans were using these preparations in effective amounts. However, the herbs being used were not random. Many of these same substances can be found as effective, if risky, abortifacients in modern herbals, such as *Natural Liberty,* a guide to self-managed abortion.[68] And as historian Laurence Totelin has pointed out, it's insufficient and condescending to consider all ancient remedies to be only symbolically effective (or to work only on the placebo effect).[69] If the ancient writers said that something worked, we have to imagine that in some sense it worked—perhaps not with the degree of efficacy that we expect from contraceptives and abortifacients today, but enough to be meaningful to people in the ancient world.[70]

It does seem that efficacy was directly related to risk. The Hippocratic writer of the medical treatise *Diseases of Women* 1 explains that "it's impossible to have an abortion without violence"—from a drink, a food, a vaginal suppository, or "something else" (perhaps a sharp object?)—"and violence does damage."[71] The writer cautions that an abortion can lead to uterine ulceration and inflammation. In one of the Hippocratic case studies, the doctor suspects that the patient, referred to as "the wife of Simus," may have taken an abortifacient, though he is not sure.[72] After four days of misery—vomiting green bile, a swollen, black tongue, red eyes—she dies.

So, it does seem that people in the ancient world were using substances that were abortive. How effective those substances were (versus how dangerous they were) is a question we do not have the sources to answer. Whether we can prove it scientifically or not, it's not irresponsible to assume that some people in some circumstances in the ancient world had successful abortions.

WHO WAS HAVING ABORTIONS?

Unfortunately, the reasons or circumstances under which a woman in ancient Rome used contraceptives and abortifacients are not fully knowable. Accounts from women themselves are nonexistent, and as the diatribes at the top of the chapter show, male writers tended to be egregiously chauvinistic when reporting on the use of both contraceptives and abortifacients. For instance, Julia, the daughter of the emperor Augustus, supposedly managed her reproduction by only engaging in extramarital affairs while she was already pregnant. She is said to have quipped, "I never take on a passenger until the ship is full."[73] There is more than a dash of misogyny here. Julia's life was never truly her own. At age fourteen, she was forced to marry her first cousin. When he died a few years later, her father married her off to his chief general, Agrippa, a man twenty-five years her senior. They had five children together and then, after Agrippa's death, Julia was married off to her stepbrother, Tiberius, with whom she had a sixth child. Throughout these nearly twenty years of dynastic unions and forced reproduction, Julia was rumored to have had several affairs. She eventually died on a small, lonely island, having been permanently exiled there by her father on charges of adultery and treason.

Male writers delighted in attacking Julia with lurid descriptions of her sexual transgressions. She was said to have "left nothing undone" when it came to extravagance and lust and to have "received herds of lovers."[74] Many seem to have been thrilled by the idea that Julia flagrantly disregarded the conservative anti-adultery laws of her own father. Unfortunately, Julia's treatment, in life and literature, seems to have been typical for women of her status. Just like her compatriot Corinna, Julia was subject to the scrutiny and disdain of the men of her social class.

Women like Corinna and Julia, who wanted to engage in sex for pleasure (including extramarital affairs), would have been using some form of birth control. So, too, would have women doing professional sex work, as well as women engaged in other types of professional entertainment work, including dancers, singers, acrobats, and actresses.

Perhaps women who had had particularly difficult or dangerous pregnancies and births in the past and who might have been reluctant to get pregnant again would have used, or even been encouraged by a midwife or doctor to use, contraceptives. Soranus cautioned against the dangers associated with pregnancy and birth for some bodies: those of women who were too young and still underdeveloped, women whose uteruses were too small to bring a fetus to full development, or those whose uteruses had knobby swellings and fissures at the cervix.[75] We can also imagine all sorts of specific and individual circumstances that might have led someone to use contraceptives: a personal, if idiosyncratic, desire to not have children (or any more children); a desire to avoid pregnancy if one's husband had been away on military or political service for a long period of time; the wish to avoid pregnancy by a particular man. When contraception failed—or failed to be used—abortion was the necessary next step.

The moralizing tirades against abortion combined with the many abortifacient methods in the medical texts have prompted some scholars to speculate that there was a glut of abortions taking place in ancient Rome.[76] Why would there be such a uniform outcry against them unless they were happening frequently? Other scholars have suggested just the opposite: given the intense antiabortion rhetoric, the dangers posed by abortifacients, and the lack of specific evidence for actual abortions (as opposed to merely recipes in medical texts), there must not have been much abortion going on at all.[77] Furthermore, this second camp asserts, we don't see any population patterns in ancient Rome that suggest widespread fertility control.[78] That is, given the rate at which the population in the Roman Empire was growing, it seems unlikely that people were practicing family planning—using birth control or abortion to limit the number of children that they had.

The issue with the first argument—that there was a lot of abortion going on—is that the antiabortion screeds have much more the flavor of a moral panic than any reflection of reality. What's important to keep in mind is that when Roman men were talking about the evils of abortion, they were talking about abortion in specific circumstances with specific consequences. They were not condemning abortion across the board for all people everywhere. Their concern was primarily with upper-class Roman women, who were being accused of shirking their responsibilities to reproduce. But there is no identifiable pattern of upper-class Roman women doing any such thing. Incentives for reproducing were high, and the social consequences of being childless could be intense. There was almost certainly no "abortion epidemic" happening.[79]

The second point—that there wasn't much abortion happening at all—may be true. Given the intense pronatalism at Rome and the many benefits that could accrue to mothers of multiple children—free, freed, and enslaved alike—it's likely that family planning more often took the form of planning to build families, not to avoid having children. But arguments built on absence require care. As the mantra of the historian goes, "Absence of evidence is not evidence of absence." The point that there isn't much specific evidence for abortions is really a non-point. There isn't much specific evidence for women doing most things in ancient Rome.

I cannot prove for certain that abortion was happening in the Roman Empire, other than to say that abortion has happened everywhere, always, in every place that humans have ever had babies. The reasons, methods, frequency, and attitude might change significantly, but the reality of it is constant. Women in ancient Rome were just as complicated and idiosyncratic as they are today. There were good reasons why individual women may have wanted to seek out abortions: fear of childbirth, previous experience with pregnancy or birth complications, indications that things were not right with the fetus, lack of legal status of themselves or their children (if they were enslaved or unmarried), lack of financial means to support a child or additional children. These reasons might have even included adultery and concern for their own bodies. We can acknowledge this reality without falling into the moralizing misogyny of men like Juvenal and Corinna's boyfriend.

What's alarming about looking at abortion in the ancient Roman world is how disconnected the different voices are from each other. On the one hand, there's a category of treatments that is important not only for healthcare, but for fertility care. Contraceptives, abortifacients, emmenagogues, and expulsives were all crucial components of reproductive health and longevity. And on the other hand, there are a bunch of men drawing lurid and salacious portraits of morally reprehensible women.

Let's imagine that while their affair was going on, Corinna regularly used birth control. Perhaps she took a monthly contraceptive drink or used a tuft of wool, inserted into her vagina before sex. But her contraceptive method failed. Then she undertook some sort of risky abortion that left her exhausted and near death. In one of the poems, Ovid mentions two types of abortion: sharp objects and herbs.[80] Perhaps she drank a potion or inserted a vaginal suppository made of effective but dangerous herbs such as rue or wormwood. Maybe someone inserted a sharp object into her uterus to destroy the fetus and she then took a powerful expulsive that induced multiple days of bleeding. In this context, her boyfriend's poems are not just over the top, they are cruel. He claims that his main concern is her health and safety, but at the same time he piles on all the classic, misogynistic ideas about abortion.

In the texts of the Roman Empire, abortion is portrayed as uniquely female. Pliny the Elder explains that while men invented every type of sexual deviance, "Women invented abortion."[81] But the reality is that Roman men would probably have been involved in the decision-making for many of these abortions.[82] Corinna's boyfriend stood to benefit as much if not more than she did from her abortion. While adultery was certainly less frowned upon for men than it was for women, men could still be brought to court on charges of seduction if they associated with the wrong man's wife or daughter. In fact, Corinna's boyfriend was eventually exiled from Rome by the emperor Augustus. The reasons remain mysterious, but from what we can reconstruct, seducing married women—and encouraging others to do the same—seems to have been one of the reasons for his punishment.

Men would have expected certain women—particularly sex workers—to limit their fertility through birth control and abortion.[83] And in the context of a marriage, decisions about reproduction may have been made jointly.[84] Just because something was left up to women to do doesn't mean that men didn't approve of it, even if only tacitly. Certainly, there would have been exceptions—situations of reproductive coercion or illicit affairs—wherein women would have procured abortions secretively. But we should not believe the likes of Ovid and Juvenal that all upper-class Roman women were vain, adulterous, and duplicitous. Antiabortion rhetoric was a way for Roman men to vent their fears and anger around women's knowledge and control of reproduction. We will see this fear and anger emerge again in chapter 8 when we look at male perspectives on female midwives. Painting women as irresponsible stewards of fertility and reproduction was a step in the direction of male control of gynecology and obstetrics.

In the next chapter, we will look at how people in ancient Rome dealt with the anticipations and uncertainties of the prenatal period. We will see that as with fertility and conception, a male medical discourse was concerned with monitoring and controlling pregnant women in the name of optimal reproductive outcomes. Pregnant women were pitted against their fetuses in an antagonistic contest in which pregnancy was imagined as a zero-sum game. At the same time, women's actual bodies—through bioarchaeological analyses of their skeletons—have given us insights into the realities that pregnant and perinatal women in ancient Rome faced. And despite new male forays into reproductive control, midwives and other experienced women still held authority in the realm of prenatal knowledge and care.

SIX

Pregnancy Problems and Prenatal Care

ON AUGUST 24, 79 CE, Mount Vesuvius in Italy erupted, smothering the surrounding area in a thick layer of ash, volcanic rock, and deadly gasses. The nearby towns of Pompeii, Herculaneum, and Oplontis were quickly buried, trapping hundreds of people and animals inside. One of the victims was a nearly full-term pregnant woman. Her bones were unearthed in 2017, along with the tiny bones of her thirty-six-week fetus, still inside her.[1] She was discovered with the remains of more than fifty other people in a room in the villa of Lucius Crassus Tertius in the town of Oplontis (about five kilometers away from the more famous Pompeii). Lucius Crassus ran a wine importing and exporting business. It seems that the people in this room were members of one or a few extended families seeking shelter from the eruption and waiting to be rescued by the Roman navy. What was going through this young woman's mind on this fateful day? Probably fear and a fierce drive to protect her unborn child. She was found lying on a piece of fabric with an oil lamp and coins nearby. She had likely gathered what she thought necessary for her evacuation.

Among the victims of Pompeii itself was a woman between sixteen and eighteen years old who was pregnant with a full-term fetus. She was found with eleven other people—perhaps members of her family or her slaves—in several rooms of a large house.[2] She was likely wealthy. The remains of her bones were stained green-blue-black, suggesting that she was wearing a lot of jewelry when she died. Her teeth and the teeth of those buried with her, including those of the young children in the group, show evidence of dental cavities. They likely ate a diet high in well-cooked carbohydrates, fruit, and honey and low in abrasive foods such as nuts and seeds. However, examination of her skeleton revealed that she had spina bifida—evidence of a folate deficiency in her own mother during pregnancy.

What stories do these bodies tell? The fact that their bones remained intact in the place where they died and that they can be securely identified as pregnant means that they provide rare opportunities to understand the conditions of pregnancy in ancient Rome. Bioarchaeologists study people through the remains of their bones and teeth in order to learn about their lifestyle and diets.[3] They can determine if a pregnant woman was getting the nutrients that she and her fetus needed and whether or not they were suffering from the negative effects of any common diseases such as malaria.[4] The women from Oplontis and Pompeii present dramatic snapshots of the problems that could befall pregnant women in ancient Rome. Certainly, most weren't fleeing from erupting volcanos. But what happened to these two may allow us a glimpse into the much more common issues that arose in the prenatal period.[5]

In this chapter we will look at the problems that ancient Roman women faced in the prenatal period and the care they received (or did not receive). We will see that while women turned to midwives and other experienced women for help, a new medical discourse was teaching men how to blame their wives if something went wrong. While the medical texts spelled out an ideal prescription for prenatal behavior and care—a prescription aimed at wealthy women—bioarcheological evidence, like that taken from the bodies of the women in Oplontis and Pompeii, gives us a better look at the real story of pregnancy in ancient Rome. Pregnant Roman women suffered from nutritional deficiencies, were subject to physical and sexual abuse, and were represented as sources of harm to their developing fetuses.

CALPURNIA MISCARRIES

In the early 2nd century CE, twenty-five years or so after the pregnant women from Oplontis and Pompeii were caught in the eruption of

Mount Vesuvius, Calpurnia had a miscarriage and almost died. There is no record of how old she was, but her miscarriage and near-death experience were attributed to her young age. Calpurnia appears in a pair of letters written by her husband, a Roman lawyer and government official named Gaius Plinius Caecilius Secundus ("Pliny the Younger" or just "Pliny"). One letter was addressed to Calpurnia's grandfather and another to her aunt. Pliny presents Calpurnia's "failure" to carry his child to term differently to his two addressees.

In the letter to his grandfather-in-law, Calpurnius Fabatus, Pliny laments that the old man's hopes for a great-grandchild have been dashed: "I know how anxious you are for us to give you a great-grandchild, so you will be very sorry to hear that your granddaughter has had a miscarriage."[6] Pliny himself was quite anxious for children. Calpurnia was his third wife and his previous two marriages had produced no children. He himself had climbed high on the Roman political ladder and had paved the way for his future son.

The second letter, addressed to Calpurnia's paternal aunt, Hispulla, a mother figure to the girl, focuses on Calpurnia's health rather than the lost child. Pliny speaks to the concerns that Hispulla must have felt on hearing that her dear niece had suffered a miscarriage: "I fear . . . while you will be glad to hear your niece is free from danger, you will be horrified to hear about the danger she was in." He reassures her that Calpurnia's "good spirits are returning" and that she feels "restored to herself."[7]

The pair of letters shows how the same event—the miscarriage of Calpurnia—is framed differently for Pliny's male and female reader. He takes the same set of circumstances and repackages them to appeal to what he assumes are the different concerns of his addressees. Each letter also allows him to express different aspects of his own emotions and concerns about the miscarriage. In both letters, Pliny attributes the miscarriage to Calpurnia's young age. She was likely about fifteen, perhaps around thirty years younger than Pliny himself. In the letter to Hispulla, Pliny explains, "The danger was indeed grave . . . through no fault of her own, but perhaps due to her young age." These are compassionate words. The miscarriage was due to Calpurnia's youth, but it wasn't her fault.

The same explanation as given to Fabatus is much harsher: "Being young and inexperienced she did not realize she was pregnant, failed to take the precautions that pregnant women should take, and did things that she should not have." Here, Calpurnia is "young and inexperienced." She fails to take necessary precautions. Rather than absolve her of blame, Pliny tells Fabatus that Calpurnia has "learned a harsh lesson and paid for her mistake" by nearly dying. In the letter to Fabatus, Pliny consoles the old man who has been "robbed of a descendant"; in the letter to Hispulla, he focuses on the great relief that she must be feeling to learn that her niece has come safely through this harrowing experience.

In both letters, Calpurnia is a source of hope for the future. As a consolation for the loss of his promised great-grandchild, Pliny tells Fabatus that he should be grateful that the gods have spared the life of his granddaughter, who will go on to have other children. So too, in his letter to Hispulla, Pliny refers to Calpurnia as the one on whom they can "build hope." As sorrowful as it is, the loss of the child is preferable to the loss of the mother. She can go on to have other children.

The sense in these letters is that Pliny was having his own complex emotional response to the miscarriage. He waffles between expressing deep affection and concern for his young wife and blaming her for her careless ignorance. The care is heartening. The blame follows a common script. Miscarriage lurked everywhere in Ancient Rome. Popular wisdom held that miscarriage could be caused by something as simple as a sneeze or the smell of a blown-out oil lamp; stepping over a viper, a raven's egg, or another woman's menstrual blood; or the mere sight of a sea hare (a type of mollusk).[8] Consuming a medicinal plant for one purpose could have unintended consequences—hulwort taken as an antidote to poison could cause a person to miscarry.[9] Medical writers cautioned women that almost anything they did—eating, drinking, moving around, and having emotions—could dislodge the embryo from the uterus.[10]

According to the medical texts, women like Calpurnia who were young and inexperienced were most at risk for miscarriage. They took longer to realize that they were pregnant and even once they knew, they weren't aware of all the things they were supposed to do and not do, eat and not eat. Gynecological texts divided women into those "with experience" and those "lacking experience."[11] Women with experience could be trusted to see not only to their own medical care, but to that of other women as well. The male medical writers relied on them for intimate knowledge of the female body and, quite practically, for physical examinations of other female patients.[12]

WOMEN'S EXPERIENCE

Women with experience—midwives, sex workers, women who had been pregnant before, or simply older women who had seen many pregnancies—knew the early signs of pregnancy.[13] They knew that it was important to not eat certain plants or use particular medicinal preparations. Or, rather, they knew the *right* way to use a substance. Many plants and minerals were useful for conflicting aspects of reproduction—contraception, fertility, miscarriage prevention, and birth. Expertise lay in knowing how to use a substance at the right time and in the right way to encourage the desired outcome.[14]

The women with experience were also keepers of religious and magical knowledge surrounding pregnancy.[15] They were aware of the elements of sympathetic magic, both positive and negative, that could affect a pregnancy. There was, for instance, a popular belief that knots tied on or worn about the body could keep the mouth of the uterus tied up and protect the developing fetus. But all knots needed to be loosened at the outset of labor or there was risk of it becoming interminable. Similarly, the so-called eagle stone—a hollow geode with a smaller stone rattling around inside (à la a fetus in a pregnant belly)—was thought to prevent miscarriage when tied to the left arm of a pregnant woman as an amulet.[16] But when the time came for birth, it had to be removed from the arm and moved either to the belly or the thigh in order to promote a quick and easy labor.[17] If left on the arm, it could prevent the birth from happening altogether.

There's a myth that circulated in different forms in antiquity about a birth that was hindered by the magical binding action of a malevolent entity.[18] Alcmene was pregnant with Hercules, the son of the god Jupiter.[19] But Jupiter's wife, the goddess Juno, was jealous of her husband's tryst with the mortal woman. When it was time for Alcmene to go into labor, Juno, in her manifestation as Lucina, the goddess of childbirth, came to the pregnant woman's door. Rather than assist with the birth pains as was her role, Juno Lucina bound up her own body in an action of cursing: she crossed one knee over the other and interlaced her fingers. With her body knotted in this way, she uttered magical incantations that prevented Alcmene from giving birth. In another version of the story, it was the Fates, at Juno Lucina's bidding, who crossed their legs and fingers and prevented Alcmene from giving birth.[20]

The knowledge of when to tie and untie knots was an important part of being experienced in pregnancy and childbirth.[21] It was general knowledge that the knots on the body of a laboring woman needed to be unbound—her hair, breast band, clothing, and sandal straps all had to be loosened. But there were more specialized manipulations of knots as well. Women who regularly miscarried were encouraged to try this solution:

> Gather the wool of a sheep eaten by a wolf and have three sisters wash it, card it, comb it, and spin it, and make a belt out of it. The woman who wears this belt on her belly for nine months, never taking it off at any point, will not miscarry.[22]

Another precaution advised the pregnant woman to take little worms that could be found in the grass and tie them around the neck as an amulet that would prevent miscarriage.[23] But the amulet had to be taken off prior to birth or its binding action would prevent delivery. A folk practice aimed at easing labor instructed the father of the unborn child to take off his belt and tie it around the pregnant woman who was about to give birth. He would then loosen the belt, saying, "He who has bound you will loosen you," and the baby could be born.[24]

Why were these practices thought to work? They operated through a kind of homeopathy. The belt of sheep's wool and the amulet of worms, tied on after conception had taken place, would transmit their binding properties to the cervix, keeping it closed and preventing the fetus from slipping out prematurely. In the case of the father tying on and then removing the belt, he who caused the successful conception had a hand in facilitating a smooth and quick labor. It was the role of experienced women to hold this sort of knowledge about when and how to bind and unbind the uterus.

Perhaps these binding and unbinding spells were analogies for broad ideas of closing and opening, tightening and loosening, difficulty and ease. One possibility is that they were related to the very real umbilical cord, which could tie and untie, bind and unbind.[25] The twists and knots of the umbilical cord could present difficulties for fetuses in the uterus or infants at birth. Although very rare, the umbilical cord can occasionally get so wrapped around the fetus that it is unable to be born. Without the possibility of a cesarean section, such a binding could mean death for the baby, mother, or both.

Something else to consider is the wisdom of modern midwives concerning the positions of the mother's body in late pregnancy. In the 1990s, midwife Jean Sutton and childbirth educator Pauline Scott observed that more and more babies were being born posterior—descending down and out of the birth canal spine-to-spine with the laboring parent.[26] This position—as opposed to the opposite one, with baby's belly toward parent's spine—makes labor longer, more difficult, and more painful.[27] Sutton and Scott identified that modern lifestyle habits—such as sitting in deep-set couches and car bucket seats—can close off the pelvis, preventing the fetus from settling down into the optimal position for labor and birth. They encouraged sitting forward on chairs, with knees below the hips, crawling around on all fours, and even doing supported, whole-body inversions in order give the fetus room in the abdomen and pelvis to find the optimal position for birth. A prenatal position that, when assumed too often, can prevent the fetus from dropping into position in the pelvis ("lightening") in the optimal "occiput anterior position"—baby's face toward pregnant parent's spine—is sitting with the legs crossed, which can extend the length of pregnancy, prolong labor, and make it more painful and difficult. Sutton and Scott didn't invent something new. They looked at the ways that pregnant people had more traditionally engaged and held their bodies in late pregnancy—for example, sitting in upright chairs, squatting, getting on all fours to scrub floors, walking places—and how those positions had changed in the 20th century. Based on the physiology of the uterus and the pelvis, they developed recommendations for how the pregnant person could better facilitate fetal positioning. While there's no direct evidence that ancient women were aware of this connection between their own positions and that of the baby, it's possible that some of it was observed and incorporated into folk practices around birth.

DIVINE ASSISTANCE

One way that pregnant women attended to their own health and that of their fetus during the prenatal period was through appeals to divinities. They prayed at temples and sanctuaries, promising to make votive offerings in exchange for healthy pregnancies and safe births. In the Greek-speaking parts of the empire, women made dedications of thanks to the goddess Hera: terracotta figurines of pregnant women (see fig. 6), uteruses, keys, and infants.[28] They also appealed to Eileithyia, the goddess of childbirth, Artemis Eileithyia ("Artemis of Childbirth") or Artemis Lochia ("Artemis of the Birth Bed"), and the healing god Asclepius, among others.[29]

Roman-Egyptian women had a whole pantheon of birth gods.[30] Isis guarded women throughout their reproductive years. The god Bes, a comic dwarf figure, would protect pregnant women from conception through birth. He had a female companion, Taweret, who assisted him. She was a cross between a hippo, a lion, a crocodile, and a woman with long, dangling breasts and a protruding, pregnant belly. The goddess Meskhenet could be called on at the moment of birth. She was depicted in the form of a birth brick with the face of a woman—the personification of the bricks that early Egyptian woman squatted on to give birth. It was her role to provide the child's soul and fix its destiny at birth (like the Fates in the Greco-Roman tradition).[31] Hathor, a love and fertility goddess, would hover around the pregnant and laboring woman as

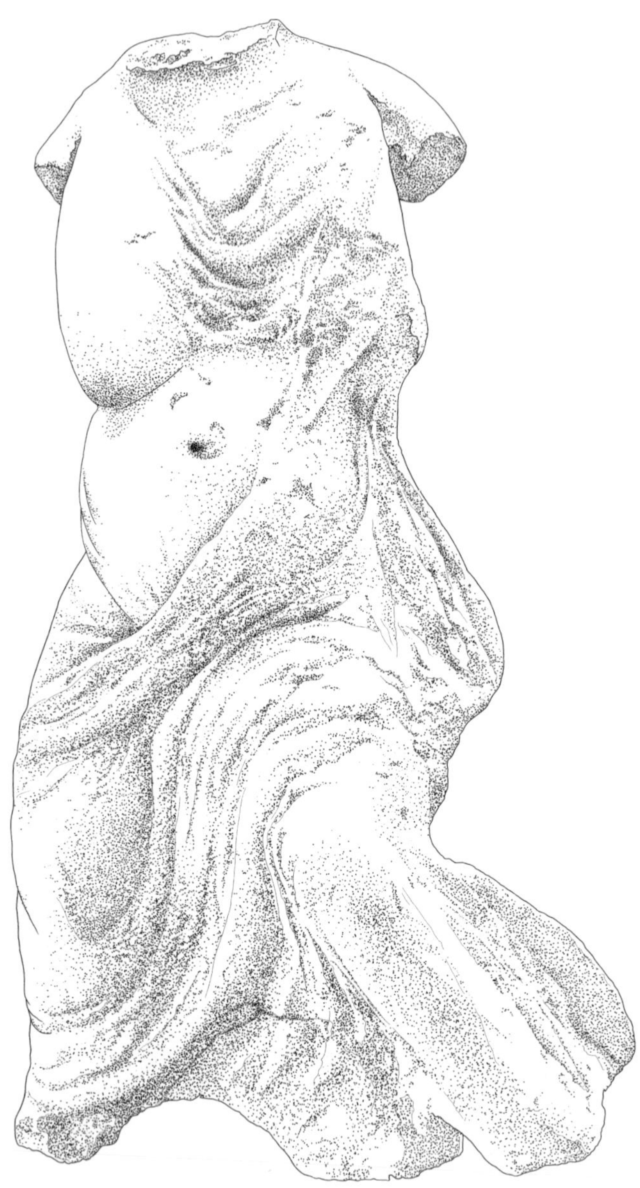

FIGURE 6. Roman terracotta votive of a pregnant woman. 100 BCE–200 CE. Science Museum Group, Sir Henry Wellcome's Museum Collection A63499. Drawing by Hayley Monroe.

another protective divine force. And the ram-headed god Khnoum was responsible for forming the child while it was in the womb.[32] Many other gods and goddesses could be called on as aides and supports during the prenatal and birth periods.

In the Latin-speaking parts of the empire, including the city of Rome itself, both women and men made supplications and offered thanks to Juno Lucina, Bona Dea ("Good Goddess"), and Mater Matuta ("Mother Matuta"), all of whom were associated with fertility, pregnancy, and childbirth.[33] People also seem to have appealed to Hercules in matters related to gynecology and pregnancy. Hundreds of clay models of breasts and uteruses have been found in a sanctuary of Hercules in Praeneste, a city about thirty-five kilometers southeast of Rome. These could have been dedicated by pregnant women, men, or other members of the household in thanks for healing, successful pregnancies, or even breast milk.[34] It's possible that this connection between Hercules and childbirth is related to the myth of Hercules's own birth. Despite Juno Lucina's best efforts to prevent his mother Alcmene from giving birth, Hercules was eventually strong enough—with a little help from a midwife figure—to make his way out of the womb, leading the way for his twin brother, Iphicles, to be born as well.

But Hercules's connections to pregnancy and childbirth go beyond his own birth. He fathered many children and so operated as an agent of fertility.[35] He also protected the pregnant uterus from miscarriage. Hercules's power is shown on a red jasper amulet, made sometime in the 1st through 4th centuries CE, that could have been worn by a pregnant woman as a protective talisman (see fig. 7).[36] We don't know where this amulet came from. Its imagery would have made sense to many women throughout the Roman Empire, since it draws on multiple mythical, religious, and magical traditions. On the front of the amulet, Hercules wrestles the Nemean lion—the first of his famous twelve labors. The fighting figures are surrounded by the protective ouroboros, the snake that eats its own tail. On the back, a pregnant woman squats down, brandishing a large club, her unbound hair falling loose over her shoulder. Below her, the amulet is broken off, but a large penis can be seen

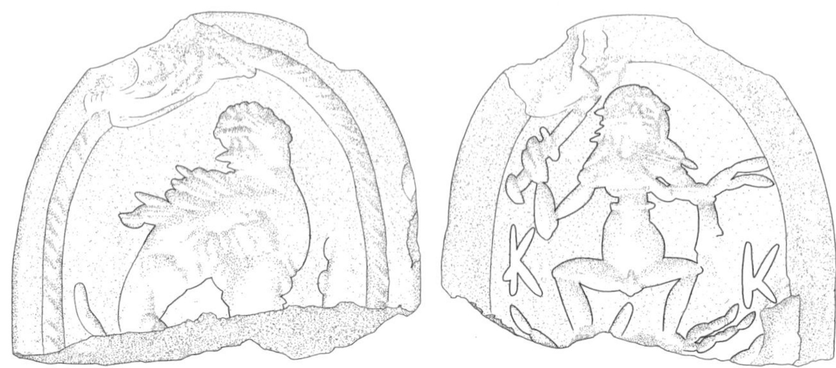

FIGURE 7. Red jasper amulet depicting Hercules wrestling the Nemean lion (front) and Omphale brandishing a club while squatting over a donkey with an erect phallus (back). CBd 760, 16 × 14 × 3 mm. 1st–4th century CE. British Museum. Drawing by Hayley Monroe.

jutting up toward her full-frontal vulva. The penis belongs to a donkey that is lying on its back. The pregnant woman is Omphale, the queen of Lydia, who kept Hercules as a (willing) sex captive for a year. The donkey with the large penis represents a malevolent entity, sometimes understood to be the Egyptian god Seth, who threatened pregnant women with rape and miscarriage.

The lovers, Hercules and Omphale, work in tandem to ward off malevolent attacks on the pregnant uterus and fetus.[37] Hercules's wresting of the lion represents mastery over the mercurial womb, itself a potential threat to the developing fetus.[38] His actions are reinforced by the protective, binding ouroboros snake. Omphale, brandishing the phallic club, wards off the giant donkey penis, protecting her unborn child from miscarriage and herself from hemorrhage.[39] The red color of the jasper stone also provided protection. In ancient religio-magic contexts, it repelled all dangerous entities from the wearer.[40] In the specific context of pregnancy, it warded off demons who could attack the womb and fetus, causing a miscarriage.

By the time Calpurnia was pregnant, in the early 2nd century CE, such amulets were ubiquitous throughout the empire. A knowledgeable

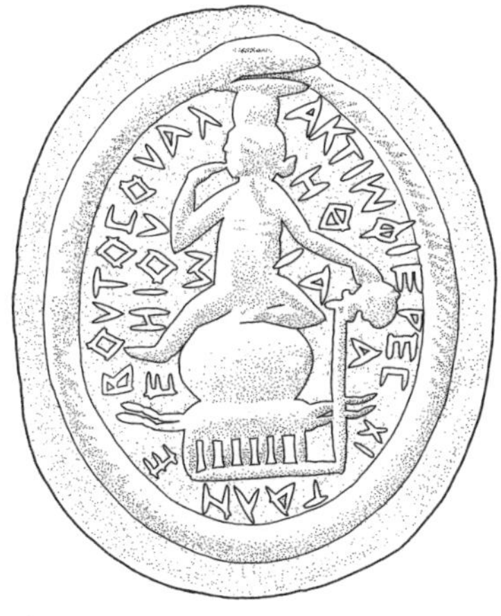
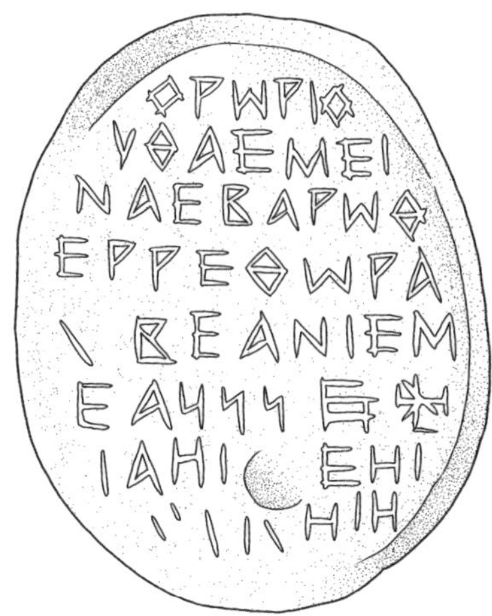

FIGURE 8. Red carnelian amulet depicting the divine infant Horus sitting on a cupping-vessel-style uterus and holding the handle of a key that is closing the uterus, surrounded by the ouroboros snake and magical formulas (front); magical formulas (back). CBd 1055, 29 × 23 × 4 mm. 1st–4th century CE. University of Michigan, Special Collections. Drawing by Hayley Monroe.

woman might have instructed the young, inexperienced Calpurnia to tie one onto her body—perhaps one of the pregnant Omphale variety. By using an Omphale amulet, she would have doubly empowered herself. First, she would have chosen to attach the amulet to her body. And second, the image of Omphale wielding her club against the threatening penis would have communicated the idea that women were capable of protecting and caring for themselves.[41]

Other amulets worked through less aggressive forms of magic.[42] On a red carnelian amulet, the divine Egyptian baby Horus sits on top of a cupping-vessel uterus, holding an oversized key (see fig. 8).[43] He is surrounded by indecipherable Greek letters—a protective magic formula—and the ouroboros snake. The amulet depicts the growth of the fetus and the hopes for a healthy pregnancy and birth. The key represents the locking and unlocking that has to happen at the "mouth" of the womb to let in semen, hold in the fetus, and release the baby at birth. Here, the strong baby Horus turns the key, ready to release himself in birth. The amulet could have been worn in a ring or pendant or tied up in a small cloth or leather pouch, providing prenatal protection to the wearer.

INTERMINABLE PREGNANCY

On the opposite end from miscarriage, women in the ancient world were concerned with how long their pregnancies would last. They knew that for the most part a healthy baby could be born between seven and ten months, but some women worried that their pregnancies had gone on for much longer than that. In a story recorded in the early 4th century BCE, a woman named Kleo traveled to the sanctuary of the healing god Asclepius in Epidaurus, Greece, looking for a cure for her pregnancy, which had gone on for five years.[44] At this sanctuary, patients would sleep inside the temple of the god, who would come to them in their sleep and provide a remedy.[45] Kleo explained her problem to the priests and spent a night in the temple. The next morning, upon leaving the sanctuary, she immediately gave birth to a baby boy.[46] The baby had continued to develop over his five years in the womb and came out as a young child. He washed himself at the sanctuary fountain and walked around with his mother. Similarly, Ithmonika was a woman who had previously visited the sanctuary asking to get pregnant with a baby girl.[47] The god Asclepius granted her prayer and she soon found herself pregnant. But three years later she still had not given birth to the child. Returning to the sanctuary to ask for the god's help again, she realized that while she asked to become pregnant, she had made the mistake of not also asking to give birth. Once she realized her error, she again spent the night in the temple. The next morning, upon leaving the temple, she gave birth to her daughter.

It's hard to say what these stories really mean. The story of Ithmonika follows a common folk motif: the hero or heroine is granted some boon by a magical entity, but it comes with a tricky catch.[48] For instance, King Midas wished that everything he touched would turn to gold, not realizing that this would include his food and his own daughter; and the goddess Eos wished that her mortal lover be granted immortality, not anticipating that she also needed to ask for his eternal youth. He lived forever, but as a shriveled old man.[49]

In the time of the Roman Empire, the stories of astonishing illnesses and miraculous cures could be seen inscribed on five-foot stone slabs in the sanctuary of Asclepius.[50] The stories of Kleo and Ithmonika were inscribed at the top of the first stone slab and were the first thing that a traveler could read (or have read to them by a temple attendant) upon entering the sanctuary.[51] Pregnant women or those hoping to become pregnant who traveled to temple for help could see them as evidence of the god's efficacy. They spoke to the powerful healing abilities of the god—similar to the stories that spread about Jesus of Nazareth healing the man with leprosy or the woman with a twelve-year bloody flux.[52] Such stories were common in the ancient Mediterranean. But they also attested to a real phenomenon of pregnancy—the feeling that it is interminable and that something will prevent the baby from being born.

One of the Hippocratic writers recorded that he had sometimes heard from women that they thought their pregnancies had exceeded ten months.[53] He explained this phenomenon as a combination of flatulence and amenorrhea (retained menstruation). A build-up of gas in the stomach, combined with lack of a period would make "inexperienced women" think that they were pregnant when they weren't. If they then got pregnant, they might think that their pregnancies had started earlier than they really had—that is, when their periods first stopped. It was their own inexperience that confused these women.

As we have seen, the male medical writers tried to set themselves apart from prenatal practices that they deemed magical or superstitious. But this separation was mostly rhetorical posturing rather than a reflection of actual practice. It was largely female practitioners who were taking care of women. There's a good chance that whatever the male medical writers had to say about prenatal care they took from knowledgeable women in their communities. The Hippocratic writer of a treatise called *Fleshes* acknowledged as much. He explained that he learned about the signs of pregnancy and the early development of the embryo from sex workers: "It is to the extent that the common prostitutes have instructed me that I know about these things."[54]

PRENATAL CARE IN THE MEDICAL TEXTS

While the male medical writers distinguished between women who were experienced and those who were inexperienced in matters of pregnancy and childbirth, little writing remains from the experienced women themselves.[55] They generally appear, like the sex workers in *Fleshes,* as unnamed authorities in the male-authored texts, providing a sense of legitimacy in the process. Male doctors know things because they have learned them from *experienced women.* It's difficult to untangle what has come into the texts from experienced women and what the male medical writers have themselves imposed by claiming that their source is some sort of experienced woman.[56] The reality was likely some combination of the two. Real women contributed to the medical knowledge that appears in the writings of the Hippocratics, Soranus, and Galen; at the same time, male doctors and medical writers were starting to impose their own ideas onto pregnancy and childbirth.

Just as with fertility treatments, the 2nd-century-CE doctor Soranus used his *Gynecology* to exert male control over prenatal care. His text was dense, full of theory as well as practical advice, and clearly aimed at a readership of upper-class Roman men who were looking to maximize their reproductive success.[57] The main goals of the text were to promote conception, prevent miscarriage, and produce the best babies possible.[58] Later versions of the *Gynecology* were pared down to the practical basics. A 5th-to-6th-century Latin version published by a North African physician named Muscio eliminated the more theoretical aspects of Soranus's work.[59] It was addressed to midwives and instructed them in the best way to care for pregnant women. Elements from Muscio's *Gyneacia* persisted into the Middle Ages. Soranus's influence was felt for centuries and anticipated the even greater control exercised by men over gynecology and obstetrics from the 15th century onward.[60]

Soranus divided prenatal care into three distinct phases.[61] These phases may have aligned with traditional prenatal care that was practiced by women, or they may have represented a medical systemization that would have been strange for the average woman in ancient Rome. For women in pre-modern periods, there tended to be just two main phases of pregnancy: pre- and post-quickening, before the first movements of the fetus and after.[62] By dividing pregnancy—and prenatal care—into three separate phases, Soranus and his later adapters created more opportunity for medical intervention. Eventually, this tripartite division was adopted by US Supreme Court justice Harry Blackmun when he wrote the majority decision for *Roe v. Wade* in 1973—based in no small part on Soranus's *Gynecology* and other ancient writings.[63]

Soranus's first phase of pregnancy came immediately after conception.[64] The goal was to keep the semen inside the uterus by avoiding any sudden change or upset to the body and psyche. Almost anything physical or mental could dislodge the semen from the uterus: vigorous exercise, holding the breath, coughing and sneezing, lifting heavy weights, sitting on hard chairs, and even strong emotion. The woman who was trying to conceive was advised to lie quietly in bed for a day or two following intercourse. She was to be given small amounts of fresh virgin olive oil and mild grains to eat and was advised to avoid wine and hot baths. After two days, she was instructed to exercise passively by being carried around in a litter. Short leisurely walks were appropriate, with the distance gradually increasing each day.

Soranus's second phase of prenatal care focused on alleviating symptoms that are often associated with the first trimester today: nausea and vomiting, strange cravings and aversions, and exhaustion.[65] Lumped together, these symptoms were collectively called *kissa,* which means "ivy" in Greek, though there is no good explanation for the name. Soranus explained that *kissa* appeared around the fortieth day and lasted for about four months. He acknowledged that it could appear earlier, be shorter or longer, or even not affect a pregnant woman at all. The symptoms could include pica—a desire to eat substances that are not usually eaten. In ancient Rome that could include dirt or clay, charcoal, vine tendrils, and unripe fruit. Soranus attributed nausea and vomiting to excess fluid in the body. Treatment involved wrapping and constricting the body with bandages. He advised the pregnant woman to fast or restrict her eating and apply ointments and astringent poultices to her body. She was to be carried around in a litter and get mild exercise by singing and reading out loud.

Care during the final phase of pregnancy—the point at which the fetus could be viable—was divided by month.[66] In the seventh month of pregnancy, the woman was supposed to avoid too much movement, so as not to trigger preterm labor. She was supposed to avoid rubbing her abdomen too vigorously and to remove her usual breast bands so that her unrestricted breasts could start to fill up with breast milk. The eighth month of pregnancy was seen as a particularly harrowing time. There was a common belief that babies could be born in the seventh month (even sometimes the sixth) and survive, but babies born in the eighth month would not survive.[67]

There are a few possible explanations for this belief about eight-month babies. One involves the mixing of medicine and numerology. According to certain philosophical schools—notably the Pythagoreans—specific numbers of days, weeks, or months had a profound effect on pregnancy and birth outcomes. These numerological schemata are quite complex, but in a nutshell, numbers could be more or less harmonious with the chords of the universe. According to these schemes, eight months was an unharmonious amount of time to spend in the uterus, while seven, nine, or ten was fine.[68]

Another explanation is a bit more straightforward. While pregnant women and those who assisted them tracked their pregnancies to the month, it wasn't always easy to know exactly how far along someone was. Given high rates of infant mortality, having a built-in belief that babies born in the eighth month did not survive offered some relief to women and caregivers when infants died unexpectedly. The death could be attributed to the baby being born in the eighth month.[69]

Wisely incorporating this widespread belief into his prenatal regimen, Soranus advised special care for the eighth month of pregnancy. He advised the pregnant woman to avoid excess movement and eat lightly. The weight of the pregnant belly could be relieved with bandages, and the woman could rub a salve made of beeswax and myrtle-infused olive oil on her belly to prevent stretch marks. Once she made it out of the tricky eighth month, the emphasis was on mechanically preparing her body for birth. Soranus instructed pregnant women to loosen the lower belly band and to tie a bind tightly underneath the breasts so as to encourage the fetus to drop down into the pelvis. He explained that the vagina should be gradually opened with herbal sitz baths and softening pessaries made of goose fat and deer marrow. He also advised pregnant women to avoid sex, noting that it is "always harmful" to them, but "even more so in the last months of pregnancy." The concern was that intercourse could break the chorion (part of the amniotic sac), which could jump-start premature labor or waste the precious, slippery fluid that would be needed later for the smooth passage of the infant. Alarmingly, Soranus advised the midwife to begin performing frequent manual dilations of the cervix—perhaps something like a modern stretch and sweep—a safe enough procedure today, but unnecessarily risky in the pre-modern, pre-germ-theory world.[70]

In the manuals of Soranus and his successors, it is midwives who are providing hands-on prenatal care to the pregnant woman. Soranus doesn't say whether he actually did obstetrical and gynecological work. That is, he doesn't insert himself into his text as a practitioner. But he exerts control in a larger way—at the societal level.[71] What his *Gynecology* does is take knowledge that was traditionally held among women and make it widely available to elite Roman men, with the addition of his own systemization and commentary. But this dissemination of knowledge was not a neutral good. It came with an increased medicalization of the birth process and, in turn, increased focus on the fetus at the expense of the pregnant woman.

What is shown repeatedly in the history of pregnancy and childbirth is that the writing down and systematizing of gynecological knowledge shifted authority from experienced women to laymen (husbands, fathers, enslavers) and male medical practitioners. In consequence, the status of the fetus was raised, while that of the pregnant woman was lowered.[72] She became alienated from her own body. This process only reversed in modern times, thanks to the rise in literacy and education among women. The writing down of gynecological knowledge as a liberatory practice for women—for example, in something like *Our Bodies, Ourselves* from 1973—is quite new. For most of human history, the dissemination of written gynecological knowledge was instead something that could be used to point a finger of blame at pregnant women when something went wrong.

It's clear from his explanations of the problems that could arise during pregnancy that Soranus thought women were largely to blame for prenatal problems. His recommendations for diet, exercise, and entertainment presupposed that anything and everything the pregnant woman did could be potentially harmful to the fetus. It was the role of the male head of the household to make sure that the pregnant woman (or even the potentially pregnant woman) was doing everything possible to avoid a miscarriage and to produce the best possible child.

The fact that our sources for prenatal care in ancient Rome are male-authored medical manuals casts the period in a particular light. The voices of midwives and other women are missing, and what is left is a record of increasing medicalization. Ultimately, Soranus, and later Muscio and others, presented prenatal care as something complex and challenging that pitted pregnant mother against unborn fetus.[73] Miscarriage and other pregnancy problems, they explained, were things caused by—and able to be fixed by—the pregnant woman. Women were told to avoid pungent foods and to incorporate mild foods into their diets. Exercise was encouraged, but only what was gentle and would not disturb the developing fetus.

NUTRITION

Soranus recommended mild foods for early pregnancy: non-oily fish, lean meats, and non-pungent vegetables.[74] The pregnant woman was to avoid garlic, leeks, preserved meat and fish, and foods that were very moist. During the *kissa* phase, after a period of fasting, she was instructed to eat easily digested foods that were good for the stomach: soft-boiled eggs, spelt groats made with cold water or vinegar and pomegranate seeds, a dry porridge of barley groats or rice, or lean fowl such as francolin, ring dove, partridge, wild duck, thrush, blackbird, pigeon, or chicken.[75] The ideal diet included an impressive variety of wild and domestic game (hare, antelope, kid, and young pigs), seafood (red mullet, crayfish, shrimp, sea snails, oysters, and mussels), and vegetables, fruits, and nuts (raw and boiled endive, parsnips, purslane, plantain, wild asparagus, olives pickled in brine, apples, boiled or baked quinces, pears, medlars, serviceberries, preserved grapes, and almonds).[76] After the *kissa* phase passed, Soranus advised the pregnant woman to eat more plentifully and drink wine—at least until the eighth month, when she might have to restrict her intake due to discomfort.[77]

A diet consisting of some combination of these foods would have been very nourishing for a pregnant woman in ancient Rome. It would have included large amounts of protein and the wide variety of vitamins and minerals that she would have needed to sustain a developing fetus. There seems to have been awareness of the importance of a rich and varied diet during the prenatal period. But who would have had access to such a cornucopia? Likely, it would have been the same women who had the means to lie undisturbed in a quiet, dark room for several days, be carried around in a litter, indulge in frequent baths, and receive massages. These recommendations are all aimed at a certain class of wealthy women who would have been tended to by households of enslaved people.[78] These enslaved people would have prepared their meals, run their households, carried them around in litters, and massaged and ministered to their bodies according to the instructions of doctors like Soranus and Galen. The reality is that the vast majority of women living in the Roman Empire would not have had access to such diets and care.[79] They wouldn't have had a choice about what they could eat while pregnant.

Bioarchaeological data, like that which has been and continues to be analyzed from the remains of the pregnant women who died in the eruption of Mount Vesuvius, shows that the diet of the majority of people living in the Roman Empire consisted primarily of cereals such as spelt, wheat, barley, and oats.[80] While these ancient grains may have been more nutritionally dense than their highly manipulated modern counterparts, they were still insufficient, particularly for the prenatal period.

Cereals are low in iron. They also contain phytates that can reduce the intestinal absorption of iron.[81] Anemia, or drastically low iron, probably afflicted many pregnant women in the ancient world.

Class, gender, and geographical location affected one's access to a varied and nutritionally rich diet.[82] Poor and enslaved people had more uniform diets with a greater consumption of carbohydrates than wealthy and free people.[83] Men in general had access to greater amounts of protein, possibly due to their higher status, or even to their occupations, which involved procuring and processing meat and seafood.[84] But along with class and gender, geographical location was a large determiner of diet.[85] Unsurprisingly, people living near the sea ate a mixture of foods from the sea and land, while those living further inland ate primarily terrestrial foods.[86] While evidence of all manner of kitchen gardens has been found—from large plots on country estates to container gardens on apartment balconies—it's unclear how much growing space would have been available for people living in crowded urban apartment complexes.[87] Cooking the food was another matter entirely. In the cities, only the more affluent houses had kitchens. Most urban residents would have cooked on small braziers or not at all. Many would have relied on the grain gruels dished up by street vendors for the majority of their meals.[88]

Skeletal remains of very young infants (under one month old) who died in Roman Switzerland in the first few centuries CE show that their mothers were likely suffering from vitamin C deficiencies.[89] Their little bones show signs of scurvy. Given that this disease emerges after a person has gone four to ten months with a vitamin C deficiency, it means that the infants were not being adequately supplied in utero and while breastfeeding. This deficiency in maternal diet may have been caused by widespread and frequent crop failures.

Soranus himself remarks on the high frequency of malformed bones in children in the city of Rome—possibly a reference to rickets caused by deficiencies in vitamin D.[90] While vitamin D can be obtained by sun exposure, the body also requires vitamin K, magnesium, and zinc to adequately absorb it.[91] Lack of vitamin D can inhibit calcium absorption, causing rickets. These deficiencies could have happened during fetal development or in early infancy. Soranus attributed the high incidence of bone malformation in children to the dubious assertion that Roman mothers cared less about their children than Greek mothers. Some of his rival physicians asserted that these malformations were caused by women having too much sex while pregnant or getting pregnant while intoxicated.[92] It's much more likely that diet—over which most women and children had little to no control—was actually to blame.

LIFESTYLE

Lifestyle recommendations for pregnant women also feature prominently in Soranus's *Gynecology.* His ideal client, again, is an elite Roman woman who doesn't work, has plenty of leisure time in her day, and has enslaved people to tend to her needs. He recommends that women engage in light exercise throughout most of pregnancy: leisurely walks, singing and reading out loud, dancing, being carried around in a litter by slaves, and receiving massages.[93] The most vigorous exercises he proposes are punching a leather bag and playing with a ball.

The reality is that the vast majority of women in ancient Rome would not have had the time or resources to engage in the activities that Soranus recommends. Some of them, enslaved or working for pay in domestic and public spaces, would have gotten far more—and far more vigorous—exercise than was recommended. As far as we know, enslaved women who were pregnant were not given reprieve from their work, nor were women who earned a living in manual labor jobs—as vegetable sellers, cleaners, cooks, weavers, hairdressers, sex workers, and more.[94]

PHYSICAL AND SEXUAL ABUSE

But even upper-class Roman women may not have been able to adhere to the final recommendation: abstinence from sex. Soranus and his successors warned that sexual intercourse during pregnancy harmed the fetus.

In the early stages of pregnancy, sex could dislodge the precariously implanted seed from the uterus. Late in pregnancy, it was thought to trigger premature labor. But women in the ancient world had little to no control over their sex lives. Upper-class women were at least nominally supposed to have sex only with their husbands, but enslaved women were subject to regular sexual exploitation and violence.[95] A Greek philosopher living in the Roman Empire at the same time as the young Calpurnia wrote an advice pamphlet for brides and grooms in which he advised men to respect their wives by having sex with slaves.[96] So while a free, married woman may have been able to avoid sex while she was pregnant, the same was not true for enslaved pregnant women.

Of course, we now know that sexual intercourse is not harmful in pregnancy, and that for the most part, physical activity of all sorts is beneficial. What's important to recognize is the significant disconnect between what Soranus advised was necessary for a healthy pregnancy and what women were actually able to do. If anything went wrong, the woman's supposed incompetence could be blamed. And while sex might be fine during pregnancy, violence is not. Today, we know that people are at greatest risk of violence from their partners when they are pregnant. As many as 20 percent of pregnant people today suffer intimate partner violence. Violence can result in serious harm to the pregnant person and the fetus, including preterm birth, low birth weight, and fetal or parturient death.[97]

In 140 CE, Appia Annia Regilla, age fourteen, was married to a prominent Roman senator, Herodes Atticus, who was forty at the time.[98] She gave birth to five children. In 160 CE, when she was eight months pregnant with her sixth child, she died from a kick to the stomach. Regilla's brother charged her husband with her murder on the grounds that Herodes Atticus had ordered one of his lackeys to beat her. Emperor Marcus Aurelius dismissed the charge and exonerated Herodes Atticus. We know about Regilla today because her brother was a prominent politician with enough power to bring charges on her behalf—even if his efforts came to nothing. The vast majority of pregnant women would not have had such an advocate.

MOTHER VERSUS FETUS

When Pliny wrote to his grandfather-in-law to lament that his young wife had lost her pregnancy, he did not specify what caused the miscarriage except to point to her young age, ignorance, and negligence. Calpurnia could have done any number of things that midwives, experienced women, or medical men like Soranus would have advised against. Perhaps she did not rest sufficiently or ate pungent foods. Maybe she inadvertently stepped over a raven's egg or smelled a lamp being blown out. From our modern vantage point, we know that Calpurnia's miscarriage likely had very little to do with whatever she herself did or didn't do. The fact that she almost died from the experience suggests that she was suffering from a rather serious gynecological condition that was beyond the scope of ancient medicine to handle.

The scant evidence we have of women's own experiences—stories, religious votives, protective amulets—suggest that they had ways of dealing with the fears and uncertainties of pregnancy. They talked with one another, and experienced women likely encouraged and reassured those who were pregnant for the first time.

But the picture we get of pregnancy from Soranus and his successors is a medical one. In these texts, pregnancy was a time for a woman to be highly monitored so that no harm would come to the fetus. In the elaborate prescriptions for diet, exercise, and lifestyle, Soranus pits the mother against the fetus. Her physical and mental choices determine the course of the pregnancy and the quality of her offspring.[99]

But how much control did Roman women actually have over their own prenatal care? Were they really the ones to blame if something went wrong? In Calpurnia's case, her husband certainly blames her miscarriage on her inexperience. She didn't know the things that she needed to know in order to keep her fetus alive. But what about other sources of blame? What factors could lead to pregnancy problems, including miscarriage, that were outside the scope of an individual woman's control?

In writing about pregnancy today, Cynthia Daniels explains her reluctance to cast fetal harm in terms of women's culpability and personal responsibility:

> It is clear that responsibility for fetal harm is so deeply shared with men, with public institutions, and with social striations, that it makes little sense to try to tease out individual from collective responsibility for fetal harm. How are we to separate poor nutrition from drug use from lead paint from poverty from genetics from chronic violence and abuse as causes of fetal harm?[100]

In other words, the well-being of a fetus does not come down only to the care or neglect of the pregnant parent. Pregnant people make choices that shape their pregnancies. But how far can these choices be separated from things over which they have no control? A pregnant person today may want to eat more vegetables, but if she works multiple jobs and lives in a food desert, her ability to eat as many vegetables as she wants or needs might be compromised. Or we might imagine a situation in which she is under the financial control of a partner who gets to decide where and how money for the household is spent. Is she then responsible for harm that comes to her developing fetus from poor nutrition? Surely she is not solely responsible.

These same considerations apply, likely even more so, to women in the ancient world. Soranus's *Gynecology* gave individualized instructions to women who were not living individualized lives. Pregnant women in ancient Rome, as today, were in relationships, communities, social arrangements, and class systems that affected their access to resources and in large part determined their ability to care for their unborn children.

There is little room in the medical texts for the journey on which women guide one another. And there is no concession to the different lifestyles that were available to different women. An upper-class woman like Calpurnia might have been able to rest, bathe, exercise, avoid sex, and eat many different foods, thus optimizing her reproductive success. But what about the enslaved women serving her—giving her massages, making her meals, doing her shopping, and taking the redirected sexual attentions of her husband? If these women were also pregnant, their prenatal experiences would have been vastly different from Calpurnia's.

Soranus's manual, which would continue to have a massive influence on prenatal care for more than a thousand years, offers a way for men—as doctors and husbands—to exert some control over the reproductive process. As with the fainting Cyrilla in chapter 1, what we hear about Calpurnia is filtered through the writing of a man. The idea that women can do things to prevent miscarriage and other prenatal misfortunes gives her husband the confidence to accuse her when something goes wrong. The bodies of women like the ones who died in the eruption of Mount Vesuvius provide more insight into the realities of pregnancy in ancient Rome.

In the next chapter we will look at the pregnancy and birth experience of an upper-class Roman woman named Petronilla. While she was pregnant, her husband died. Her pregnancy then came under suspicion as her in-laws tried to cut her unborn child out of her husband's will. In Petronilla's story we will see just how scrutinized and monitored a birth in ancient Rome could be. We will also see that midwives played key roles as expert witnesses to pregnancy and birth. Their judgments held medical and legal authority, even at a time when they were being increasingly denigrated in male-authored texts.

SEVEN

Petronilla Petitions the Magistrates

AROUND 147 CE—about fifteen years before Cyrilla was fainting in the bath—a woman named Petronilla was pregnant. But she had a problem. Her husband had died and his relatives were claiming that she wasn't actually pregnant. This was a problem because at the time, wives did not generally inherit from their husbands. The only way that Petronilla could access the resources from her deceased husband's estate was if she could prove that she was having his child and needed child support. If people believed her in-laws, she would get nothing. She had to find a way to prove that she was pregnant and that she had gotten pregnant while her husband was still alive. So Petronilla, who was living in Roman Egypt, wrote letters to the chief magistrates of the province, explaining her situation and asking for their help. Portions of two of her letters, written after her son's birth, have survived.[1]

The magistrate, Calvisius Patrophilos, had apparently recommended that Petronilla follow the legal procedure called "inspection of the womb" (*de inspiciendo ventre*). It outlined the steps to take if there was any doubt surrounding a pregnancy. It stipulated that the woman be examined by midwives and then give birth in front of observers to prevent her from faking her pregnancy and birth or from substituting someone else's infant—called a "suppositious child"—should her baby be stillborn. Calvisius Patrophilos advised Petronilla to go to the home of a respectable woman in the community, whom he recommended, and be examined by midwives. He suggested that she give birth at that respectable woman's house with birth observers present, who would be sent by her in-laws. This way, Petronilla could prove that she was pregnant with her husband's child.

It seems that Petronilla was able, for the most part, to follow the magistrate's instructions. In the surviving portion of her second letter, Petronilla writes of "the woman to whom you ordered me to go":

> She reported to you that she had examined me in the company of the midwife; she acknowledged that I was pregnant, but that it was not possible for me to give birth at her house; instead, she promised that she would watch over me, if I continued until all my time was fulfilled and nothing happened that was my fault. May I be benefited. Farewell.[2]

From this letter we learn that Petronilla was examined by the respectable woman and a midwife, who both acknowledged that she was pregnant. And although she was not able to give birth at the respectable woman's house, as the magistrate had recommended, the respectable woman agreed to watch over her until she gave birth. The matter was decided in Petronilla's favor.[3] In a second letter, this time to the governor of the province, Petronilla requested a guardian for her son, Lucius. It seems that her husband's relatives were still questioning the boy's paternity and seeking to have Petronilla convicted of *calumnia*, "false allegations." The guardian's job would have been to ensure that little Lucius's inheritance was protected from his litigious relatives and to dole out child support from that inheritance until Lucius came of age.[4]

What we see in this case is a situation of pregnancy in doubt. The cause for the doubt was the death of a wealthy man, Herennius Valens. His relatives, wanting to inherit his estate, claimed that his wife was not pregnant. Multiple authorities were called in to handle the matter. First, Petronilla appealed to the provincial magistrates as legal authorities. Second, the magistrates deferred to the expertise of a midwife. This midwife performed a physical examination to determine whether or not Petronilla was pregnant. Her expertise in matters pertaining to women's bodies gave her legal authority. Finally, the legitimacy of the birth depended on it taking place under the watch of a respectable woman in the community. As a woman of experience, she too held legal authority in the matter.

Doubt around pregnancy in ancient Rome manifested as doubt that a person was pregnant and doubt about the parentage of the unborn child. These doubts were handled both legally and medically. Although male writers of medical texts asserted themselves as experts in these matters, it was women—midwives and respected women in the community—who were called in as expert examiners and witnesses.

DOUBTING PREGNANCY

There were, of course, important medical reasons to want to identify a pregnancy. As we saw in chapter 4, identifying and purging a uterine *mole* was necessary for restoring a woman's health and for making space for an actual fetus. Being able to tell that something was mimicking a pregnancy helped preserve a woman's current and future fertility. But the doubt around Petronilla's pregnancy was primarily a social and legal matter. The problem wasn't that Petronilla might be pregnant with a *mole,* but that she might not be pregnant at all. She stood to gain—and others stood to lose—if she was pregnant.

In the 2nd century CE, a legal right enjoyed by certain legitimate children—the right to inherit from the father's estate—was for the first time extended to fetuses. Practically speaking, what this meant was that a *curator ventris*, "guardian of the womb," would be assigned to the pregnant woman.[5] He was responsible for supplying the expectant mother with food, drink, clothing, and shelter at a standard allowed by the resources and social rank of the deceased husband. There seems to have been a lot of concern among the jurists that women would abuse this privilege—that they would lie about being pregnant to get more child support. One jurist warned of women who "litigated in bad faith."[6] So the male authorities came up with legal mechanisms for determining pregnancy. These were the procedures that the magistrates used in Petronilla's case.

In a related but opposite case, sometime in the 160s in the city of Rome, a divorced woman named Domitia had a conflict with her ex-husband, Rutilius Severus. The dispute was over whether or not she was pregnant. Rutilius claimed that she was; Domitia said that she was not. Rutilius appealed to a Roman magistrate, who referred the matter to the emperors, Marcus Aurelius and Lucius Verus. Rutilius asked for official examiners to be appointed to settle the matter. The emperors directed Domitia to go to the home of a "very respectable woman" and be examined by three "skilled and trustworthy" midwives. If two out of three of the midwives said that she was pregnant, then she was legally considered to be pregnant, and it was the ex-husband's right to send observers to the birth.[7]

What was going on here? It's possible that Domitia really wasn't pregnant, and Rutilius was using the legal arm of the state to harass his ex-wife. The emperors' decision acknowledges this possibility, stating, "If she does not give birth, the husband should be aware that his reputation and honor are involved, and he will quite rightly be held to have devised this to injure his [ex-]wife."[8] But there is no indication of what the punishment—if any—would have been if a husband claimed his ex-wife was pregnant and she wasn't.

Another possibility is that Domitia was pregnant but had her own reasons for wanting to distance herself and her child from her ex-husband. Maybe she wanted to keep the child with her instead of sending it off to be with her husband or his family. A child only belonged to its mother up until the point of birth. After that, it was under its father's control. Although it went against law and custom, it's possible that Domitia had quickly remarried and wanted the child to belong to her new husband, since children were considered to be the offspring of their mothers' husbands. It's also entirely possible that Domitia was escaping a situation of domestic violence and didn't want her child to end up a victim as well.

DOUBTING PARENTAGE

Like Petronilla's case, Domitia's case gets at the issue of doubtful parentage. One of the overblown fears among upper-class Roman men was of "suppositious children." A suppositious child was an infant that was substituted in at the moment of birth—if the pregnancy was faked or if the infant died at or near the time of birth. Roman men imagined that another infant would be brought in—generally from an enslaved woman in the household—and passed off as the wife's, so they asked for birth observers. This fear was, at its root, eugenic. One jurist wrote, "It is in the public interest that there should be no substitution of a child, so that the dignity of social classes and families can be preserved."[9] A suppositious child wasn't just bad because of the duplicity of the mother and the cuckolding of the father, but because of the tainting of supposedly superior bloodlines. Of course, other children and relatives who stood to inherit were also concerned about suppositious children. An unborn fetus could hold up the distribution of the estate in the case of a father's death or cause the shares to become diluted.[10]

The procedures for avoiding a suppositious child were elaborate.[11] A woman whose pregnancy was in doubt had to give birth in a room with at least three lights (so nothing suspicious could happen in the shadows) and only one door. All other doors and windows had to be boarded up. Thirty days before she thought she might give birth, the woman was supposed to alert any interested parties. In Petronilla's case these would have been her in-laws. Then, those people could send observers to stand outside of the birth room for those thirty or so days. There could be up to three free men and three free women with up to two companions each—potentially as many as eighteen observers. They could search anyone entering or leaving the room, including the pregnant woman—they could search her every time she went to the bath or to a different room in the house. The woman had to make an announcement at the start of her labor. The interested parties could send up to five birth observers—like those who were supposed to be present at Petronilla's birth—and the birthing woman could have five of her own observers. In addition, there could be two midwives and up to six enslaved women present—bringing the total number of observers and attendants up to, again, eighteen. When the baby was born, if they wanted to, the observers could examine the newborn. This is an enormous number of people to be involved in the birth of a child, even an elite child. It's hard to say if this procedure was ever followed precisely. It could be that rather than reflecting reality, this law shows how obsessed elite Roman men were with property, legitimacy, and inheritance—and how distrustful they were of women.

There's a recorded case in the late 3rd century of a man called Legitimus accusing his aunt—the wife of his father's brother—of using a suppositious child. Presumably if there had been no child, Legitimus would have been his uncle's heir. Legitimus was instructed to prove his claim to the governor of the province.[12] "Legitimus" must be a pseudonym assigned to the man by himself, since it means, literally, "the legitimate one." Such substitutions are the subject of Roman comic plays, where stock characters fight for control in farcical domestic situations. In one play, a sex worker passes off another woman's baby as her own so that she can extract child support from three separate clients—each under the impression that the child is his.[13]

However, it wasn't just men who made allegations of child substitution. In another case from Roman Egypt, in 120–121 CE, a man named Herakleides was accused of substituting a child after his wife Apia's death. The accusation was that Herakleides and Apia's baby had died and that Herakleides had found another infant to take its place. His motive was to inherit from Apia on behalf of their child. Who made the accusation? It was Apia's mother, who stood to regain Apia's property barring the existence of the child.[14]

MIDWIVES AS EXPERT WITNESSES

In cases of doubtful pregnancy, it was midwives who served as expert witnesses. When the pregnancy of an elite woman was contested, as in the case of Petronilla, it was midwives who were called in to perform a physical examination. Roman legal statutes were quite clear on this matter. As in the case of Domitia, if there was a question about pregnancy, the woman was legally obligated to submit to examination by three midwives.[15] If at least two out of three of them declared her to be pregnant, then her ex-husband or other interested parties could send birth observers to the birth to take possession of his child once it was born. If the woman failed to submit to medical examination, she could face seizure of her property or a fine.[16] If upon examination by midwives she was found not to be pregnant, the only punishment an ex-husband suffered was a possible ding on his reputation. If a woman falsely claimed that she *was* pregnant (and she was found not to be upon examination), she could be punished for *calumnia*, "false allegations."[17]

Although there is no record of the procedures, the midwives' examination likely involved an assessment of external and internal signs.[18] Based on the medical texts, it likely involved visually assessing her face and breasts, palpating her abdomen, and inserting fingers into the woman's vagina—perhaps to feel for changes in the cervix and cervical fluid. Perhaps these midwives combined their visual and tactile assessments with diagnostic questions. In the medical and scientific texts, pregnant women's embodied perceptions and feelings were important tools for determining the moment of conception and for distinguishing between a pregnancy and a *mole*.

What if the midwives were wrong? While a woman could face consequences for falsely claiming to be pregnant—or claiming not to be pregnant—nobody else, including the examining midwives, could be prosecuted on this charge.[19] Midwives had legal immunity if they turned out to be wrong. The woman could get some protection, too, if the midwives were wrong. If their assessment led her to a false belief of pregnancy—or non-pregnancy—then she could be relieved from penalty too. Midwives were endowed with expert authority in the case of doubtful pregnancy. They were legal actors to whom judges and elite Romans were compelled to listen. But they were also protected from consequences if they erred in their assessments.

It matters that the experts in cases of doubtful pregnancy were midwives because it means that despite all the ink spilled by male writers enumerating the signs of pregnancy, midwives were ultimately still in charge. While physicians and medical writers were starting to encroach upon reproduction via fertility treatments and prenatal prescriptions, birth was still very much in the hands of midwives. Just as Galen consulted with midwives on matters pertaining to reproduction and the female body, so too the Roman legal system relied on the expertise of midwives in cases of doubtful pregnancy.

. . .

Petronilla was savvy enough to realize that her unborn infant would only be able to inherit from her deceased husband if her pregnancy was announced and confirmed. Waiting until she gave birth to declare her son's existence would have thrown suspicion and doubt on his parentage and given her husband's relatives a reason to deny his claim, so she got the local legal authorities involved. She declared her pregnancy. She submitted to examination by midwives, who acted as expert witnesses. Finally, she agreed to give birth at the home of a specific woman and to allow interested parties and competing claimants to witness the birth. All of these steps were necessary because Petronilla was a woman of high social status who had been married to a wealthy man. Her unborn child mattered because it was potentially its father's heir. Since her husband was dead, Petronilla likely could have had an abortion with little fanfare and no social or legal repercussions. From a legal standpoint, nobody besides her cared about her baby. In fact, given the competing claims on the inheritance from her in-laws, she likely would have pleased a number of people by having an abortion.

In another legal document from Roman Egypt, after a man named Hermias died, his mother and his pregnant widow came to an agreement.[20] His widow, Dionysarion, agreed to waive her rights to child support and his mother, Hermione, agreed to let her daughter-in-law expose the baby (leave it outside to die or be picked up by strangers) when it was born and to not prevent her from remarrying. For these women it was mutually beneficial to rid themselves of the deceased man's child and to move on with their separate lives.

We cannot say how widespread situations like those of Petronilla, Domitia, and Dionysarion were. Domitia's case was recorded by the jurists as a guiding example for cases of doubtful pregnancy. Records of Petronilla's and Dionysarion's cases survive because of where they happened to live. Egypt was different from other provinces in that due to the arid climate, documentary evidence preserved on papyri is much more likely to have survived there than in other places. The few census documents that we have from the empire come from Roman Egypt, as does much of the direct evidence for the everyday lives of non-elite women.[21] From Roman Egypt there are preserved letters, sent between family members, discussing upcoming or recent births. There are legal petitions from women like Petronilla, discussing matters of inheritance and familial relationships. There is also a significant collection of wet-nursing contracts, legal documents drawn up between wealthy households and the women they hired to breastfeed their children.[22] The documents from Roman Egypt also give the most realistic look into infant exposure. It's possible that cases like Petronilla's were happening in other provinces throughout the empire but that evidence of them did not survive.

A collection of legal documents from another wealthy woman in the 2nd century suggest that it may have been a standard occurrence for courts to appoint guardians for children. In 132 CE, a woman named Babatha died in a cave near the Dead Sea, fleeing, along with twenty other people, from the violence of the Bar Kokhba revolt, an uprising of Jews against the Roman Empire in the Roman province of Judea. She had lived in the Roman province of Arabia, which was annexed to the empire in 106 CE. A leather pouch of papyrus documents was found along with her skeleton. The documents attest to the impact of the Roman legal system on her life. They include marriage contracts, property transfers, and guardianship appointments. They reveal that after her first husband died, a council of men appointed guardians for her son; the guardians were to pay for her son's care and maintenance out of his deceased father's estate. In 124 CE, Babatha petitioned the provincial governor, and in 125 she sued one of the guardians. She had the same complaint each time: the stipulated allowance of two *denarii* (Roman silver coins) a month was not enough for her son's care (one *denarius* was a little more than the daily wage of a Roman soldier). Her legal actions seem to have been unsuccessful. A third document from 132 shows that she was still receiving only two *denarii* a month.[23]

Babatha's dossier of legal documents, like Petronilla's, survives because the conditions were right. The caves around the Dead Sea have preserved many papyri and scrolls that offer insight into the lives of people from two thousand years ago. Babatha's documented disputes with the provincial governor and her son's guardian about her son's inheritance and the management of her deceased husband's estate suggest that these sorts of legal procedures may have been common for wealthy Roman women. Arabia had been a Roman province for fewer than twenty years, and yet Roman legal procedure had already had a major impact on Babatha's life.

Both Petronilla's and Babatha's cases show wealthy, propertied, free women in the Roman Empire legally advocating for themselves and their children. Babatha's case shows the benefits that wealthy women in the empire stood to gain from having a child (even if her child's inheritance was not doled out as she wished). Petronilla's case shows the legal and social procedures that came into play when women of a certain status had doubtful pregnancies. What is most striking is that doctors play no role here. Midwives, presumably paid for their labor, come in to offer expert testimony on pregnant bodies. They perform as much a legal and social function as a medical one. Despite doctors' claims to prenatal expertise, and despite increasing efforts to medicalize fertility and prenatal care, it is still female midwives who are called in to settle disputes around pregnancy.

In the next chapter, we will see who these Roman midwives were, what their training and scope of practice was, and how they were viewed by their communities. Perhaps unsurprisingly, we will see that men and women had very different attitudes toward midwives. While men were suspicious of the expert women who took care of their wives, women depended on midwives for their well-being and survival. Midwives themselves were proud of their profession, taking steps to be remembered for their work.

EIGHT

The Real Midwives of Ancient Rome

SCRIBONIA ATTICE WAS A MIDWIFE. She lived and worked in Ostia, a port city thirty kilometers southwest of Rome. When she died around 140 CE, she commissioned a small mausoleum to house her ashes and those of her husband, her mother, and other members of her household. We know she was a midwife because she decorated the entrance to her mausoleum with a terracotta relief of an active birth scene (see fig. 9).

A second relief on the mausoleum shows her husband, Marcus Ulpius Amerimnus, working as a physician (see fig. 10). The reliefs of Scribonia and Ulpius—as wife and husband, midwife and doctor—show some parallelism in their work. Both are depicted sitting on low stools while tending to a patient who sits on a higher seat in from of them; they wear the garments of working-class professionals. But beyond these similarities, the differences are striking. While Scribonia's relief focuses solely the hands-on aspect of her work, her husband's accentuates his use of tools.[1] Scribonia's relief shows her in the dynamic act of midwifing, crouched in front of a laboring woman, ready to catch the baby. The only "tools" in the scene are the birth chair on which the laboring woman sits and Scribonia's hands. Ulpius's relief, too, shows him in the process of treating a patient: he holds a sponge or poultice to the leg of his patient, whose foot rests in a small shallow bowl.[2] But half of his relief is taken up with an oversized display of his physician's tools—several types of scalpels and spatulas. The contrast between midwifing and doctoring is clear.[3]

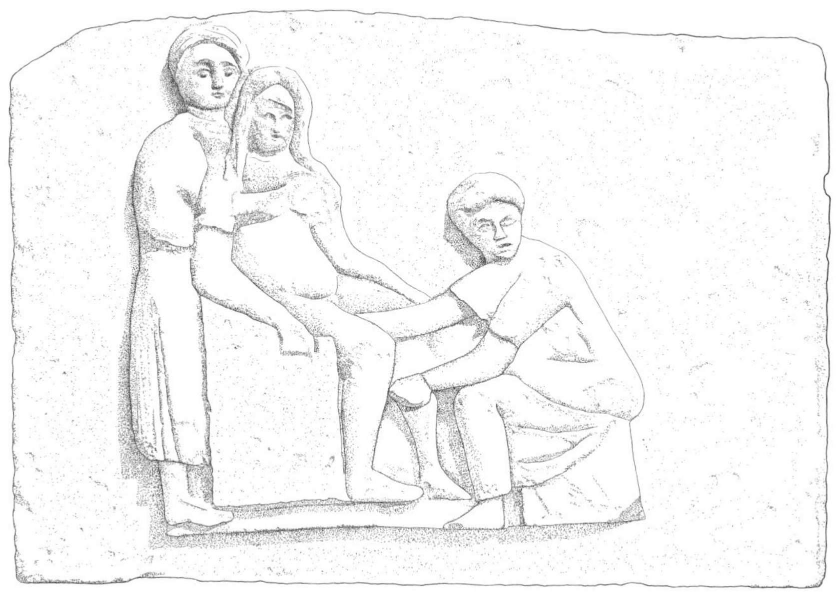

FIGURE 9. Terracotta relief depicting a childbirth scene on the tomb of Scribonia Attice and Marcus Ulpius Amerimnus (Tomb 100), Necropolis of Isola Sacra, Ostia Antica, Italy. 2nd century CE. Museo Ostiense 5204. Drawing by Hayley Monroe.

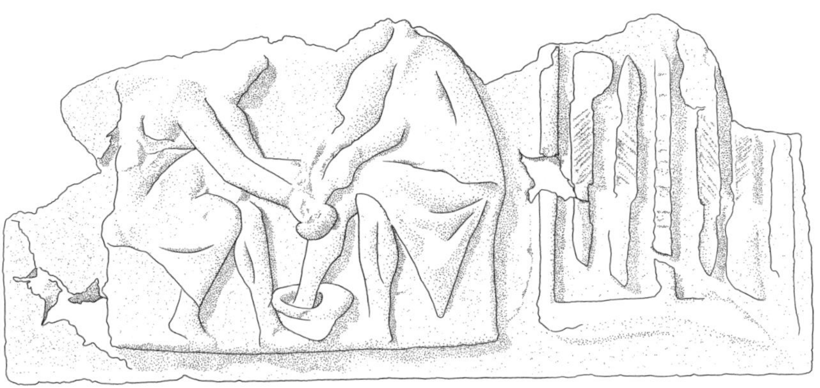

FIGURE 10. Terracotta relief depicting a doctor treating a patient's leg with oversized surgical tools to the right; from the tomb of Scribonia Attice and Marcus Ulpius Amerimnus (Tomb 100), Necropolis of Isola Sacra, Ostia Antica, Italy. 2nd century CE. Museo Ostiense 5203. Drawing by Hayley Monroe.

Scribonia achieved the upper limit of what was possible in terms of wealth and status for a midwife in ancient Rome. Her second name, Attice, tells us that she was probably of Greek origin and that she, along with her husband, may have been formerly enslaved. Perhaps they earned enough from their work to purchase their freedom. The inscription on their mausoleum also tells us that they themselves were enslavers. It indicates that the mausoleum should also house the ashes of Scribonia's freedmen and freedwomen and their descendants—people that she had enslaved and then manumitted, perhaps upon her death.

Most of the real midwives of ancient Rome survive only as names on spare tombstones: Hygia, Volusia, Maria Peregrina, Julia Primigeneia, Sallustia Imerita, Antonia Thallusa, Irene.[4] Around forty names in all, spanning seven hundred years from the 4th century BCE to the 5th century CE, their graves scattered from modern Belgium to northern Algeria to the western coast of Türkiye (Turkey).[5] They were commemorated by husbands, partners, children, enslavers, and occasionally themselves. What they all had in common was their desire—or someone else's desire on their behalf—to be remembered as a midwife—*obstetrix* in Latin or *maia* in Greek. Most of these women were either enslaved or formerly enslaved.[6] Midwifery was an honorable and potentially lucrative way for formerly enslaved women to provide for themselves and their families and to socially advance within their lifetimes.

Hygia was an enslaved midwife married to an enslaved man named Apollonius.[7] She lived in the second half of the 1st century CE in the city of Rome. When she died at the age of thirty, Apollonius had a funerary plaque carved in her honor (see fig. 11), to mark the final resting place of her ashes in a columbarium (see fig. 12) near one of the eastern gates into the city. Hygia was enslaved to and provided midwifery services to the household of a woman named Flavia Sabina—such a common name for free women in ancient Rome that we cannot identify exactly who she was. Hygia's name, too, hides more than it reveals. The mythical Hygia was the Greek goddess of cleanliness and health, the daughter of Asclepius, the god of medicine. It's a fitting name for a midwife.[8] If Hygia was born into slavery, she may have been given this name by her

HYGIAE
FLAVIAE·SABINAE
OPSTETR·VIXIT·ANN·XXX
MARIVS·ORTHRVS·ET
APOLLONIVS·CONTVBERNALI
CARISSIMAE

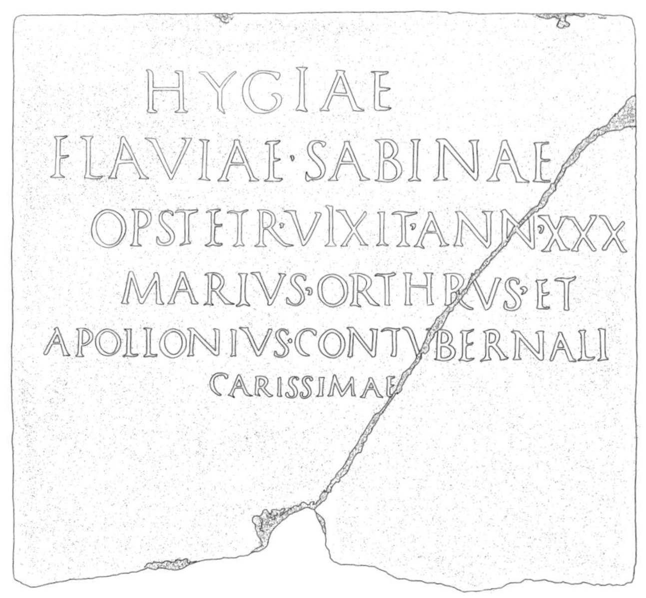

FIGURE 11. Funerary plaque for the midwife Hygia. The word used for midwife here is *OPSTETR,* a variation and abbreviation of *OBSTETRIX.* Late 1st century CE. Sepulcher R of Porta Maggiore, near the Statilii columbarium, Rome. *CIL* 6.6647. Drawing by Hayley Monroe.

enslavers with the intention that she train to be a midwife or provide services as a wet nurse. If she was captured and enslaved later in her life, she may have been assigned this name to reflect skills she already possessed. If she had lived longer, she may have been able to save up enough money from her midwifery work to buy her own freedom and even that of her husband—perhaps as Scribonia Attice did.

What were the lives of Scribonia, Hygia, and their fellow midwives like? What was their training and scope of practice? How were they viewed by their communities? In the first place, we should beware of applying our own modern perspectives and definitions to the ancient world.[9] Today, "obstetrician" is a title that denotes a highly trained, licensed physician and surgeon. But the Latin word from which it derives, *obstetrix,* literally meant "a woman who stands in front" and it

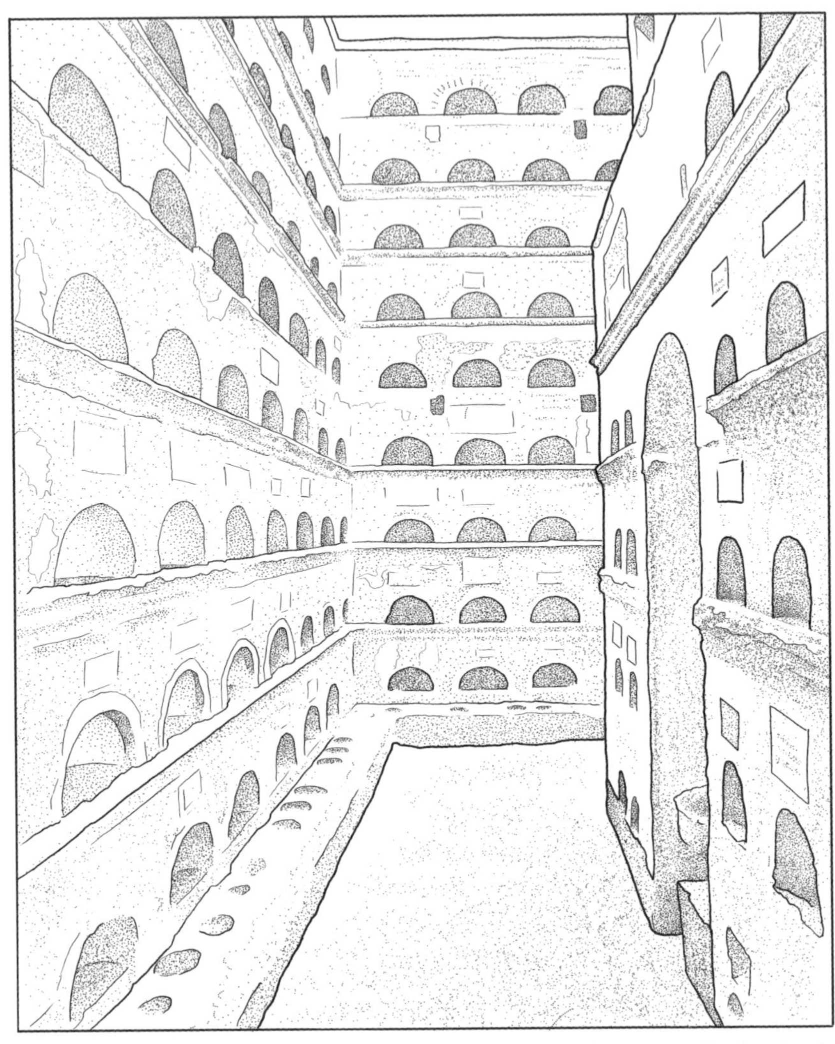

FIGURE 12. Columbarium (Columbarium 1 of the Vigna Codini: west gallery) under the Via Appia, Rome, Italy. These underground structures had niches that held urns with the ashes of many members of a household, including enslaved people. The ashes of the midwives Hygia and Secunda were displayed in columbaria like this one, with simple inscribed plaques below the niches. 1st century CE. Drawing by Hayley Monroe.

referred to the position that a midwife took in front of the laboring woman. It's akin to someone calling themselves a "baby-catcher" today.

So too, the title "midwife" today can designate many different types of practitioners. In the United States alone there are Certified Nurse Midwives (CNMs), who are trained as nurses and primarily attend births in the hospital, often in coordination with or under the direction of obstetricians; Certified Professional Midwives (CPMs), who often train through an apprenticeship model with a national credentialing board, are variously licensed state-by-state, and attend birth at home or in other out-of-hospital settings such as free-standing birth centers; and unlicensed midwives, who have no particular training or licensing.[10] This is to say nothing about how midwifery care functions throughout the rest of the world. In the United States, only 12 percent of births are attended by a midwife, whereas in some European countries, such as Denmark and the UK, midwives are the first point of contact for all pregnant people.[11] In Canada, there is one credentialing stream and midwives have admitting privileges in hospitals, so they can facilitate births in any setting—at home, in a birth center, or at a hospital—and can change setting mid-labor if necessary.

As with every other part of this ancient Roman birth story, we are looking at realities filtered through the cloudy lenses of time, patriarchy, misogyny, and, in this case, a long history of denigrating and suppressing midwives. It can be difficult to look back to the practice of midwifery in ancient Rome through the medieval and early modern periods when midwives were increasingly restricted in their scope of practice and replaced by man-midwives and doctors;[12] through the 19th and early 20th centuries, when midwives in the United States were criminalized and birth moved largely into the hospital;[13] and from the vantage point of today, when midwifery is variously vilified or romanticized. In this chapter I try to break through these accreted layers of history to see what midwives and midwifery were actually like in ancient Rome. At the same time, the long history of midwifery can also offer important points of comparison and contrast for when our ancient sources fail us.

Midwives, like most skilled tradespeople in ancient Rome, probably trained through an apprenticeship model. Healing occupations tended to run in families.[14] Women probably learned midwifery starting at a young age from mothers, grandmothers, aunts, and older women enslaved in the same household. Scribonia Attice's mausoleum was also the resting place of her mother, Scribonia Callityche. It's possible that the elder Scribonia was also a midwife and taught her daughter the trade. Aside from the tombstones, we have no written record from the midwives themselves, so it's likely that they shared knowledge and expertise orally. Some of their practices and theories have come down to us via citations in male-authored medical texts.

Midwives seem to have all been women, in contrast to physicians—*medicus/medica* in Latin and *iatros/iatra* in Greek—who could be men or women, though most of them were men.[15] We know that midwives were distinct from physicians because a few practitioners have identified themselves as both on their tombstones. Phanostrate, a Greek woman practicing in the mid-4th century BCE, provides the earliest record we have of a person identifying herself as a doctor and a midwife (*iatros* and *maia*).[16] Notably, she used the masculine form of the Greek word for doctor (*iatros*), though what this was meant to signal we don't know. Perhaps it indicated that she was a physician for all people and all conditions, not just a physician treating female ailments.[17] Or perhaps she learned her doctoring from a male relative or mentor and simply adopted the same title that he held. A woman named Valia Callista who lived in Rome in the 2nd century CE is remembered on a tombstone set up by her husband as a physician-midwife (*iatromea*).[18] And yet another Roman woman, Publicia Procula, set up a tombstone for herself on which she referred to herself as "a doctor as well as a midwife" (*medica idem obstetrix).*[19] But most practitioners referred to themselves as either "midwife" or "physician."[20]

What the distinction was between the scope of practice of a midwife and a female physician isn't clear. It's possible that a midwife was expected to deal with gynecological and obstetrical issues with a particular focus on birth and the early care of the newborn, while female physicians dealt with the entire body and people at all life stages, just like male physicians.[21] In terms of social status, some female physicians seem to have been free born, whereas midwives were largely enslaved or formerly enslaved.[22] The tombstone inscriptions for some of the female physicians emphasize their education and learnedness.[23] A female physician named Naevia Clara, who practiced in Rome sometime between the 1st century BCE and the 1st century CE, was commemorated as "a physician and a person of letters" (*medica philologa*), implying the she was literate and trained in medical theory.[24] Another woman named Scantia Redempta was twenty-two years old when she died sometime in the 2nd century CE in Capua.[25] She was commemorated by her parents, Flavius Tarentinus and the elder Scantia Redempta, as being an outstanding student in the study of medicine. This memorial suggests that Scantia was undertaking some sort of formalized medical training when she died.[26]

A difference between midwives and female physicians may have been how and by whom they were trained. Whereas our scanty record for midwives leaves no secure indication of their training, some of the female physicians show connections to male practitioners. In 1st-century-CE Rome, a formerly enslaved physician named Restituta set up a memorial for her teacher and patron, a formerly enslaved physician of the emperor Tiberius named Tiberius Claudius Alcimus (freedpersons took on the names of their former enslavers).[27] It may be that midwives learned from other women and female physicians learned (and took their titles from) male physicians.[28]

The most important thing to keep in mind is that physicians in ancient Rome were not necessarily more trained, learned, or respected than midwives. There were no credentialed medical practitioners in the ancient world. Like midwives, physicians largely trained through an apprenticeship model.[29] There were a few medical centers where they could train in anatomy and surgery, but these institutions did not award diplomas and there was no such thing as a medical license.[30] Physicians made their reputations by their practice. If their practice wasn't going so well, they would pack up and move on to another town.[31] General attitudes toward physicians in Roman literature reflect this reality. There were jokes about doctors murdering their patients.[32] They were accused of being greedy and unscrupulous—for instance, giving a patient a "medication" that would keep him sick so that he would need to keep paying the doctor for treatments. But doctors who were successful could win great accolades and rewards.[33] As we saw in chapter 1, Galen—who famously did not charge a fee for his service, so that he could avoid any accusation of being greedy—received a reward of 400 gold pieces for curing Boethus's wife. Successful doctors were celebrated by grateful communities and rewarded with money, land, and immunity from taxes.[34] Midwives received similar treatment on a smaller scale. We don't see evidence for midwives moving around in the same way that physicians did. It's likely that on the whole, they were more tied into and fixed in their communities than were doctors.

MIDWIVES AND MEDICINE

It's possible that the relationship between midwifery and medicine in ancient Rome has been overstated. The impression we have that midwives were less-educated doctors whose scope of practice was limited to women's issues comes from a handful of male doctors who wrote about medical complications in prenatal, laboring, and postpartum women. Perhaps the main reason that we categorize ancient Roman midwives among medical professionals—aside from the influence of our modern perspective— is because of the distinct push by male practitioners of the time to bring midwifery within the scope of medicine. Today we might call this "medicalization," but at the time it was more about which types of practice were part of a written, literary tradition and which were not. This distinction between literary and non-literary practices broke along gender lines. On the whole—with some exceptions—men were writing and women were not.[35]

The Hippocratic medical writers, who were active starting as early as the 5th century BCE, began to turn obstetrics—the work that midwives did—

into a written literary tradition. But they did not bring the midwives themselves along. Although the Hippocratics explained how to assist a woman giving birth, they never used the word "midwife" (*maia*) in their writings.[36] A few female practitioners make brief appearances in their texts—"female healers" (*akestrides*), an "umbilical cord cutter" (*omphalētomos*), and a "female doctor" (*iētreuousa*)—but never a midwife.[37] This omission is not because there were no midwives in ancient Greece—we know from inscriptions and from other written sources that there were.[38] I suspect what may have been going on is that the Hippocratic doctors were starting to bring childbirth—even normal, uncomplicated childbirth—into their scope of practice. In the competitive medical marketplace of antiquity, laboring women could be paying customers. But perhaps midwives were not—as far as the Hippocratic doctors were concerned—medical practitioners, and so they were left to the wayside of the written tradition.[39]

By the 2nd century CE in Rome, Soranus was taking a different tack. He aimed to write down, codify, and control not only gynecology and obstetrics, but the midwife herself. At the start of his *Gynecology,* he outlined the characteristics and practices of what he considered to be the "best midwife."[40] Around the 1st century, a practice of enumerating professional standards for medical practitioners had begun to emerge.[41] Physicians like Galen who were trying to distinguish themselves from other practitioners published treatises in which they laid out the method for distinguishing the best doctors from the mediocre ones.[42] In doing the same thing for midwives, Soranus signaled that midwifery should be considered a medical practice and midwives should be grouped among the medical practitioners.

Similarly, an imperial decree from the early 3rd century CE put midwives in the category of medical practitioners. It concerned the professions that were deemed important enough to have their salaries set by the provincial governors, including different types of teachers and doctors. Midwives were included among these practitioners, because, as the decree reads, they "seem to practice a sort of medicine."[43]

What is notable about Soranus's criteria for the "best midwives" is that in addition to the physical, mental, and habitual characteristics that made for an excellent practitioner—physically robust, well-disciplined, sober, discreet, free from superstition, and having soft hands—he insisted that the best midwife know how to read and be versed in medical theory. He wrote, "She must be literate so that she can learn the art [of midwifery] through theory [as well as practice]," and "we call someone the best midwife if she is trained in all branches of therapy"—that is, diet, surgery, and drugs.[44] Soranus was asserting that writing and reading were essential to the exemplary practice of midwifery— almost certainly excluding many practicing midwives.

In outlining his criteria for the "best midwife," Soranus paved the way for male takeover of birth. He wrote, "It is not absolutely essential for her [the best midwife] to have had children, as some people say, so that she can sympathize with the mother because of own experience with labor pain; for those who have given birth do not necessarily have more sympathy."[45] By saying that the best midwife did not have to have given birth herself, he downplayed the significance of embodied experience. In doing so, he created an opening for the man-midwives of later centuries.

It's almost certain that among Roman midwives there was a range of practitioners with varying levels of expertise and investment in their work. There were likely midwives who thought of themselves as members of the medical profession, offering services similar to those of doctors. Perhaps these were the self-proclaimed midwife-physicians. Maybe, like Soranus's speculative "best midwife," they could read and write and were well-versed in medical theory. Then, perhaps there were other midwives like Scribonia Attice, who defined themselves by their profession but were not interested in making the same claims to learned medical authority that a physician would. And finally, there is evidence for part-time midwives.

A 4th-century-CE story featured a brief encounter with one of these part-time birth attendants.[46] An unnamed woman was running a tavern in Rome; she also happened to be "good at helping women in labor." As she was in the middle of pouring a drink for a customer, a neighbor ran in to fetch her on behalf of her friend and relative who was having a difficult labor. The barkeeper hurried off to help her relative and to do "all the things that are usual in childbirth." A little while later she returned to the tavern and picked up where she left off, after, we are told, washing her hands. It seems that her paid work was running the tavern, maybe a family operation. Perhaps, like many shop owners, she lived above the bar. Midwifing seems to have been something she did on the side, for friends and relatives. The context of the story implies that she was not paid for the work; it was something she did as part of an extended community and network of women.

But if there was a range of midwives, we should not necessarily assume that doctor-midwives, or midwives that were trained like doctors—Soranus's "best midwife" and the like—were better at their work than midwives such as Scribonia Attice or the anonymous barkeeper. There is no reason that they would have been more sought out by clients, paid more, or had better outcomes than less medically inclined midwives. There is also no reason to assume that because a midwife was illiterate she was ignorant, ill-trained, or not versed in theory.[47] Doctors were no more respected and trusted than midwives, and when it came to birth, they were probably respected and trusted significantly less than midwives.

ENSLAVED MIDWIVES

Midwifery was one of a number of skilled professions in ancient Rome that were done largely by enslaved and formerly enslaved people. It can be hard to understand the dynamics of a slave society from the vantage point of a modern, (ostensibly) free society.[48] In ancient Rome, anyone who had the means to do so outsourced labor of all sorts to enslaved workers, even labor that required a great deal of training and skill, such as that performed by midwives, physicians, and scribes.[49] For example, the prolific orator and politician Cicero, who authored dozens of philosophical treatises, letters, and speeches, did not actually *write* most of them. He dictated his words to enslaved or formerly enslaved scribes, who wrote them down and read them back to him. The fact that this meant that enslaved people could read and write did not concern the enslavers. If it was work, enslaved people were doing it.

Some of these enslaved laborers could earn money from their work—sometimes enough to purchase their own freedom.[50] But this did not mean that they were completely free. Formerly enslaved people were called *freed* and they were socially and legally bound to their former enslavers. This ongoing relationship of subordination was the reason why Scribonia Attice made provisions for her former slaves to be buried in her family tomb.

To understand what life and work might have been like for an enslaved midwife like Hygia, it can be helpful to look at working conditions in pre–Civil War America. Although there were significant differences between ancient Roman and American slavery—not least the fact that American slavery was racialized in a way that Roman slavery was not—the comparison can bring out aspects of enslaved midwifery in ancient Rome that would otherwise be impossible to see.

Historian Sharla Fett has written about the "remarkable cultural and social versatility" of enslaved Black midwives in the antebellum South. These women worked both in slave quarters and in the homes of wealthy white enslavers; they "routinely crossed lines of class, community, and race in ways that were unusual, especially for enslaved women."[51] These enslaved midwives were privy to the most private and vulnerable spaces and experiences of the slaver class.

We can imagine that enslaved midwives in ancient Rome also crossed physical and social boundaries of space and class. One of the spare columbarium plaques that survives from the city of Rome commemorates "Secunda midwife of Statilia Maior."[52] Secunda was a midwife enslaved to a woman named Statilia the Elder. She managed the births of Statilia and likely all the other women in the household, free and slave alike. It may also be the case that Secunda traveled to tend to other free and enslaved women in nearby households. She would have witnessed intimate intrafamily interactions and been privy to household secrets. It's likely for this reason that Soranus emphasized the need for discretion in his "best midwife."[53]

Fett has also highlighted the access that enslaved African American midwives had to elite modes of transportation.[54] The need to have the midwife arrive quickly meant that enslavers would often send a horse, or horse and buggy, to pick up an enslaved midwife from another plantation. How might this access to elite transportation have functioned in ancient Rome? Perhaps an enslaved midwife like Secunda traveled in a sedan chair carried by other slaves in order to quickly reach a woman in labor.

This cross-cultural comparison also provides a note of caution. Fett notes that enslaved midwives in the antebellum South probably did not have as much access to their wages as it may seem.[55] They labored for the financial increase of their enslavers, who took either all or a large share of the profits from their outside work. In ancient Rome, Scribonia Attice was probably the exception rather than the rule. If she was a freed woman, then it is striking that she was able to establish a lucrative enough practice to pay for her and her family's burial and to own her own slaves. We may be able to see the slightest glimpse of a different experience on the inscription that accompanies Scribonia's grave relief. The inscription asks for divine help protecting the family grave from evil. It indicates that the burial space is intended for Scribonia, Ulpius, Scribonia's mother, and her freedmen, freedwomen, and their descendants, "except for Panaratus and Prosdocia." Historian Molly Jones-Lewis has suggested that Panaratus and Prosdocia, who have been eternally cast out from the tomb, may be freedpersons whom Scribonia and Ulpius trained while they were enslaved.[56] Perhaps upon being freed they set up rival practices to those of Scribonia and Ulpius. If so, what we see here is Panaratus and Prosdocia being subject to what Jones-Lewis calls "social violence." Professional competition between former enslavers and enslaved may have led Scribonia to cast Panaratus and Prosdocia out from the household tomb. This is a speculative, unprovable interpretation, but it aligns well with the dynamics of medical practice and enslavement in ancient Rome.

COMMUNITY PERCEPTIONS

Midwives in ancient Rome operated in an environment that was deeply hierarchical and patriarchal. While supporting birthing people through pregnancy, labor, and the postpartum period, they also had to deal with the many negative perceptions that the men in their communities had of them. The male writers who have left us records of midwives and their work portray these women as greedy, inebriated, superstitious, incompetent, and ignorant.[57] In a male-authored comic play from the 2nd century BCE, a young woman is pregnant and about to the give birth. An enslaved woman is sent to fetch the midwife. She is reluctant to go because, she explains, the midwife is "drunken and indiscreet" and it's a bad idea to entrust a first-time mother to her care.[58] In another comedy, an old man complains of being fleeced by the midwife, who charges an exorbitant fee.[59] (Perhaps the charge of being greedy came from Roman men who had to pay the midwife but who may not have been aware of the full extent of the her work.)

Many midwives were foreign, enslaved, formerly enslaved, and elderly. These were all strikes against them. Although midwives in ancient Rome were not explicitly connected to witches, there were some associations between the two.[60] In the ancient Roman imagination, witches were hideous, fearsome old women. They had claw-like nails, long stringy hair, putrid breath, and foul body odor.[61] They knew secret spells and powerful potions, deriving their power from the gods of the underworld. In particular, they were thought to steal babies for use in their magic rituals.[62] Midwives, because of their unique access to babies, were suspected of harboring similar nefarious intentions.[63] They held the power of life and death over fetuses and very young infants—a power that was supposed to belong to the male head of the household. A story that was told about the 4th-century-CE Roman empress Helena involved sabotage by a greedy Gallic midwife. When Helena gave birth to a baby boy while traveling in Gaul (modern-day France), the local midwife was allegedly bribed—by Helena's rival empress, Eusebia—to cut the umbilical cord "more than was right," killing the baby.[64] In another salacious history of the Roman emperors, midwives were represented as selling amniotic sacs to lawyers, which supposedly brought them good luck in their cases.[65]

Pliny the Elder, writing in the 1st century, went so far as to say that midwives knew about using the torn-up limbs of stillborn fetuses for wicked practices.[66] He cites them as experts in the use of human body parts and fluids for medical and magical purposes—a dubious honor they shared with sex workers. Pliny tells us that "the most celebrated midwives" swore by human urine as a cure for skin irritation and sores.[67] He writes that a midwife named Salpe used a fomentation of human urine to strengthen the eyes and also mixed it with egg white to treat a sunburn.[68] Then there were ingredients taken from female bodies.[69] According to Pliny, a midwife named Sotira advised using menstrual blood to treat certain types of fever as well as epileptic seizures.[70] She supposedly instructed the woman to rub her menstrual blood on the feet of the suffering patient without his knowledge. And Pliny reports that a sex worker named Lais and the midwife Salpe agreed on an amulet for curing the bite from a mad dog or malarial fevers: smear menstrual blood on wool from a black ram and wear it enclosed in a silver bracelet.[71] These uses of menstrual blood, although for healing purposes, are akin to the dark magic of witches. Pliny calls menstruation the "plague of the female sex" and explains that it can be used for harm as much as for healing: a smear of menstrual blood on a pregnant woman can cause a miscarriage, as can stepping over it.[72]

The midwives in Pliny's text are also associated with male magicians; they both know how to use animal body parts and fluids as aphrodisiacs, fertility aids, contraceptives, and gynecological treatments. The midwife Salpe appears alongside the magician Osthanes, both prescribing donkey parts as aphrodisiacs: Osthanes recommends the fluid from a donkey's vagina after copulation, collected in a red cloth, enclosed in silver and worn as an amulet; Salpe's method involves plunging a donkey's genitals into hot oil and rubbing the man's or woman's genitals with it.[73] The midwife Olympias of Thebes cures barrenness with a mixture of bull's gall, serpent fat, copper rust, and honey, smeared on the genitals before intercourse.[74] Unnamed male magicians (*magi*) give bloody pus from a rabbit to the male partner (to drink?) in order to promote conception.[75] Unnamed midwives give women with vaginal flux (like Cyrilla from chapter 1) the urine of a she-goat to drink, or they apply goat dung to her vagina.[76] The magician Osthanes uses the urine of a he-goat in an anti-aphrodisiac drink for women.[77] These remedies skirt the line between medicine and magic. While there may be therapeutic qualities to the treatments, they also work through sympathetic manipulation. Donkeys and rabbits are virile animals—their fluids imparted procreative potency to the patients. Goat urine is smelly and off-putting. Drinking it was thought to stop whatever needed stopping—a vaginal flux or unrestrained erotic desire.

So in Pliny's depiction, midwives were associated with sex workers and magicians. They had access to witchy ingredients such as fetuses and bodily fluids, and they knew how to use magical amulets and potions to manipulate reproduction. Midwives and sex workers both had proprietary knowledge of the inner workings of the female body and human reproduction.[78] Men were suspicious of the way they thought both midwives and sex workers could manipulate reproduction through the use of fertility treatments, aphrodisiacs, contraceptives, and abortifacients.

Soranus leaned into these stereotypes as well, even as he directed his treatise at midwives and those who hired midwives. He drew a contrast between himself—a practitioner of rational medicine—and superstitious midwives, who might be led astray by a dream or omen and so overlook the necessary remedy.[79] Bad outcomes in childbirth, he explained, were caused by incompetent midwives. Soranus accused them of causing infection by cutting the umbilical cord with a piece of glass, a reed, a pottery fragment, or even a thin crust of stale bread, since superstition led them to avoid using a proper iron knife.[80] Modern scholars of ancient childbirth have, in some cases, replicated these negative portrayals of ancient midwives. They have taken Soranus's injunction that midwives not be superstitious to indicate that they *were* superstitious, in contrast to the supposedly rational medicine being practiced by male doctors and surgeons.[81]

But there is equally strong evidence that midwives were valued members of their communities. The Roman legal system trusted midwives as expert witnesses in cases of contested pregnancy and birth. As we saw in chapter 7, midwives examined Petronilla to confirm that she was pregnant when competing heirs accused her of faking her pregnancy to get a portion of her dead husband's estate. Similarly, in apocryphal accounts of the birth of Jesus of Nazareth, it was female midwives who were called to the scene to verify Mary's virgin birth.[82] Their authority carried weight in religious as well as legal contexts.

The Roman legal system also distinguished midwives from witches and magicians. The imperial decree that claimed that midwives "seem to practice a sort of medicine" contrasted midwives and doctors with "people who make incantations or imprecations, or to use the common expression of imposters, exorcisms."[83] Another Roman legal text put an exact amount on the worth of an enslaved midwife. Cataloging the going rates for slaves, it set the price of a child or unskilled adult at ten *solidi*, of skilled artisans at thirty *solidi*, and of physicians and midwives at sixty *solidi*.[84] Midwives were considered quite valuable to the enslavers of ancient Rome.

Women also clearly trusted their midwives. As we saw in chapter 1, when Cyrilla was experiencing the vaginal flux, she called on her "usual midwives" for help.[85] Soranus wrote that "people are accustomed to call in midwives when women are sick and suffering something unique that they do not have in common with men."[86] The male medical writers noted that women preferred to be treated by other women. There was a mythical story, circulating as early as the reign of the emperor Augustus, that explained the origin of the first midwife.[87] She was a woman named Agnodike who trained under a male doctor and came to be very popular with her clients because they were not ashamed to present themselves naked to her like they were to the male practitioners. It's not a true story about where midwives came from, but at its root it shows the appreciation that women in antiquity had for their midwives.

Then, of course, there is the fact that midwives were proudly commemorated as such on their tombstones. Even when the profession of her husband or other family members is not given, the woman is commemorated as a midwife. A tombstone with a pair of inscriptions for a midwife and her husband from the province of Africa Proconsularis reads, "Consecrated to the spirits of the dead, Caelia Bonosa Mazica, midwife, very pure and virtuous wife, she lived 42 years and 3 months, here she lies"; and "Consecrated to the spirits of the dead, the pious Publius Flavius Cornelius Felix, son of Publius, he lived 75 years and 6 months, here he lies."[88] Even assuming a large age gap between the spouses, it seems that Caelia died before her husband. He probably purchased the gravestone and had it engraved with her epitaph. Then after his death, someone else completed the stone with his epitaph. While Publius's profession is not stated, in the precious space available on the stone, it was important to him to communicate that Caelia was a midwife.

SCRIBONIA GETS CALLED TO A BIRTH

Any midwife will tell you that babies come at night. They come especially when the moon is full, or new, and the seasons are changing at the solstice and the equinox. So we must imagine Scribonia asleep in her home. In 2nd-century Ostia, most people lived in rented apartments in two- to five-story brick buildings.[89] Given her rising social status, Scribonia may have lived in a large multiroom ground-level apartment built around a central living room. Her apartment may have included a bathroom with piped-in water, as well as a kitchen. Let's imagine her asleep in one of the side rooms, on a wool-stuffed mattress on a wooden bed. Perhaps one of her slaves comes and shakes her awake. Let's say it's Prosdocia, before she and Scribonia have had their falling-out.

> A man is waiting outside with a donkey-drawn cart. Scribonia rouses quickly from a light sleep. Prosdocia gathers supplies—herbs and medicaments, a wool cloak for Scribonia, a birth chair, a portable bronze lantern. The two women climb into the back of the cart. They bounce as the cart clatters over the cobbled streets, which are paved with large lava stones. The cart is stopped by a *vigilis*, a night policeman, whose job it is to patrol the streets and make sure they are sufficiently lit. The cart driver starts to explain that the mistress of his household is in labor, but the *vigilis* recognizes Scribonia and Prosdocia. They helped his wife a month ago. The cart rumbles on. Scribonia feels the aches in her back and legs from too many late nights, too much squatting and crouching. Tomorrow, or the next day, after the birth is over, she will go the *balnea*, the small neighborhood bath complex near her apartment. She will relax her body in the warm steam room.

Prosdocia lets her thoughts drift to dreams of freedom and her own midwifery practice. She has been enslaved to Scribonia since she was a small girl, sold away from her mother in Rome. She learns all she can from Scribonia and in the little free time she has, she does jobs for people in the community. They know she is the midwife's assistant and they will pay her for fertility treatments or to tend to a sick child.

The cart slows and pulls up to a large, five-story apartment building. From a small window on the second floor a voice cries out, "Juno Lucina! Help me!" The driver assists Scribonia and Prosdocia down from the back. He will wait outside in case he needs to fetch anyone else, or to take the women home when the birth is over. Prosdocia raises the bronze lantern up to a wooden door, illuminating a sign with a loaf on the front. An enslaved woman opens the door and the women enter the dark, quiet bread shop. They make their way to a stairway at the back and up to the living quarters of the baker and his wife.

NINE

At the Birth

AROUND 70 CE, Empona gave birth to twin boys. She was a Gallic woman (from modern-day France) whose husband, Julius Sabinus, had recently attempted to lead a revolt against the Romans. When the revolt was tamped down and most of the rebels killed, Sabinus faked his own death and went into hiding in underground caves. He lived there for almost a decade, while his wife led a double life—spending her days aboveground, in "mourning" for her husband, and her nights underground with him. During this time, Empona became pregnant. She had to hide the pregnancy from her friends and family, since, as far as they knew, she was widowed. When she went into labor, the 2nd-century biographer Plutarch writes, "She endured her labor alone, descending like a lioness into a den to be with her husband; in secret, she raised the male cubs that were born."[1]

Plutarch tells the story of Empona at surprising length because to him, she is the model of conjugal love. The only reason we get to hear anything about her labor is because of the extraordinary circumstances in which it took place. Plutarch explains that Empona kept her pregnancy secret by rubbing an ointment all over her body that caused her body to swell up. This swelling hid her growing belly from the women that were closest to her, "even though," as Plutarch writes, "she bathed with them" (presumably in the nude). Of course, she could not have any birth attendants. So, like a lioness, she labored alone. And, most extraordinary of all, she gave birth to living twin boys, both of whom grew to adulthood.

. . .

There are so few accounts of the birth moment from ancient Rome. Some scholars have suggested that this is because birth was women's business. Since men weren't there, they didn't write about it. This may be partly the case. (Although, as we will see, there were men at births.) But I think the larger issue is that men didn't see the average birth as a moment worth recounting. It was just what women were expected to do. To be worthy of commemoration a birth had to be—like Empona's—extraordinary.

But what about all the ordinary births? In a way, these were the most consequential. They comprised the vast majority of births. And for each woman who gave birth, it was a potentially transformative and life-altering experience.

THE BIRTHING SPACE

Most ancient Roman women gave birth in their homes, whether that was a one-room apartment in a crowded city like Ostia or a multiroom villa at Pompeii. There were no hospitals or birth centers. Many of the "tools" of natural childbirth—soft cloths, clean hands, warm compresses, encouraging words—are the same 2,000 years later. But there were ritual, magical, and religious elements to Roman childbirth that may seem at least bizarre, if not off-putting, to us: red wine mixed with frankincense and ground-up snakeskin to make childbirth easier; vaginal fumigations of fat from a hyena's loins to aid a difficult birth; and prayers to a pantheon of gods and goddesses.[2]

The physician Soranus wrote that the ideal birthing space—what may have been available to some upper-class women, but few others—was neither too big (drafty) nor too small (hot and cramped). It included two beds, one firm for the labor and one soft for resting on afterward, a pillow, a birthing stool, and a bedpan. It was supposed to be supplied with soft stacks of wool, strips of linen bandage, soft sea sponges,

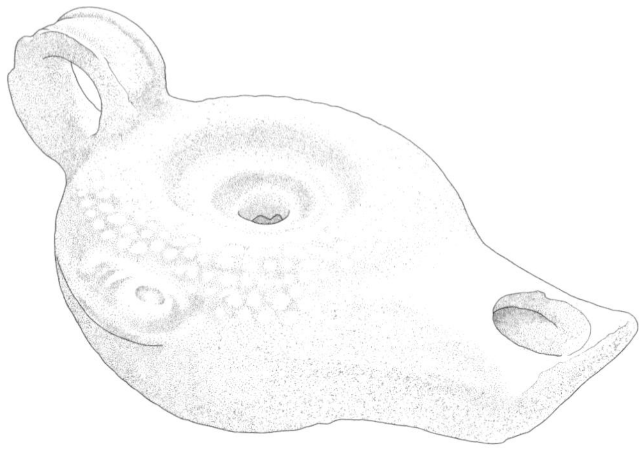

FIGURE 13. Roman terracotta oil lamp. 1st century CE. J. Paul Getty Museum. Drawing by Hayley Monroe.

and warm water. Heat would have been supplied by coal braziers and light by hanging and table-top oil lamps. Enslaved people were expected to function as human tools, providing physical support to the laboring woman.[3]

The birth space would have been filled with all kinds of pungent smells: burning oil lamps, herbal fumigations, offerings of meats, grains, and wines to the gods, plus the human smells of sweat, blood, and feces. "Well-lit" in the ancient world would not have come close to the bright lights available in a hospital birth ward today. Roman oil lamps used a fibrous wick, such as linen, to burn fuel made from animal fat, beeswax, or olive oil (see fig. 13). They gave off the amount of light of a large candle flame. But these lamps would likely have created a pleasant atmosphere—much like the candles that some people burn at home births today. The midwife and other birth attendants had low stools to sit on or just kneeled on the floor. In some parts of the empire—perhaps Egypt, where this practice still happens in rural areas today—the midwife stood in a pit in the ground with the laboring woman squatting above her.[4] Other observers at the birth might have had low couches to recline on, like at a dinner party.

BIRTH ATTENDANTS

The birth attendants at a wealthy woman's birth could have comprised a professional midwife and assistants or members of the woman's own household, including relatives and enslaved women. They might have included neighbors or friends. In some cases, a male or female doctor may have been present, as well as men of the household.[5] As we saw in chapter 8, midwives were professional working women. They were trained and charged a fee for their services, so there would not have been a midwife at every birth. People who could not afford to hire a midwife or people who lived in rural areas with no midwife nearby would have relied on other experienced women in their vicinity. Much of the physical work at an ancient Roman birth would have been done by enslaved people.

Sometimes family members planned to travel from far away to assist each other at births. In a 2nd-century letter from Roman Egypt, a woman writes to her sister, Tinarsieges, to let her know that she intends to come help her with her birth: "If you are coming to your days of giving birth, write to me so that I may come and perform your delivery."[6] She asks Tinarsieges to send her leaves so that she can weave her a basket. She also mentions that when she comes, she will bring jars and lupines for the birth. Lupine had many medicinal uses. At a birth, it could be made into a pessary with myrrh and honey to help the fetus down the birth canal.[7] Lupine root boiled in water and drunk helped to promote urination after birth.

In another letter from the 2nd century, Thermouthas tells her mother Valerias about her pregnancy and asks her to send supplies: "Send me the blankets at the price [we agreed upon] and fine quality wool, four fleeces. . . . Also, I am at the moment seven months pregnant."[8] Thermouthas does not say whether or not the wools and fleeces were intended for her birth, but they could have been.

MIDWIVES AND DOCTORS

A question that emerges out of our modern birth practices is whether doctors or midwives attended women in labor. Simply put, if there was a practitioner at the birth, it was usually a midwife. Even at the highest levels of society, midwives managed the births. The imperial household and other wealthy families had enslaved midwives to serve them or kept freed midwives on retainer. Antonia Thallusa was a midwife who served the imperial family, as indicated by the simple inscription on her columbarium plaque, which records that she was a freedwoman and that she worked for the household of the empress.[9] At least ten other funerary inscriptions for midwives indicate that they were slaves or former slaves of wealthy and elite families at Rome.[10] As we saw in chapter 8, it's likely that these midwives provided care for not only the free women in their household, but for their fellow slaves and former slaves.

In the few visual depictions of birth that survive from ancient Rome, it is always midwives or other women who attend the laboring or postpartum woman. There are a handful of birth scenes that appear on sarcophaguses for elite Roman men. These stone coffins were elaborately decorated with scenes from the deceased man's life—his birth, education, and political and military accomplishments. The birth scenes follow a typical pattern.[11] In one from the late 2nd century CE, the newly postpartum mother rests on a birth chair, looking down toward her feet, where a midwife is bathing the newborn in a basin (see fig. 14).[12] Three assistants stand nearby. One of them holds a large cloth with which to swaddle the infant after the bath. Two others consult a globe on a pillar. While this scene almost certainly does not represent the specific events surrounding the birth of the man buried in the sarcophagus (consulting a globe, in particular, is quite unusual), it does provide something perhaps equally useful—an image of an idealized birth scene.[13]

The postpartum woman is wearing a long, draped dress and slippers. Her hair is veiled. This is the typical dress of an upper-class Roman woman. It's possible that someone of her station would have worn clothing like this during labor, but she could also be dressed this way because

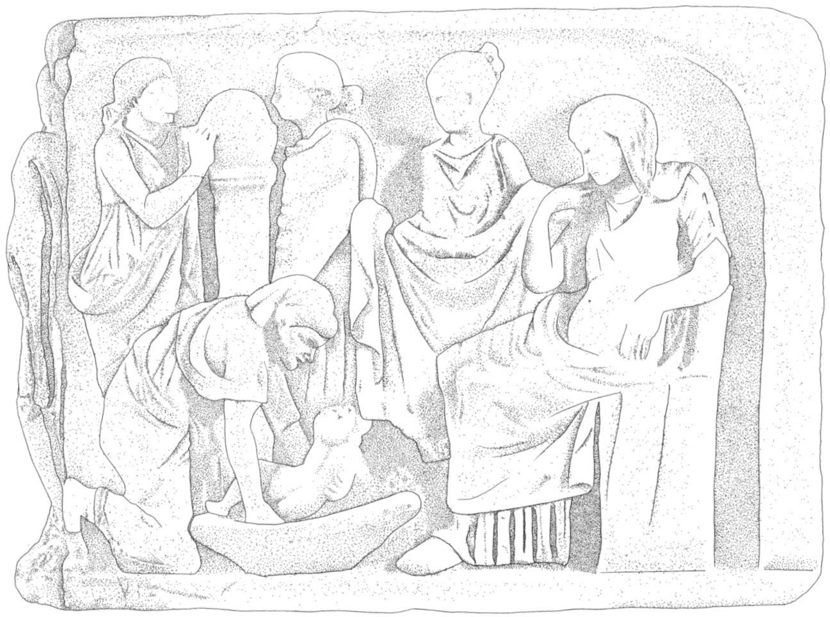

FIGURE 14. Scene of a newborn's first bath on the side panel of a Roman marble sarcophagus. Late 2nd century CE. Los Angeles County Museum of Art. Drawing by Hayley Monroe.

the focus is more on the infant (and the man he will become) than on his mother in the act of giving birth. Some laboring women might have worn an outfit similar to the midwife's. Her much simpler garb and short, practical head covering signal that she is of a lower class than the postpartum woman. Or, like the laboring woman on the tomb of the midwife Scribonia Attice in chapter 8, many women probably wore nothing at all while they were giving birth.

The other three women in the scene represent the many assistants that would have been at a rich woman's birth. But they also represent the Fates—a group of three goddesses who determined each person's time of birth, length of life, and time of death.[14] The globe they consult likely refers to the child's horoscope—predicting the sort of person that he will be and the sort of life he will lead based on the position of the planets, sun, and moon at his exact moment of birth.[15] This connection between the birth attendants and the Fates was common throughout the ancient Mediterranean. In the Greek-speaking parts of the Roman Empire, the Eileithyiai, the goddesses of childbirth, decided a child's fate: they ensured a successful birth or caused the child to stay trapped in the womb.[16] In Roman Egypt, the four Meskhenets—personified birth bricks and goddesses of destiny—oversaw labor and birth. This connection between midwives and Fates was probably related to the midwife's role in cutting the umbilical cord. Just as the Fates measured and cut the thread for a person's length of life, so too the midwife held an infant's fate in her hands as she cut the umbilical cord. Significantly, there is no doctor in the scene. If it was more prestigious to have a doctor than a midwife, then this idealized birth scene would almost certainly have included a doctor. But this sarcophagus and others like it show what would have happened at an ideal upper-class birth.

Doctors may have come to the birth if something went wrong and the midwife needed medical assistance, but care did not transfer from midwife to doctor. Rather, the belief was that a difficult labor called for more attendants.[17] The doctor and midwife would work together. In the gynecological manuals, doctors treat women in the prenatal and postpartum periods, providing fertility treatments and dealing with postpartum issues like perineal tearing or a retained placenta. But at the birth itself, the doctor's assistance would have been primarily surgical. The addition of a doctor at a difficult birth scene would not have brought a sense of relief like it might today. It was a harbinger of doom. The expertise that physicians could offer largely involved extraction of a dead or impacted fetus. If the doctor was coming, either someone was already dead or someone was about to die.

There is some evidence that there were male doctors at uncomplicated births, but they are clearly secondary medical personnel. In one of his treatises, the physician Galen describes a typical birth:

> Midwives do not make the laboring woman get up right away and sit on the birth chair. They start by palpating the cervix as it dilates little by little and first they say, "It's opened enough to let in the little finger,"

> then "It's bigger now," and in response to us asking questions periodically, they say that size of the opening is increasing. And when it is big enough for the fetus to get through, they make the laboring woman get up and sit on the birth chair and encourage her to push vigorously.[18]

According to Galen, midwives manage the labor, checking on cervical dilation. Once the cervix is fully dilated, the midwives make the woman to get up onto the birth chair from where she has been laboring, perhaps on a bed or the floor. Galen asks about the progress of the labor, but does not perform any manual examinations himself.

As we saw in chapter 8, not all doctors were men. There were female doctors as well as midwives. They seem to have taken care of women and children, holding particular expertise in gynecology and pediatrics, but they also treated people, including men, for more general complaints.[19] But there were far fewer female doctors than male doctors and, importantly, it was primarily the male doctors who were writing things down. Consequently, though medicine was not a strictly gendered occupation in antiquity, it largely became so by the Middle Ages, when women were explicitly barred from attending most medical schools and from practicing medicine.[20] A dichotomy and a conflict eventually emerged, with male doctors on the one side and female midwives on the other, even though that's not how it was in antiquity.

So most births were managed by female midwives, some births were managed by female doctors or female doctor-midwives, and some births had a mix of male and female practitioners in attendance. A short letter preserved on a scrap of papyrus from Roman Egypt describes a woman's birth that is going to be managed by a doctor. A young man named Phanias writes to his friend Harthonis, asking him to take care of some of his affairs while he's out of town—pop into the bag maker to see if his saddlebag is ready, and see whether some wool that he is owed has been processed. He also asks his friend to check in on his mother, who has either just given birth or is about to. He says, "Watch over my mother, and the house, and the doctor, and the things related to the birth."[21] The word he uses for doctor is the masculine *iatros*, but as we saw with the doctor-midwife Phanostrate in chapter 8, this word could refer to a male or female practitioner. A millennium later, in medieval Italy, doctors provided fertility treatments and prenatal care to wealthy women and arrived at births when their surgical expertise was needed—usually if the mother or fetus had already died.[22] Midwives attended the vast majority of births, even at the highest levels of the social strata. It's possible that this practice was the continuation of what was going on in the Roman empire.

MEN AT BIRTH

Male relatives, though, had important roles at the time of the birth. Sometimes they were the ones fetching the midwife. In the 1st century CE, the Stoic philosopher Seneca wrote about a stereotypical grandfather-to-be who was so excited and anxious for the birth of his grandchild that he did not pay attention to the news or the sports schedule for the day as he went to fetch the midwife for his laboring daughter.[23] Men might also have had to dash out to get last-minute supplies—cloths, herbs, or quick-birthing amulets.

While the birth space was usually filled with women, that wasn't always the case. Some fathers were intimately involved in the births of their children. In a long and heartbreaking funerary inscription from 3rd-century-CE Rome, parents Lucius Minicius Anthimus and Scribonia Felicissima commemorate their four-year-old son Lucius Minicius Anthimianus, who died after a series of debilitating illnesses.[24] The inscription is composed from the point of view of the young Lucius, who informs passersby of his fate. As an expression of his parents' enormous grief, Lucius describes his birth, in which his father played the role of the midwife:

> When the Hours brought me into the light from the birthing pains of my mother, my father rejoiced to take me up from the earth in his hands and washed me clean of the blood of the womb and himself placed me in swaddling clothes. He offered prayers to the immortals which were destined not to be, for the Fates were the first to have made all the judgments about me. And my father picked my mother as nurse and reared me.[25]

In the story of little Lucius's birth, it is his father who receives him from his mother's womb, gives him his first bath, and swaddles him—all tasks usually performed by the midwife.[26] Instead of picking a wet nurse to breastfeed and care for Lucius, the inscription explains that the elder Lucius chooses his own wife for this role. This family was clearly invested in doing their own care work. The inscription is written in Greek and the names suggest that Lucius and Scribonia were freed. As formerly enslaved persons lacking any legal relationship to their own parents, their son represented their chance for a multigenerational family legacy.

The long inscription detailing the younger Lucius's illnesses is saturated with the language of fate. The Hours were the goddesses of time and the seasons. They were often associated with birth, since it was a uniquely consequential moment in time. And just like the Fates that stand watch over the first bath on the sarcophagus, the Fates here are the "first to have made all the judgments" about young Lucius. The immortal birth attendants were just as, if not more, important than the human ones.

WELCOMING IN HUMAN AND NONHUMAN FORCES

In the pre-Christian polytheistic Roman empire, many deities hovered around the birthing space. Some—like the Hours and Fates at young Lucius's birth—were there to set the infant on its life course by determining its time of birth and death. Other divinities were there to aid the mother—by promoting a quick labor, supporting her through her pains, and preventing hemorrhage. In the western part of the empire, Juno Lucina—"Juno of the light" or "Juno who brings to light"—protected women as they were giving birth.[27] In the few fictional depictions of childbirth from ancient Rome, women cry out to Juno Lucina in the most intense parts of their labor.[28]

In chapter 6, we saw the role that amulets played in promoting fertility and protecting pregnancies. Amulets were also important at the birth itself. Foremost among these were *okytokion* ("quick birth") amulets (*okytokion* gives us our word "oxytocin"). Like amulets to restrain the

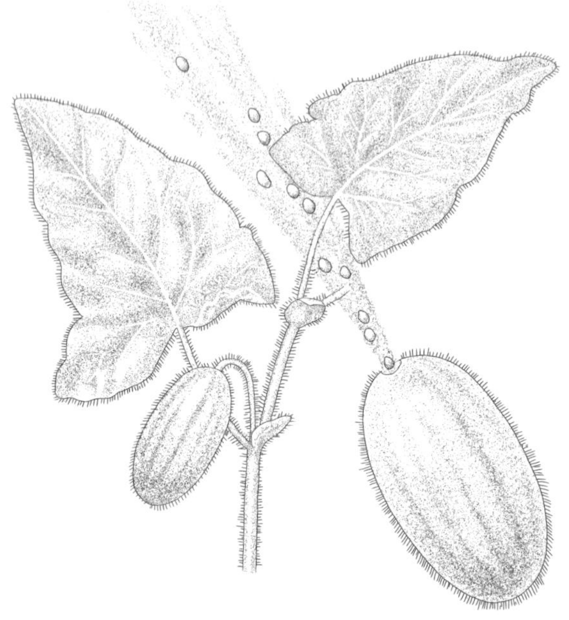

FIGURE 15. Squirting cucumber, *Ecballium elaterium* (L.) A. Rich. When the ripe fruit of the plant is touched it expels a viscous, seedy liquid. Because of this property, it was used in a variety of medical and magical recipes to promote conception or to expel things from the body, including menstrual fluid, fetuses, and placentas. Drawing by Hayley Monroe.

wandering womb, *okytokion* amulets could be made out of many different perishable and nonperishable materials. The ones that survive are made from semiprecious gemstones and have writing on them telling us what they are. Herbal handbooks and medical texts contain recipes for cheaper, temporary ones. One recipe "to speed up birth" calls for squirting cucumber to be plastered with wax, wrapped in a piece of red wool, and placed on the upper thigh.[29] Ingredients, color, and location were all important to the charm's efficacy.[30] Squirting cucumber is a plant that dramatically ejects its seeds when touched (see fig. 15). This exploding property of the plant was thought to help expel things from the body. It was an ingredient used in expulsive remedies (as discussed in chapter 5) and also to help deliver a full-term fetus. The red color of the wool was intended to attract the blood of childbirth, causing it to speed up. And the amulet was placed on the upper thigh so that it would be closest to where it was needed on the body.

Other amulets made from perishable materials relied on similar principles of homeopathic manipulation—the idea that like attracted like or that some property of the substance would transfer over to the laboring woman. The placenta of a dog, laid on a laboring woman's lower abdomen, was thought to draw the fetus out.[31] As a substance that had been expelled from a body in birth, the dog's placenta was thought to transfer its expulsive property to the laboring woman. Similarly, a sloughed-off snakeskin wound around the loins was thought to make childbirth easier—the cast-off skin would help to cast out the fetus.

Like the red wool amulet, reddish stones such as jasper and chalcedony were used as *okytokion* amulets to protect pregnant and laboring women and promote speedy labor. These amulets could be carved with magical and religious symbols, increasing their power and permanence.[32] A red jasper amulet with a pregnant woman squatting on a birth stool was probably an *okytokion* amulet (see fig. 16).[33] Later versions included invocations to the fetus to "come out!"[34] These also morphed into Christian versions of the same thing: "Come out like Christ!"—exhorting the fetus to emerge from the womb just like Jesus of Nazareth had, famously causing his mother Mary no pain.

As we saw in chapter 6, the laboring woman and her attendants also had the responsibility of managing knots in the birthing room. It was thought that these could hold up labor and make it more difficult. When a woman went into labor, it was important that her hair and garments be unbound. If she was using any knots to magically retain the pregnancy, such as an amulet knotted around her neck, that needed to be released as well.

While all of these elements—vocal appeals to childbirth deities, *okytokion* amulets, and knot-untying—might seem superstitious to us today, we should not underestimate the effect these labor management

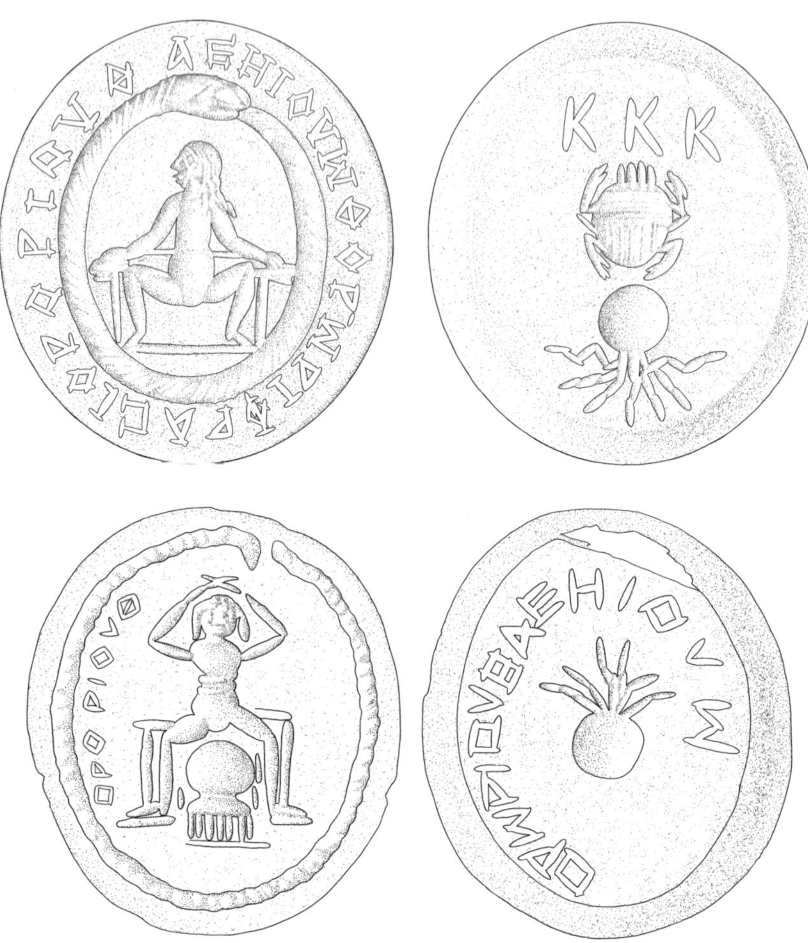

FIGURE 16. Amulets depicting women on birth chairs (front), and octopus-like uteruses (back). Top: red jasper, CBd 759, 17 × 15 × 2 mm. Bottom: hematite, CBd 758, 16 × 13.5 × 3 mm. 1st–4th century CE. British Museum. Drawings by Hayley Monroe.

techniques would have had on the experience of the laboring woman. Today we know that ritual and rhythm are important to the management of unmedicated childbirth. Childbirth educator Penny Simkin explains that the intensity and pain of labor is managed through the adoption of planned and spontaneous rituals that are repeated at every contraction, often involving sacred or profane talismans.[35] In the 2nd century CE, Soranus wrote that the use of amulets "should not be forbidden" because even if they did no good directly, they might, by inspiring hope, "cause the patient to be more cheerful."[36] He recognized the positive psychological effect that an amulet could have.

In modern women's circles, as a practice of preparing the expectant mother for birth, friends and relatives often gift her beads and charms to make a birth necklace. When she is in labor, by looking at and touching the necklace, she can be reminded of all the people who are supporting her. *Okytokion* amulets could have served a similar purpose. The magical tradition underpinning the amulets worked through matrilineal identification. Whenever a woman's name was inscribed on a birth amulet (to personalize it), she was identified as the daughter of her mother. For instance, an amulet made out of a thin gold sheet from Roman Britain addresses a series of magical names, entreating them, "Make it so, with your holy names, that Fabia whom Terentia her mother bore, being in full fitness and health, shall conquer the unborn child and bring it forth; the name of the Lord and Great God being everlasting."[37]

Fabia, the intended user of the amulet, is identified as the daughter of Terentia. The fact that Terentia made it safely through Fabia's birth contributes to the amulet's power, along with the beginning invocation of the magical names and the ending appeal to "the Lord and Great God." Amulets without personalized inscriptions could be reused and passed down through the generations.[38] An amulet, particularly one that had gotten a mother, sister, or grandmother through labor, would have been extraordinarily powerful and meaningful.

But the power of a Roman birth amulet was not just in its psychological effect. Historian Anna Bonnell Freidin has shown how amulets "participated in a birthing network," bringing together "both human and nonhuman actors" in support of the laboring woman and newborn.[39] That is, in a very real, concrete way, amulets brought together the elements—humans, divinities, and the invisible push-pull forces of the universe—that were needed to facilitate a positive birth experience.

Here's how it might have worked. To begin with, the amulet brought other people into the birth space. Let's say a mother wanted to pass her *okytokion* amulet on to her daughter. Maybe she brought the amulet to her daughter when she went into labor. Now the mother was at the birth. Then there needed to be people to "operate" the amulet—to hold it against the lower belly or thigh of the laboring woman. This might have been done by one of the midwife's assistants or an enslaved person in the household. Here, timing was key. Extractive amulets were believed to radiate their power indiscriminately. The same forces pulling the fetus down and out of the womb could also dangerously dislodge the uterus.[40] Whoever was managing the birth amulet had to make sure to leave it in place long enough to bring down the fetus and placenta but to remove it promptly before it could trigger a uterine prolapse. Such an operation would have required intimate attentiveness to the laboring woman.

Amulets also called nonhuman forces into the birth space. Many were inscribed with tiny images of traditional Egyptian birth deities: Isis, protector of women and children; Khnoum, the ram-headed fashioner of fetuses; Bes, the comic dwarf who watched over the birth moment.[41] Many amulets also had magical formulas for opening, closing, and harnessing the uterus. These tiny images and words were not just metaphorical representations. Used properly in the moment, these amulets were thought to bring the divine entities into the birth room and extend the "community of care" around the laboring woman.[42] And finally, the material of the amulets was an animate force at the birth. As we saw before, the red color of the *okytokion* amulet—whether from dyed wool or jasper stone—was intended to attract the red blood of birth. Stones such as magnetite, which could pull objects toward itself, gave proof to the idea that stones had a life force. The use of stones as birth amulets tapped into this force, making it another nonhuman actor at the birth.

Amulets, then, were more than just psychosomatic placebos promoting cheerfulness (as important as that function was as well). They worked to gather a group of supportive human and nonhuman participants at the birth. These supportive agents countered the potential negative effects of the Fates or the goddess Fortuna, "chance" (Tyche in Greek)—another capricious entity hovering around the birthing space.[43]

THE TOOLS OF BIRTH

Birthing women and their attendants used a variety of tools and materials besides amulets to facilitate labor and birth. One of these was the birth stool. Depending on where in the empire the birth was happening, this stool could be simple or elaborate. In Egypt, a flat U-shaped seat supported by four legs was popular, while people in the western empire favored a birth chair with a high back and arms rising above an open semi-circular seat.[44] On these birthing chairs, wood panels extended down from the seat on either side, while the areas below the seat in the front and back were open to allow for catching the baby as well as for the application of fumigations, ointments, pessaries, and other medicaments during labor.

It's possible that midwives in ancient Rome traveled with small portable birth stools. Otherwise, the household of the laboring woman had to supply one. A birth stool is one of the goods that appears in a 2nd-century-CE marriage contract from Roman Egypt.[45] The red jasper *okytokion* amulet that we saw earlier shows the laboring woman seated on a birth stool with wide arms on which she can rest her hands (see fig. 16). Another birth image from a wooden label that was attached to the outside of a mummy in Roman Egypt shows a woman squatting on a simple stool (see fig 17). Both of these women appear to labor naked. The woman on the mummy label wears a double-stranded necklace—perhaps a birthing necklace with an *okytokion* amulet in the center.[46]

Midwives and their assistants used wool cloths to cover the laboring woman for warmth and, Soranus explains, for modesty.[47] Sea sponges came in handy for applying warm water and olive oil infusions to the vulva and perineum. Wool tampons could be smeared with unguents or soaked in herbal infusions and inserted into the vagina to dilate the cervix, counteract inflammation, or provide pain relief. Assistants also

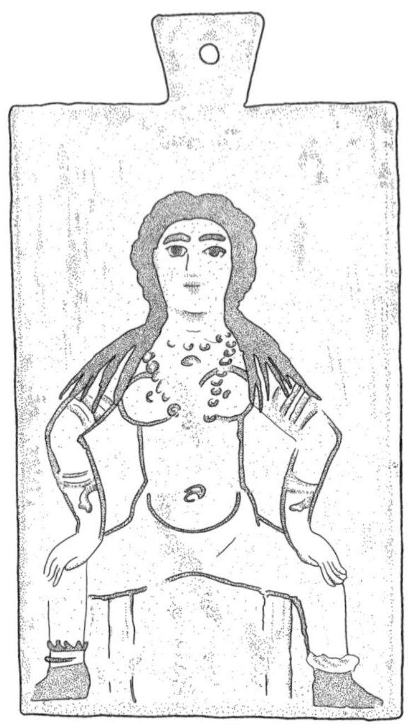

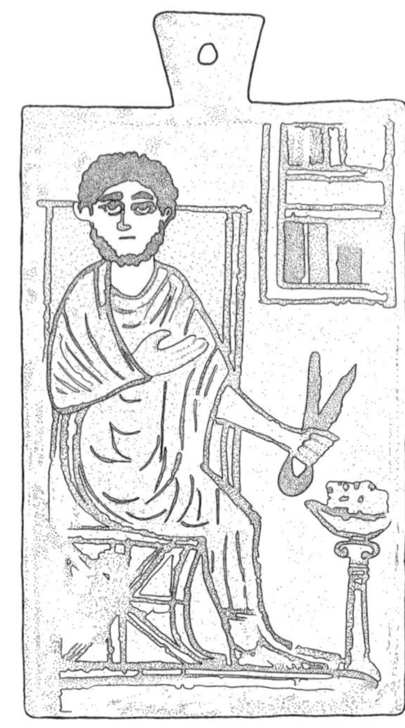

FIGURE 17. Mummy label from Roman Egypt depicting a laboring woman on a simple birth stool (front) and a man holding a pair of scissors—perhaps a doctor or the father of the baby, prepared to cut the umbilical cord (back). 2nd century CE. National Museum of Scotland. Drawing by Hayley Monroe.

inserted these wool tampons into the anus to prevent hemorrhoids and prolapse. Small pots with reed straws were used to hold burning herbs and direct smoke up into the vagina in fumigations. Pillows and wool blankets could be used to prop up the laboring woman's hips for certain manual procedures.

Soranus advised that the birth attendants should softly press on the laboring woman's upper abdomen, helping to move the fetus down toward the birth canal.[48] He instructed the midwife to cover her hands with pieces of cloth or with scraps of thin papyrus to catch the baby so that it did not slip. One of the Hippocratic texts explained that after the birth, the infant could be placed below the laboring woman on stacks of soft wool. It remained there, still attached to its mother, until the placenta was born.[49] As the wool compressed slowly under the infant, the weight and movement provided light traction on the umbilical cord. The effects of the wool stack could be enhanced by a bladder filled with air and punctured with a pin. As the air in the bladder leaked out, the placenta was gently tugged from the mother's body. Once the placenta was born, the midwife would cut the umbilical cord. Anything sharp would do: a knife, a broken piece of pottery, or a crust of stale bread. Soranus advised using a clean iron knife.[50] The other side of the mummy tag with the laboring woman shows a man holding a pair of iron sheers. He could be a doctor, or perhaps the baby's father, who is about to cut the umbilical cord. Specialized medical instruments such as speculums and hooks would only come into play if something went wrong in the course of the birth.

LABOR MANAGEMENT AND PAIN RELIEF

Management of the birth involved the use of herbs, oils, wine, and other medicaments. Many of these were for the purpose of accelerating labor: teas made out of laurel root and dittany; wine mixed with juniper berries and anise; recipes such as the drink that called for turpentine and honey to be mixed with olive oil and wine.[51] Another treatment called for the laboring woman to drink olive oil and pour warm olive oil and marsh mallow tea over her vulva and to inject goose fat and olive oil into her vagina.[52] This injection was thought to lubricate a dry vulva and vagina and help the passage of the fetus.

Cervical ripening teas are still popular today. They are often the first way to try to stimulate labor when a pregnant person has gone past their due date or is impatient to have the baby. Drinking oil—typically castor oil—is another popular way to get labor going or to accelerate a slow or stalled labor. Wine, too, is still used today, though it generally has the effect of slowing down or temporarily stopping labor rather than speeding it up. Drinking spiced wine may have helped women in ancient Roman relax and manage the intensity and pain of birth.

Other treatments may seem more bizarre, such as drinking dried deer penis in white wine for a quick birth.[53] In this category are vaginal fumigations and vapor baths. Strong smelling—though not necessarily unpleasant—substances such as resin, cumin, and pine bark could be steamed or burned to produce a thick vapor or smoke that would be directed up the woman's vagina.[54] Other substances, like hyena fat, might not have been so pleasant.[55] However, these remedies were not used routinely, but only when a woman was having difficulty giving birth.

The Romans recognized that an upright position was best for birth. In the absence of a birth stool, Soranus explained that the same position could be achieved by having the laboring woman sit on the lap of another woman who was seated on a chair or couch.[56] If the laboring woman was weak or tired, a lying-down position could be adapted to take advantage of gravity: she was advised to lie on her back on a firm bed with her feet together and thighs apart, her hips elevated on a bolster so that her vagina pointed downward.[57] In a well-known mythological birth story, the goddess Leto kneeled while holding onto a palm tree over her head to birth the god Apollo.[58] Women in ancient Rome may have held on to trees, posts, or other vertical supports while laboring and pushing. In cases of difficult labor, position changes could help. Soranus advised that putting the laboring woman on her hands and knees or on her knees leaning forward was thought to allow the uterus to fall forward in the abdomen, putting it in line with the vagina and allowing easier exit of the fetus.[59]

The midwife and her assistants had a variety of methods for helping the laboring woman cope. The first line of care was touch with warm hands.[60] Birth attendants applied cloths drenched in warm olive oil to the abdomen and labia, frequently refreshing the oil so that it stayed warm. Bladders from animals such as goats, sheep, or pigs could be filled with warm olive oil and applied to the lower back for pain relief. Sacks of warmed grain could be used similarly.[61] The assistants used their bodies to physically support the laboring person. Ideally, Soranus wrote, there were three assistants, two to support the laboring person at her sides and one from behind.[62] That way they could relieve some of the weight and strain through the contractions.

According to Soranus, birth pain was a positive sign. It meant that labor was proceeding as it was supposed to and that the fetus was alive and well. He wrote, "If [the fetus] is alive, the woman has labor pains and the urge to push . . . but if the fetus is dead, she does not have these pains."[63] A lack of pain—particularly a failure of the pain to intensify—indicated that the fetus had likely died. The midwife and her assistants coached the laboring woman not to succumb to her labor pains but to work with them to bring the baby out. Soranus explained that one of the causes of difficult labor, especially in first-time mothers, was that the laboring woman did not cooperate and work with, rather than against, her labor pains.

While pain was a positive sign, fear was a negative one. Just as failure to cooperate with the labor pains could lead to a difficult birth, so too could fear.[64] For this reason, one of the most important jobs the midwife had was to allay the anxieties of the laboring woman, telling her, as Soranus put it, that "there is nothing to fear and that the birth will be easy . . . she is in no danger and should be brave."[65] Similarly, the assistants were supposed to dispel fear with verbal encouragement.

We should not see these beliefs and practices as misogynistic and barbaric. In a time before nitrous oxide, saddle blocks, and epidurals, labor could only be managed in the way these women did it—guiding the laboring woman to work with the labor pains, while physically and psychologically supporting and uplifting her. It is also important to realize that our understanding of birth pain as pathological—that is, as something that needs to be eliminated—only emerged in the mid- to late 19th century with the introduction of anesthesia—ether and chloroform—into birth.[66] Before that time, birth management practices did not focus so much on alleviating pain as on hastening labor and coaching the laboring woman to work with the pains.[67] Labor pain had a positive and functional role: the crescendoing responses to pain from the laboring woman allowed midwives to track the progression of labor.[68]

Today, unmedicated physiological birth is managed in much the same way that it was in ancient Rome. Some birthing people today find these natural methods of labor management and pain relief to be better for them than more invasive pain-management strategies. When a laboring person is in a calm, supportive environment, receiving attentive, hands-on support, the pain and intensity of labor can often be bearable. Soranus's account of a birth scene shows the birthing woman being supported continuously throughout her labor and birth by a midwife and several other female attendants. This physical, emotional, hands-on support, when and where it was available, would have increased the chances of a positive outcome for mother and baby. Compared to the way that many women were left to labor on their own in hospital wards in the mid- to late 20th century—hooked up to electronic fetal monitors but with no care provider in sight—a typical ancient Roman birth scene seems much more humane in many respects.[69]

But we shouldn't imagine that Roman women gave birth in an unmedicalized utopia full of ancient wisdom. Many Roman birth practices were quite dangerous. The degree to which, according to Soranus, the midwife manually intervened in the birth canal is alarming. In order to encourage labor to begin, Soranus advised the midwife to dilate the cervix with an oiled finger.[70] Then, once labor had started, he instructed her to continue dilating the cervix with her finger until the bag of waters fell out. The midwife was supposed to place the laboring woman on the birth chair once the protruding part of the amniotic sac was about the size of a chicken egg. At this point, she was to reach up inside the cervix and gently pull the fetus down in coordination with the contractions. The later, 5th- or 6th-century adaptation of Soranus's *Gynecology,* Muscio's *Gynaecia,* advised the midwife to break the bag of waters using her fingernail—the flush of water was supposed to help the head emerge.[71]

These manual interventions sound similar to those used today: a cervical sweep performed on a ripe cervix can stimulate labor, as can breaking the bag of waters. But in the ancient Roman world, these maneuvers carried great risk. Anytime hands, herbs, and oils were introduced into the birth canal, it could also mean the introduction of pathogens and the chance for laceration and other physical trauma. There does seem to have been some attention to cleanliness. Soranus instructed midwives to make sure to use clean olive oil that had not been previously used for cooking, and when wool cloths were used for the woman or infant, they were supposed to be "soft clean cloths."[72] But there were no explicit instructions about handwashing. And even today, with all of our attention to antiseptic sanitation, the insertion of a (sterile, gloved) hand and instruments into the vagina increases the risk of infection for the laboring person and the baby. In the Roman world, the less manual intervention, the better a birth would have gone, especially if it was proceeding normally.

The main source for normal childbirth practices in ancient Rome is, as we've seen, Soranus's *Gynecology*. It's not clear if his text is descriptive or prescriptive—describing what *is* done by midwives, or prescribing what *should* be done. Were midwives and attendants providing the kind of attentive care (and performing the invasive manual procedures) that appear in Soranus's texts? Or is his *Gynecology* one of the first examples of medicine trying to give the provider something to do in a process that largely proceeds on its own?

Soranus's contemporary, the doctor Galen, had very little to say about childbirth. In his one description of normal birth, from earlier in this chapter, he does describe the midwife performing manual cervical checks on the laboring woman. But these seem to be more about monitoring the progress of labor than trying to speed it up through forcible dilation or breaking of the amniotic sac. In another treatise, Galen gives a lengthy description of birth. To him, the human body is the marvelous construction of a creator god, whom he alternately describes as Nature (female) or a divine Craftsman (male). One of the remarkable constructions of Nature is the cervix, which, he explains, is "constricted and closed during pregnancy" and "opens to its greatest extent during birth." During pregnancy, he writes, it is closed so tightly that it's not even possible to stick a probe through it, "but at birth a whole living being comes through it."[73] In his estimation, birth is a process that largely works without the need for medical intervention:

> She [Nature] took great care to make sure that the fetus approaches the cervix in the right direction [head first] and comes out without hurting or dislocating any limb. . . . If this process were to be impeded one out of every three or four times, then one hundred in four hundred births

> would be difficult. But since this happens only once in many thousands of births, it serves as a reminder of the good things that we enjoy from the Creator who formed us.[74]

This passage veers uncomfortably close to certain modern fundamentalist religious approaches to childbirth that discourage any interventions into birth on the grounds that whatever happens is God's design and plan. (Or that, in its most extreme form, sees labor pains as woman's punishment for the sins of Eve.) But at the same time, Galen is probably communicating something true: as unpredictable as birth could be, the vast majority of births, even in the ancient world, would have proceeded without complication. More insidiously, though, this perspective discounts the vital work of the midwife and attendants in even normal childbirth circumstances. It doesn't acknowledge that in many cases, these births seemed to go well all on their own because other women (and sometimes men) were there to lay supportive hands on the laboring woman, to apply warm bladders of oil and sacks of grain to her back and hips, to tell her that she was strong and everything was going to be okay, to encourage (or force) her to change positions, and to help her assume an upright posture at the moment of birth.

• • •

When Empona gave birth to her twins alone, she must have felt the lack of care. There was no one to press on her back or to hold an *okytokion* amulet up to her thigh. She may not have known she was having twins, since she had to keep her pregnancy secret from everyone she knew. No midwife palpated her belly to feel her babies' positions. Imagine the despair she felt when she realized, after the birth of one child, that her labor wasn't finished. When the thought came to her that she might die, there was no one to encourage her and bolster her spirit. The extraordinariness of Empona's birth and what she lacked shows what was expected at an ordinary birth—a supportive community of human and nonhuman forces gathered around the laboring woman.

TEN

Difficult Birth

December 15, 34 CE

A contraction seized Agrippina as she lay on the hard bed. She cried out to Juno Lucina for help. The midwife matched her vocalization, drawing it down from a high shriek into a low moan. The other women in the room joined in. Agrippina gave a guttural grunt and water gushed onto the bed.

The midwife gently slid her oiled hand into Agrippina's vagina. She could feel a small foot already partway down the birth canal. A slight expression of concern crossed her face, which she quickly masked. She ordered the assistants to fold thick wool cloths and place them under Agrippina's hips. She motioned for an oil lamp to be brought closer. Two assistants on either side held Agrippina's knees open as the midwife reached up into her vagina, running her finger around the opening of the cervix. She gently pushed the little foot back up through the cervix, caught the second foot and guided both legs down together. Agrippina let out an involuntary shriek.

Two enslaved women helped Agrippina out of bed and onto a birth chair. One of the midwife's assistants hurried over with a pot billowing thick, fragrant vapor. Placing it under the opening in the birth chair, she directed it up toward Agrippina's vagina. The midwife rubbed a rich, greasy unguent on her vulva and perineum. Agrippina leaned into the sturdy body of the woman standing behind her, who gripped her firmly under the arms. A doctor readied his tools on a nearby table, speaking in low tones to the midwife.

With each contraction, the two enslaved women pressed down on Agrippina's belly from above. The baby descended quickly. Very soon, everyone in the room could see that it was a boy. A flutter of excitement and nervous anticipation went through the room. A look of grim determination passed over Agrippina's face. With one final long push and a high shriek from Agrippina, the baby turned, and his head was released. As the sun rose on a crisp December day in the year 34 CE, the future emperor Nero slipped into the waiting hands of the midwife.

AGRIPPINA'S BREECH BIRTH

Julia Agrippina was twenty-two years old when she gave birth to her first and only child on December 15, 34 CE. We know one tantalizing detail about the birth: it was a footling breech. Agrippina, as she was known, was the younger sister of the emperor Caligula. Her baby boy would grow up to become Nero, the fifth emperor of Rome and last in the Julio-Claudian dynasty. We know about her breech birth because she wrote memoirs of her life in which she described it. Unfortunately, these memoirs do not survive. We only know about them because a few contemporary male historians mentioned them in their own writings.[1] I have embellished the rest of her story based on what we know about breech birth in the ancient and modern world.

In this chapter, I use Agrippina's birth story as a starting point to discuss the births in ancient Rome that did not proceed normally—those that were termed "difficult." First, I put breech birth in both its ancient and modern contexts, since it is something that is poorly understood even today. We will see that while breech birth was, and still is, classified as a type of difficult birth, it was—and is—also a type of birth that can proceed safely with a recognizable pattern of movements. Next I examine the variety of difficult births in ancient Rome and how they were managed by practitioners. Difficult birth provided the inroad for the male medical takeover of birth. It was the introduction of doctors' tools into the birth scene that promised to save women and infants from death, but that also led, eventually, to the loss of time-tested, effective, and low-intervention birth-management techniques. Finally, I end by looking at the incidence of maternal mortality and the memorials for ancient Roman women who died in childbirth. An outsize focus on the dangers of birth in antiquity has led to overemphasis of these stories at the expense of others. Ultimately, I show how looking at ancient birth from our modern perspective has clouded the way we see it. Far from being common, difficult birth—and, especially, maternal death in childbirth—would have been an uncommon experience.

A breech birth like Agrippina's could have been tricky. It may have required expert skill on the part of the practitioner. Today, breech presentations are classified into three types: Frank breech (baby's buttocks pointed downward with legs extended up toward its head), complete breech (baby's buttocks pointed downward with knees bent and feet also pointed downward), and footling breech (feet pointed downward). According to the Cleveland Clinic, today, about 3 to 4 percent of full-term births (those past 36 weeks) are breech.[2] Of these, Frank and complete breech are the safest in vaginal birth because the buttocks are able to mimic the action of the head in a normal cephalic (headfirst) presentation. The footling breech position presents more risks. When the feet come out first, the baby can get stuck at the buttocks or head. Also, the umbilical cord has a greater chance of prolapse—falling out of the cervix and getting compressed, cutting off the oxygen supply to the fetus.

Today most breech births are done via cesarean section.[3] As c-sections have become more common, the skills to manage a vaginal breech birth have been lost.[4] There are a few midwives and obstetricians who are willing to manage vaginal breech births, but for the most part it is avoided. If the breech position is known prior to birth, everything is done to try to turn the baby to a cephalic presentation.[5] If the breech presentation is a surprise at the time of birth, a laboring person giving birth in a hospital will generally be transferred to an operating room. Someone laboring at home may opt to stay at home if their provider is trained in breech birth. In the ancient world, c-section was not an option. Every effort had to be made to ensure a successful vaginal birth.

In ancient Rome, according to popular imagination, a footling breech was "against nature."[6] A common saying went, "It's natural to be born head first, and customary to be carried to burial feet first."[7] More complications could arise from a feet-first birth. One of the Hippocratic writers warned that a feet-first presentation was "difficult" and "often either mothers have died from this, or children, or both."[8] He recommended that the birth attendant push the fetus back up inside the uterus and try to turn it to a headfirst position.[9] This maneuver sounds similar to a modern external cephalic version (ECV), where an obstetrician attempts to manually turn the baby around via manipulations on the outside of the abdomen. But this ancient version would have been much more dangerous. Internally rotating a breech baby from inside would have been highly risky. It could have introduced life-threatening pathogens into the vagina and uterus. It also could have caused damage to the body of the mother or the baby. Thankfully, this procedure seems to have fallen out of favor by the 2nd century CE.

Multiple gynecological texts from the 1st century CE onward indicated that a feet-first breech presentation could be almost as safe as a head-first presentation.[10] In the 2nd century, Soranus explained that next to a headfirst presentation, a feet-first presentation was best.[11] He advised the practitioner to intervene only if one leg came out before the other. Then, as I have imagined in Agrippina's story, the practitioner was supposed to push the one leg back up inside and guide both feet out together. One of the later Hippocratic texts advised an even less invasive intervention. For both headfirst and feet-first births that had stalled, the practitioner was advised to use a vaginal vapor bath to loosen the stuck fetus.[12] If this did not work, the practitioner was advised to use ointments, foods, and drinks that helped to stimulate descent—for example, an ointment of thickened squirting cucumber.[13] He or she was to apply salves to moisten the perineum.[14] If a feet-first fetus was still stuck, the practitioner was advised to move their finger around the body of the fetus in a circle, moisten their hands and pass them up through the cervix, finding traction on the shoulders to pull the fetus's head down and out.[15] While very painful for the laboring woman, such a maneuver had a chance of resulting in a living mother and baby.

Best practice for vaginal breech births today is to refrain from intervening unless absolutely necessary. Midwife Mary Cronk recommends, "Keep your hands off, sit on them if necessary."[16] Most vaginal breech births will proceed normally, though differently from a headfirst birth. Part of being a skilled practitioner is knowing how a normal breech birth differs from a normal headfirst birth. It is the job of the practitioner to recognize potentially harmful deviations from normal and do the minimal intervention necessary—generally, manual repositioning of the limbs, shoulders, or head. What's interesting about footling breech births in the ancient world is that they seem to have become safer over time. It was probably midwives who noticed that if they did less manual intervention, they had better outcomes. The male medical writers picked up their information from talking to midwives or from observing births that were managed by midwives. By the 2nd century CE, the recommendation to perform an internal cephalic version turned into a recommendation to perform minimal manual intervention.

In Agrippina's case, things turned out all right. She and her baby lived. The only indication that something may have gone wrong during the birth is that Agrippina did not go on to have any more children. But there could have been many reasons for that. Although married at thirteen, she did not have her son until she was twenty-two. Perhaps she was using an effective method of birth control, or maybe there was already some issue with her reproductive system that made it difficult for her to get pregnant. Of course, the problem could have lain with her husband as well.

CAUSES OF DIFFICULT BIRTH

Ancient medical writers thought that difficult labor could arise from an issue with the maternal body, the fetal body, or the interaction between the two.[17] They explained that the fetus might be of such a size that it could not fit through the woman's pelvis. While this is extremely rare today, it is more common in very young women. Given the young age at which many Roman women first got pregnant, it may have been more common then than it is now. Also, given the ill health and low nutrition of many pregnant women in antiquity, it's possible that their bodies were not in great shape for giving birth. The medical writers point to scar tissue and infections on the cervix or in the birth canal as factors in difficult births. They also identify malposition of the fetus in the uterus—posterior, transverse, and breech—as sources of difficulty.[18] Twins and triplets were understood to be harder to birth than single babies. Finally, there was much concern over the condition of the waters and when they broke. It was believed that the slipperiness provided by the amniotic fluid was key to lubricating the fetus's passage out of the womb. If the sac broke too soon or if there was not enough fluid in it, it was thought to prevent birth. The quality of the fluid was important too. The medical texts mention amniotic fluid that is too pungent, too mild, and too thick. It is possible they are referring to conditions such as meconium in the waters or polyhydramnios—the condition of having too much amniotic fluid.

The age and lifestyle of the laboring woman could be blamed for her difficult labor. Medical writers attributed difficult labor to long widowhood, advanced maternal age, poor diet, lack of exercise, and a propensity for drinking and staying up late. As reported by Soranus, the Alexandrian physician Herophilus claimed that accumulation of fat around the abdomen and hips could cause difficult labor because it squeezed the uterus.[19] The Syrian physician Demetrius likewise attributed difficult labor to "excessive fleshiness." He further claimed that "extreme indulgence" could hinder labor since "some women are self-indulgent and do not exert themselves [in labor]."[20] Demetrius also blamed excessive slenderness, tallness, and body types with wide shoulders and narrow pelvises for difficult labor. Of these, the only that are known to contribute to difficult labor today are excessive slenderness from malnutrition and a body type with a narrow pelvis. Fat in the abdomen and hips does not squeeze the uterus, but anti-fat bias in modern healthcare still causes trouble for fat people who are pregnant and giving birth.[21]

Issues with the birthing space and inexperience of the practitioner were also thought to cause problems.[22] If the birth room was not prepared beforehand, it could limit the resources and tools available to the midwife. A space that was too cold or too hot could stall or impede labor.

Inexperience of the midwife or doctor could introduce risks into the birth that would not be there under a more experienced practitioner.

The medical sources have a lot to say on difficult birth. They give the impression that many births in ancient Rome were difficult. But on average, in pre-modern societies difficult births accounted for about 5 to 6 percent of births.[23] It's possible that there were more difficult births in ancient Rome due to factors such as early age at first pregnancy, closely spaced pregnancies, and nutritional deficiencies. Bioarchaeological data from the remains of bones and teeth in cemeteries from ancient Rome attest to high incidences of scurvy, rickets, and anemia caused by deficiencies of vitamin C, vitamin D, and iron, respectively.[24] Rickets causes softening of the bones, which can lead to rachitic pelvis—malformation of the pelvic opening that renders it too narrow to admit the fetal head during birth.[25]

MEDICAL SOURCES, MIDWIFERY CARE

The medical sources on difficult birth were all written by men, but most of these births were managed by female midwives or doctor-midwives, if by anyone at all. The men who wrote about these births learned what they knew from talking to women (or from reading the writing of other men who had talked to women). They spoke to female midwives, female doctors, and women who had given birth—the "women of experience" we met in chapter 6. Sometimes male doctors learned from working alongside female practitioners at normal and difficult births alike.[26] We know this because when the male doctors wrote about birth, even difficult birth, the practitioners doing the hands-on work were women.[27]

But while these male doctors were learning from female practitioners, they were also writing extensively about difficult birth and citing the writings of other male doctors. By the 2nd century CE, there was a robust citational practice for difficult birth that involved *only* these male writers. We can see this practice in Soranus's *Gynecology.* In his section on difficult birth, he cites the writings of fifteen male physicians, going back to the Hippocratic doctors in the 5th century BCE. He refers to all these men by name: Demetrius the Herophilean, Diocles the Carystean, Cleophantus, Andreas, Euryphon the Cnidean, and so on.[28] He engages in robust dialogue with the writings of these other medical men, supporting or refuting their diagnoses and treatments of difficult labor. But when Soranus mentions female practitioners, he refers to them only as "midwives." They are not individuals. For the most part, he only mentions them as practitioners in order to disagree with them. Midwives, he tells us, are "superstitious": they refuse to cut the cord using an iron blade and they believe that knots on the body of the pregnant woman will impede labor.[29] They tear off umbilical cords "inexpertly."[30]

Soranus's writing contributed to the masculine-feminine divide of ancient medical practice. On the whole, women participated in an oral tradition; men wrote things down. This divide, however, was not strict—some female medical practitioners *did* write things down.[31] But Soranus made a conscious choice to exclude their voices from his work, as did the Hippocratic writers before him. Reading between the lines of these male-authored texts, it's clear that female practitioners had comprehensive empirical as well as theory-based knowledge of the many permutations of childbirth, including difficult birth. By excising these female practitioners from their works, the ancient male medical writers started the process of encroaching on female management of birth.

MANAGING DIFFICULT BIRTH

Practitioners diagnosed the cause of difficult birth by questioning the laboring woman, observing her body externally, and examining her body internally. The midwife would ask the patient if anything was troubling her, since adverse emotional states such as grief could make labor difficult.[32] She would also observe and palpate her abdomen. By inserting her fingers into the birth canal and the cervix, the midwife could tell if the fetus was in a transverse position or had a nuchal hand (up alongside the head).[33] Manual examinations of the abdomen and birth canal could also let the midwife know if the fetus was alive or dead. If the fetus was alive, the thinking went, the laboring woman would have labor pains and the urge to push. Her abdomen would be warm and internal examination would find the fetus warm as well. But if the fetus was dead, then the woman would not have the same labor pains or urge to push and an internal examination would reveal a cold fetal body. Breath and pulse were key signs of the health of the mother during labor. They indicated whether she was doing okay or was in danger.[34]

Midwives knew that the psychological dimension of birth was just as important as the physical one. According to Soranus, for every cause of difficult labor, the first job of the practitioner was to "promote ease and relaxation."[35] It was the role of the practitioner and attendants to make the laboring woman feel safe and supported. If the issue was in the psyche—excessive grief, fear, anger, or even denial about what was happening—this supportive and authoritative attention might be enough to get the labor running smoothly again. If that did not work, it was time to resort to physical and mechanical measures.

The midwife and her assistants could change the temperature of the birthing space—warming up a cold room or cooling down a hot one.[36] If she was faint or weak, they could revive the laboring woman with pleasant smells and give her mild, nutritious foods to eat—bread, melon, barley gruel, apples. They could help her urinate or give her laxatives. Full bladders and bowels were known to slow down or impede labor. The midwife could also help the laboring woman breathe and vocalize effectively.

Midwives could advise movement and position changes to help a difficult labor. They could put the laboring woman on her hands and knees or on her knees leaning forward. The thinking was that these positions would cause the uterus to fall forward and put the cervix in a straight line with the birth canal.[37] This is not true, but a kneeling position does create more space in the pelvis, speeding up labor and helping a malpositioned fetus get into a better position. Similarly, for a stalled labor, midwives would have the laboring woman walk around or climb up and down steps. These methods are still used today to accelerate labor and to get the fetus in the right position.

Soranus was critical of these movements, instead preferring that a laboring woman be carried around on a litter with her head slightly raised in order to stimulate expulsion.[38] Any change of location and position may have helped labor, but walking around and climbing steps would have been much more effective than riding in a litter. Also, walking around and going up and down steps would have been available to almost anyone in labor, while riding around in a litter was only accessible to the richest women in Rome. Doctors like Soranus were in the business of convincing women and, especially, their husbands that they needed specialized medical care for pregnancy and birth. Midwives, though, based on Soranus's criticisms of them, seem to have been providing the more effective care.

In one of the Hippocratic medical texts there is a description of a procedure that sounds quite similar to what midwives do today to turn a malpositioned baby prior to birth.[39] The pregnant woman was laid on a bed with her legs higher than her head. Several women took hold of her legs and shook them toward her shoulders. The intention was to jiggle the fetus up into open space in the uterus so that it could adjust itself into a better position for descent. Today, midwives use similar measures that combine gravitational pull with shaking or jiggling to get the fetus to spin around to a more favorable position before it is born. One involves the pregnant person getting into a hands and knees position and lowering her chest to the bed. The midwife wraps a rebozo or a large shawl around her hips and shakes them vigorously from side to side. The position and movement can give the fetus enough space to correctly position its head in the pelvis for an easier exit.

Other methods for dislodging a stuck fetus involved the aid of men in the household. One of the medical texts described strapping the laboring woman firmly to a hard bed and having strong men repeatedly lift the foot of the bed up high and drop it down.[40] The theory was that the sudden jolt would dislodge the fetus. This is similar to the shaking movements performed by the female birth attendants, but much more extreme. It probably would have been quite unpleasant—if it was ever performed—and not any more effective than the leg jiggling. A similar effect might have been achieved with a simpler method whereby a strong man lifted the laboring woman up under her armpits and shook her vigorously.[41]

To encourage the cervix to open, the midwife could use an infusion of warm olive oil and herbs such as linseed, fenugreek, and mallow, either in a sitz bath or applied directly to the cervix with a sponge.[42] If these did not work, the midwife might have had to forcibly dilate the cervix with her fingers or push a lip of cervix out of the way to allow for the passage of the fetus.[43] If the fetus was stuck in the birth canal due to a breech position, shoulder dystocia, or other malposition, the midwife could manually reposition it, turning the head and shoulders or straightening and aligning limbs.[44] These procedures would have been quite painful. They would also have significantly increased the risks associated with birth. Introducing hands and herbal medicaments into the birth canal greatly increased the risk of infection. Manually turning or pulling on the fetus could have caused physical trauma to the woman or baby. There are several infants buried in a Roman-era cemetery in Egypt whose bodies have fractured arm bones and collarbones. It is possible that these infants were injured by being forcibly twisted or pulled out of the birth canal.[45]

DOCTORS AND THEIR TOOLS

In the medical texts, it is female practitioners who use their hands on the laboring patient. For instance, Soranus tells us that when a fetus is in a transverse position, it is the midwife who uses her hand to rotate its body into a headfirst or feet-first position.[46] Male practitioners come on the scene when surgical tools are needed to remove a dead fetus. In many of the male-authored medical texts, this surgical birth is the *only* birth that appears.[47]

Soranus gives an idea of what an interaction between a midwife and a male doctor might have looked like. When the doctor arrived, he was supposed to question the midwife. She could tell him what was happening and what the cause of the difficult labor was. Then there was a negotiation.

Soranus advised that the doctor "should not immediately resort to surgery, but he should also not allow the midwife to take too much time dilating the uterus with force."[48] Here, as on the tombstone reliefs for Scribonia Attice and her husband Marcus Ulpius Amerimnus, the dichotomy is clear: midwives use their hands, doctors use their tools.

A gruesome comment from Soranus attests to the role doctors played at births. He explained that a doubled-up infant was in the worst position, especially if it had its hips down. These infants could take three positions at the cervix: legs and head first, abdomen first, or hips first. Of these, he wrote, it was best to have the abdomen towards the cervix because "after we have opened the abdomen and removed its contents, the body collapses and it becomes easy to change the position."[49] The assumption was that a doubled-up infant had no chance of being born. The best-case scenario was simply that it was lying in the uterus in such a way that the doctor could easily perform an embryotomy, cutting up and removing the fetus from the uterus piece by piece.

Several texts show that male doctors performed these embryotomies from at least the 5th century BCE onward.[50] There is an early Hippocratic text called *Excision of the Fetus* that dealt explicitly with the subject. It described how to use a knife to collapse and segment the fetal body and extract it piece by piece from the uterus.[51] Specialized tools were devised for this purpose. One of these was a "claw"—a ring with a blade mounted on it that a surgeon wore on the thumb.[52] There are no surviving examples of this tool, but it seems likely that the blade would have had a slight curve at the top, which would have allowed the surgeon to insert it safely into the vagina and uterus before using it to dismember the fetus.

It was also at about this time that the trivalved vaginal speculum appeared (see fig. 18).[53] The smaller bivalved rectal speculum had been around for centuries and had also been used for vaginal procedures, but in the 1st century CE, a larger speculum emerged with a unique shape and design specifically for the vagina.[54] A few of these survive from the house of a doctor in Pompeii that was buried under volcanic ash in the eruption of Mount Vesuvius in 79 CE.[55] The vaginal speculum was used exactly as it is now, to hold open the vagina and give the practitioner a

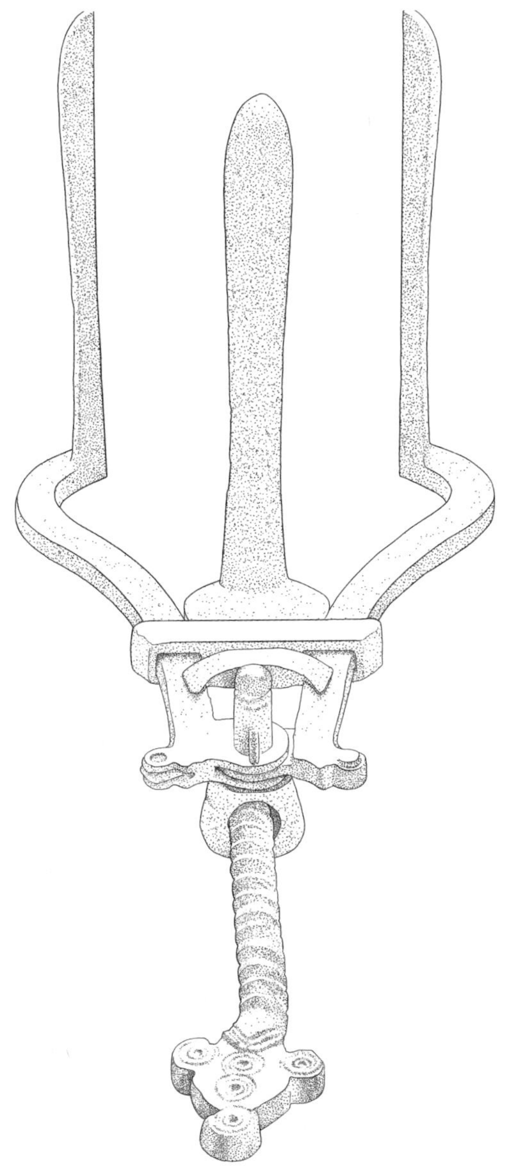

FIGURE 18. Roman bronze trivalve vaginal speculum. Lebanon. 1st–4th century CE (screw is modern). Science Museum Group 1979–327. Drawing by Hayley Monroe.

clear line of sight to the cervix—though unlike today, one medical text mentions that it was pleasantly warmed over hot coals before insertion.[56] The surgeon used the speculum during fetal extractions.[57]

The main tool for extracting the fetus was the traction hook.[58] This was a long, straight piece of metal with a smooth metal hook ending in a short, sharp point. One or two of them could be hooked into the body of the fetus in order to draw it out slowly with the contractions, along with the guiding hand of a practitioner. Other small knives, lancets, and scalpels were used to perforate and reduce the skull for easier extraction.[59] A cranioclast ("skull crusher") could be used to break up the skull before extracting the fragments with a bone forceps.[60] According to Soranus, some practitioners outfitted their birth stools with a projecting axel, windlasses, and a knob.[61] They would wind ropes around the limbs of the impacted fetus and turn the knobs to pull its body out of the birth canal. Soranus advised against this method, cautioning that extraction was better done with the woman lying down.

It's clear from descriptions of how these instruments were used to extract fetuses that the embryotomy operation had more in common with other surgical procedures than with childbirth. The obstetrical tools that doctors used were variations on the surgical tools they used for other kinds of operations, such as the extraction of tumors and cancers from the body. Sometimes they were the very same tools. Soranus explained that a knife for removing polyps should be used to split the fetal head that is too big and causing impaction.[62] Similarly, he recommended crushing the fetal skull and removing the fragments with forceps normally used for extracting teeth or bone splinters.[63] The same technique used for extracting teeth—pulling from side-to-side and not in a straight line—was supposed to be used in the extraction of the fetus. At the point that a doctor came in to extract a dead fetus from a pregnant woman, it had ceased to be a birth and turned into a medical operation. The fetus was no longer a baby that could be born, but something that could putrefy and harm the woman if left inside.

The importance of saving the mother's life was recognized by the early Christian theologian Tertullian, as well as by the Greco-Roman doctors.

While Tertullian lamented the death of the fetus in the embryotomy operation, he saw it as a "cruel necessity."[64] Nowhere do we see a deliberation over saving the life of the mother or the life of the baby. Simply put, if the baby could not be born, it had to be surgically removed before the mother died as well. Infant mortality was substantially higher than maternal mortality. Estimates based on records from other pre-industrial societies suggest that upward of a third of infants died before their fifth birthday.[65] But this does not mean that people in ancient Rome did not care about babies who died from the embryotomy operation. Burial evidence shows that they cared a great deal. In an ancient Roman cemetery at Poundbury Camp near Dorset in England, the remains of a full-term infant were buried in a wooden coffin.[66] The infant's skeleton is all there, but it has been divided into many pieces, with cut marks on the bones of the torso, arms, and legs. This baby seems to have been removed from its mother via embryotomy sometime between thirty-eight and forty weeks' gestation. It was then given a proper burial according to local custom. Clearly, this was a baby that was cherished and mourned. The fact that it was buried alone suggests that its mother may have survived the operation.

SURGERY AND CONSENT

Soranus advised doctors who were about to perform an embryotomy to warn the birthing woman about the potential consequences: subsequent fevers, inflammation, and damage to nerves.[67] They were to be transparent about the fact that if a gangrenous infection set in, she would likely die. At the same time, he encouraged doctors to not withhold care. They should not avoid the operation because of fear that it would not be successful. In the 1st century, the doctor Celsus recounted the case of an upper-class woman with a gangrenous genital prolapse. "The most prominent doctors" refused to operate on her because they feared that her inevitable death would be blamed on them. Celsus believed that had they been less timid, they could have saved her life.[68]

But while physicians might have hesitated to operate on elite, wealthy individuals for fear of reputational consequences, they had no such qualms about operating on enslaved people. While Soranus does not distinguish between enslaved and free or poor and wealthy women in his *Gynecology,* evidence from his contemporary, Galen, shows that enslaved people, like animals, were used to trial and perfect new surgical techniques. In one of his medical treatises, Galen described performing what amounted to open-heart surgery on an enslaved boy.[69] He explained that other physicians refused to operate given the great risk involved. But Galen, having practiced such an operation on hundreds of animals, was bold enough to give it a try. The boy survived the operation and was still living several years later, but it was almost certainly his enslaved status that allowed Galen to perform a highly risky, untried—at least on humans—surgery and write about it.

Although there is no way to confirm it, it would not surprise me if, as in later periods, Roman doctors practiced their obstetrical surgeries on enslaved and other marginalized women before performing them on elite, upper-class women. The surgery to repair a vesicovaginal fistula (a hole in the flesh separating the bladder and the vagina) was trialed and perfected in the 19th century on the bodies of enslaved Black women in the United States—the best-known of whom were named Anarcha, Lucy, and Betsey.[70] And when doctors were performing cesarean sections on living women in the 19th-century United States, they sought consent for the highly risky procedure—carrying a death rate of 50 percent—from their free patients but not from enslaved women.[71]

CESAREAN SECTION

There is a popular idea that the term "cesarean section" comes from the surgical birth of the famous Julius Caesar. This is not true. Julius Caesar was born vaginally; his mother survived his birth and went on to live until her son was a grown man.[72] An alternate story suggests that it was actually a distant ancestor of Julius—the first Caesar—who was cut from his dead mother's womb. "Caesar" comes from the Latin word meaning "cut," and so folk etymology has it that the cesarean section was the source of the family name.[73] That may have been the case, but it is likelier that both of these stories sprang up in the medieval period, when doctors in Italy did start performing c-sections, first on dead women and then, in the 16th century, on living women.[74] The story about the origin of the cesarean section was made popular by woodcut illustrations in medieval manuscripts that showed the "birth of Julius Caesar"—a baby being pulled from the abdomen of his dead mother.[75] These woodcuts reflected what was going on in the 13th through 16th centuries, not what happened in ancient Rome.[76] In addition, there is no evidence that obstetrical forceps were ever used in ancient Rome.[77] The only forceps the ancient Romans had would have been used to extract pieces of the fetus in an embryotomy operation. The Romans did not use medical instruments to try to deliver living fetuses.

THE MEDICALIZATION OF BIRTH

Throughout the history of childbirth, the invention and addition of tools into the birth room has had mixed results. In antiquity, doctors came into birth rooms primarily when their surgical tools were needed. These surgical interventions brought consequences not just for the individual births at which they were used, but for childbirth on the whole. Introducing obstetrical tools medicalizes birth. It takes what is fundamentally a physiological process and makes it a medical event. When used judiciously, this medicalization has been good for some birthing people. The scalpels, claws, hooks, and speculums of the ancient Roman doctors probably saved some women. If a fetus was stuck in the birth canal, doctors could perform an embryotomy. They had a chance at rescuing a laboring woman even if her fetus was lost. Similarly, the obstetrical forceps, invented in the 17th century, the first vacuum extraction device, used in 1849, c-sections that reliably resulted in living mothers and babies starting in the mid-20th century, and the Doppler fetal monitor, invented in 1964, have all saved the lives of birthing people and babies.[78]

However, the biggest advances in childbirth safety did not come from these medicalized interventions, but advances in all areas of medical practice: adoption of antiseptic practices in response to germ theory, development of antibiotics, and widespread use of blood transfusions.[79] Prior to antisepsis, the use of invasive obstetrical tools added many risks to birth. Embryotomies performed in ancient Rome may not have had a high success rate. Even if women survived the operation, many probably died from infections afterward. After the adoption of antiseptic practices, many of the gains from these regimens were mistakenly attributed to the birth tools and not simply to the routine use of soap and other disinfectants. In tandem, medicalization combined with patriarchy, misogyny, and the proto-capitalist medical marketplace has historically been bad for many birthing people. The introduction of male doctors and tools into the birthing rooms of ancient women paved the way for more widespread and systematic takeovers of birth by male practitioners in later periods.[80] Respect for the expertise of midwives and of birthing people themselves was repeatedly lost in the process. At different points in obstetrical history, doctors have misused and overused their authority and their tools in ways that have hurt birthing people and babies. The forceps is a good example.

The invention of obstetrical forceps by the Chamberlen family in the 17th century provided something that had never been available before: the ability to consistently manage difficult births in a way that saved the mother and the child.[81] As the forceps became widely known in the 17th and 18th centuries, it allowed not only for the delivery of stuck and impacted fetuses, but for the quicker delivery of *any* fetus. Male doctors now had a way of precipitating any labor they thought was proceeding too slowly. Overuse and inexpert use of the forceps led to many negative and avoidable outcomes for birthing people and fetuses, including bruising, nerve damage, broken bones, and permanent impairment for the babies, and bruising, lacerations, long-term injury, and incontinence for birthing people. The overuse of forceps in the United States reached its peak in the mid-20th century, when the introduction of strong analgesics and sedatives such as Nisentil (nicknamed "Nice-n-still"), scopolamine, and Demerol—substances that induced "twilight sleep" in laboring people—impeded their ability to push their babies out on their own.[82]

A study published in 2023 shows that Canada (where I was living and working while writing this book) has abnormally high levels of injuries following operative vaginal delivery—the use of forceps or vacuum extraction to assist during the pushing stage—when compared with twenty-three other high-income countries.[83] One in four forceps deliveries and one in eight vacuum deliveries results in severe trauma to the birthing person, including tearing of the anal sphincter, pelvic prolapse, long-term pain, and sexual dysfunction. In Canada, up to 15 percent of births involve the use of forceps or vacuum. The study found that birthing people are not being adequately informed of the risks to themselves and their babies of operative vaginal deliveries. Some people attribute this high level of forceps and vacuum use in Canada to efforts to reduce the skyrocketing c-section rate. In the United States, the c-section rate is about 32 percent, and in Canada it is about 34 percent.[84] The World Health Organization recommends a c-section rate of between 10 and 15 percent.[85] But this explanation does not take into account the likeliest cause of the high use and high injury rate in forceps and vacuum deliveries: overuse of medical instruments. While continuous fetal monitoring has been shown to have no positive effect on birth outcomes relative to intermittent monitoring with a handheld Doppler, it is general practice in Canadian hospitals, by midwives and obstetricians alike, to strap birthing people into fetal monitoring belts that give constant updates on the fetal heart tones.[86] This continual stream of information can lead practitioners to intervene sooner with medical instruments when they see fluctuations in the fetal heart tones. The use of these instruments, in turn, can have lasting physical and emotional consequences for birthing people.

The urge to hurry along the birthing process is very old and very human. In the ancient Roman world, laboring women and birth attendants used herbs, amulets, spells, prayers, baths, movement, and manual interventions to accelerate a labor that they thought was proceeding too slowly. Since at least the 17th century, doctors have used forceps, vacuum extractors, cesarean operations, and now inductions and synthetic oxytocin (Pitocin or Syntocinon) to manipulate the speed of labor. But in many cases, the best thing that a birth practitioner can do is have patience. A midwife or doctor in the ancient world—just as today—needed to have experience with the many variations of normal, physiological birth. Any attempts to hasten along the delivery with manual interventions or the use of instruments would have been extremely dangerous for baby and birthing woman alike. Agrippina probably survived her breech birth because she was attended by midwives who had experience with breech birth. They would have known that footling breeches proceeded best with as little intervention as possible. In her birth story as I have imagined it, there is a doctor on the scene. He prepares his tools in the event that he will need to perform an embryotomy. But he does not jump in to hasten along or manage the birth. He defers to the expertise of the midwife. I do not know if this is what actually happened, but given the many risks associated with manual and instrumental interventions in the ancient world, it's likely that Agrippina had a low-intervention breech birth. Even the manual interventions that I have imagined the midwife performing—informed by descriptions in Soranus's *Gynecology*—would have been highly risky. Inserting oiled hands into the vagina and cervix could have introduced pathogens or caused physical damage that may have been deadly in the weeks following birth. The practitioner had to continually balance the risk of doing nothing to assist in a difficult labor with the risks of introducing further complications via manual or instrumental intervention.

DEATH IN CHILDBIRTH

What about the women who weren't as lucky as Agrippina? A 2nd-century-CE tombstone in the ancient Roman city of Salona (modern-day Solin, Croatia) memorializes Candida, an enslaved woman who died giving birth: "To the spirits of the departed. Candida, a well-deserving wife aged about thirty, who lived with me for about seven years. She was in agony for four days trying to give birth. She could not give birth and so she died. Her fellow slave Iustus erected this stone."[87]

Candida is remembered by her partner and fellow slave, Iustus, who explains that she died after nearly four days of excruciating labor. We do not know what the problem was; those attending to her may not have known either. But they knew that try as she could, the baby did not come, and finally, due to exhaustion, blood loss, injury, or infection, Candida and the baby both died. Another tombstone from the 1st or 2nd century in Tusculum (twenty-five kilometers southeast of Rome) commemorates Rhanis Sulpicia, a freedwoman who was formerly enslaved to a man named Trio. Rhanis was "snatched away because of childbirth" at age fifteen. The inscription on her tombstone laments, "This parental tomb holds two corpses in one body; now the single (pile of) ashes holds the remains of two people."[88] Like Candida, Rhanis died in the act of giving birth. Her baby died along with her. Rhanis's body became her fetus's tomb.

There are several memorials to Roman women who died in childbirth or shortly after.[89] They attest to the worst outcomes of difficult births. A tombstone from Salaria in Hispania (Roman Spain) commemorates Gemina, an enslaved woman who died in childbirth at age twenty-five.[90] Her husband, Gaius, was a coppersmith who was freed (formerly enslaved). It's possible that he was saving up money to purchase Gemina's freedom and instead spent it on her memorial after she died trying to give birth to their child. Gaius's grief fills the monument. He beseeches the gods of the underworld, "Take me away"; he begs Gemina from beyond the grave, "If you loved me, take me away!" Her death is devastating to him. Similarly, another woman in Salona was mourned by her parents, husband, children, and son-in-law when she died in childbirth at age forty. They write, "Pregnant, alas, she experienced a fatal labor and, exhausted, was not able to drive out from her womb the wretched fetus, which, destroyed, passed away not yet in the light."[91]

One rare monument gives more detail. On the island of Paros, in the Greek-speaking part of the empire, a gravestone honors the thirty-six-year-old Sokrateia, who died giving birth to her third child. Her husband, Parmenion, commissioned a poem that graphically dramatizes Sokrateia's last moments. Speaking from Sokrateia's point of view, the gravestone exclaims, "The unstoppable Fury of my newborn infant took me, bitter, from my happy life with a fatal hemorrhage. I did not bring the child into the light by my labor pains, but it lies hidden in my womb among the dead."[92] Sokrateia left behind her father, her husband, and two boys. Her tombstone laments that she lies dead "because of the third child." According to Sokrateia's loved ones, her baby was responsible for her death.

These monuments are heartbreaking and, for a historian, frustrating. Most of them omit specific details. As a collection, they give the impression that birth in the ancient world was inherently dangerous. Perhaps the mourners thought there was no need to give details because it made sense that the birth itself was the cause of death. But we should resist that assumption. The monuments do not give details because they are not medical documents. They are heartfelt but formulaic memorials. Just as on gravestones today, there were conventions about what kind of information was shared and how. Ancient gravestones generally illustrated the positive qualities of the deceased and emphasized her connections to her family members. It's likely that death in childbirth was seen as especially worthy of commemoration precisely because it was so rare.[93] It would have been a tragic event to lose a young mother, especially together with her infant. Lamenting that a young woman died giving birth was a way to honor her, just as a man might have been honored for dying in battle.

Another reason the Romans emphasized maternal death in childbirth may have been because they considered it a good omen if a man's mother died giving birth to him. Legends were told about Scipio Africanus and Manius Manilius, two heroes of the Roman wars with the North African city of Carthage in the 3rd and 2nd centuries BCE. Both of their mothers died giving birth to them, and both men went on to have illustrious military careers.[94] For the Greeks and the Romans, childbirth was imagined as a struggle between the woman and the fetus.[95] They thought that the fetus pushed and kicked its way out of the womb. It was believed that women generally had an easier time giving birth to male fetuses than female fetuses because their maleness made them stronger and more vigorous.[96] Sluggish female fetuses, they thought, would cause long labors and more difficulties for their mothers. If a male fetus was especially strong and vigorous—an indication of his future greatness—he might destroy his mother in the process of his birth.

For Agrippina, writing about her difficult breech birth served to showcase her strength and vigor.[97] It connected her to her grandfather, Marcus Vipsanius Agrippa, who himself had been born feet first. According to folk etymology, his name, "Agrippa," referred to this fact of his birth.[98] Agrippa means something like "born with difficulty." Marcus Agrippa was the trusted general and right-hand man of the emperor Augustus. In addition to sharing the feminized version of his name, Agrippina also drew a connection between the way that Agrippa was born and the way that she birthed her own son. Emphasizing her breech birth showed that she was strong enough to handle the birth of a strong and vigorous son.

This is not to say that there weren't real risks to giving birth in ancient Rome. Maternal mortality was certainly higher in ancient Rome than in developed countries today. We do not have data to know exactly how high, but one scholarly estimate puts the number at somewhere between 5 and 20 maternal deaths per 1,000 live births.[99] For comparison, according to the World Health Organization, in the United States in 2020, .021 birthing people died for every 1,000 live births; in some countries today, the number is as high as 1 per 1,000 live births.[100] Functionally, this means that most women in ancient Rome knew someone, or knew someone who knew someone, who had died in childbirth. Based on data from other preindustrial societies, it's possible that an ancient community of 1,000 people would see one woman die in childbirth approximately every three years.[101] Historian Anna Bonnell Freidin has written about the "ripple effect of grief" that would have been felt from such a death—the impact on the woman's family members and community and the way the news of her death would have traveled through letters and word of mouth.[102]

Elite Roman men wrote with deep sadness about their wives, daughters, and sisters who died in childbirth or in the critical days and weeks afterward. In 54 BCE, Julia, the daughter of Julius Caesar and wife of his friend and then rival Pompey, died giving birth to her and Pompey's child. The baby also died. Caesar and Pompey—the two most powerful men in Rome—grieved the loss of mother and baby. Historians see this moment as a turning point in the dissolution of the two men's relationship and the subsequent civil war that tore Rome apart.[103]

There was also certainly fear surrounding birth, felt by the pregnant woman as well as her friends and family. Birth was a transition— from inside to out, from watery womb-home to dry world-home—that rocked mother and fetus in a moment of limbo between life and death.[104] In a letter from the 2nd century CE, a new grandmother wrote to her daughter, expressing her joy at receiving the birth announcement. She had been praying daily and she was glad to hear that her daughter had "escaped" from the labor.[105]

Freidin has written persuasively about how people in ancient Rome would have perceived the risk of dying in childbirth as being "*in addition*" to an overall high mortality regime.[106] That is, on the whole, people in ancient Rome were dying at much higher rates of more things than they are today. Tuberculosis, for one, was probably a big killer of women of childbearing age, as it was for people generally.[107] Malaria was another. And pregnant women would have been seen, by themselves and their communities, as taking on an additional risk to their lives going into birth.

We should not, however, let these fears and perceptions of risk—or even the fact of higher maternal mortality—determine entirely the way that we understand and describe birth in ancient Rome. While there is certainly evidence of fear and a sense of risk, it's also very hard for us to look back objectively from our modern perspective. Societal shifts in the 20th century contributed significantly to how we view birth and our tolerance of risk around it. For instance, Jacquline Wolf has shown how throughout the 20th century, the idea developed that birth should be made as safe as possible for babies.[108] Obstetrical practices changed to accommodate this goal, such as favoring cesarean sections over vaginal delivery for breech births. But these changes have, in many instances, led to more risks for birthing people.[109] It's very hard, especially from the vantage point of the modern United States, to imagine a world in which everything would have been done to protect and save a laboring woman, even at the expense of a fetus.

We are also quicker to identify risk factors that *could* lead to the death of the birthing person. A common refrain you will hear from people who have had a c-section today is that one hundred or two hundred years ago—before c-sections became relatively safe—they would have died giving birth. But this perception of danger and risk is false. As we have already seen, the c-section rate in the modern United States is about 32 percent. Conversely, even the highest estimates for the ancient world only put maternal mortality at 20 out of 1,000, or 2 percent. And even if we assume that a c-section would have helped in every case of difficult birth throughout history, recall that in the pre-modern world, the rate of difficult birth was 5 to 6 percent. [110]

So where is the disconnect? The reality is that we have many more ways of monitoring and intervening in birth—and doing so earlier—than they did in ancient Rome. We are much less risk tolerant and have much more faith in medical interventions and surgical births. As we have seen, this is not entirely a bad thing. I'm sure the birthing women who died or whose babies died in ancient Rome would have loved to have had the option of a (modern) c-section. But this misperception about what c-section does—the idea that it always saves birthing people from death—does impact the way that we understand the dangers and risks of birth in ancient Rome. Why the c-section rate is so high today is a matter of contentious debate, but in broad strokes, it can be attributed both to the dramatically increased safety of the procedure in the 20th century and to changing perceptions of the risks posed by surgical versus vaginal birth. That is, people today often *believe*—and are often led to this belief by medical professionals—that c-section is as safe as, if not safer than, vaginal birth—for the birthing person, the baby, or both—regardless of evidence to the contrary.[111]

As for ancient Rome, memorials to women who died in childbirth and accounts of maternal death in ancient literature, combined with our skewed understanding of birth risk today, have made it seem like birth back then was a terrifying, death-dealing experience. But like Agrippina, the vast majority of women giving birth in ancient Rome—even those who had difficult births—survived. Scholarly focus on maternal mortality has obscured the other important aspects of birth in ancient Rome—birth as transition, transformation, and source of power and community for birthing women. Even if birth was scary in ancient Rome, we have to imagine that for many women, conquering that fear and coming safely through birth would have been an extraordinary experience.

. . .

As we turn to the final stage of our birth story, we will look at the first few days and weeks after birth. We will see how women of different economic and social positions managed the care of themselves and their newborns. Mothers, midwives, and wet nurses came under the scrutiny of Roman men—doctors and laymen alike—who saw these women as potentially corrupting influences on vulnerable new infants. The reality, though, was that in a society blighted by high rates of infant disease and death, these early caretakers provided the best chance of infant survival.

ELEVEN

After Birth

PERPETUA NURSES HER SON

In 203 CE, in a prison cell in Carthage (modern-day Tunisia in North Africa), twenty-two-year-old Perpetua nursed her infant son.[1] A recent convert to Christianity, she had been arrested along with several of her fellow catechumens and was being held captive. Her offense was failure to make ritual sacrifices on behalf of the emperors, Septimius Severus and his son Caracalla. When she was brought before the prefect of the province and asked to recant her Christian beliefs, she refused. Her father, who was not a Christian, brought her infant son to the trial and begged her to think of the boy. He lamented that the child would not be able to live on after the death of his mother. Unmoved, Perpetua was eventually thrown to the wild beasts in the Carthage arena and ultimately killed by a gladiator.

Perpetua's story is presented as a rare firsthand account from an early-3rd-century Roman woman, though it may actually have been composed by someone else a few centuries later.[2] It imagines the experiences and emotions of a nursing mother about to face death in the Roman arena. Perpetua describes breastfeeding while in prison. When she is first arrested, her son is not with her. Her mother and brother bring the baby to her regularly so that she can nurse him. At one point she goes some time without access to her son, and she laments the physical discomfort of her engorged breasts and the lethargy of her hungry infant. After a while, the guards allow her to have the baby with her in the prison. She rejoices at this turn of events, enthusing that this reunion has turned the prison cell into a governor's mansion for her.

We are meant to understand that it is no easy feat for Perpetua to reject her infant son at her trial. But God has a uniquely maternal miracle in store for her. After Perpetua affirms her Christianity and ensures her all but certain death, her infant marvelously no longer needs her breast milk. We don't know how old the boy is, but it seems that this is an unusual development, suggesting that he is under a year. And perhaps even more miraculously, Perpetua herself experiences no consequences from the sudden cessation in nursing. As she tells it, there is no pain or engorgement. Perpetua goes to her martyrdom assured that her infant son will face no consequences from missing his mother's milk. Her own miraculous lactation cessation is her sign from God that she is on the righteous path.[3]

AFTER BIRTH

In ancient Rome, the period following the birth was as critical if not more so than the birth itself. There was the delivery of the placenta, recovery from labor, management of the lochia and breast milk, and the care and feeding of the new infant. When women died from childbirth it was often in this period, when any difficulties or anomalies with the birth or mismanagement of the afterbirth could lead to hemorrhage or childbed fever.[4]

The message conveyed by the medical texts—the main source for the postpartum period—is that the days following the birth required specific and attentive care. Every action was consequential. The reality, though, was that only the wealthiest women could have afforded the care that was advised. And if something went wrong, the child's earliest caretakers—mother, midwife, and wet nurse—were blamed. The mother's supposed threat to the newborn lay, as it did during pregnancy, in the corrupting influences of her body. At the same time, she could also harm her infant by withholding her care, if she, say, hired a wet nurse. The midwife and wet nurse were blamed if they botched some aspect of the postpartum and newborn care—the cutting of the umbilical cord, the extraction of the placenta, and the feeding of the infant. Wet nurses were enslaved, formerly enslaved, or poor free women. In a society with high infant mortality, culpability for infant morbidity or death was placed on the most vulnerable women.

• • •

On October 15, 64 CE, in Roman Egypt, a woman named Thaubas wrote a letter to her father, Pompeios, conveying the sad news of her sister's death following childbirth. She wrote,

> Please come home as soon as you receive my letter, because your poor daughter Herennia has died. And she already came safely through a premature delivery on the ninth of Phaophi. You see, she gave birth to an eight-month child, dead; she lived on for four days but then died herself.[5]

Herennia's difficulties, Thaubas indicates, stemmed from her "eight-month child," whom she delivered stillborn. Recall that children born in the eighth month of gestation were thought to die and, often, to take their mothers with them. Perhaps Herennia's delivery involved manual or instrumental intervention and infection had set in. Or maybe she had retained some part of the placenta.

The birth of the placenta was a great concern in the ancient medical texts. In most cases, the placenta emerged on its own. If it did not, it could be removed manually or through the action of amulets and herbs. If the cervix was still open and the placenta had detached from the uterine wall, then the practitioner was supposed to reach a hand, anointed with olive oil, up into the uterus and pull it out.[6] If the placenta was still attached to the uterine wall, then they had to try to gently detach it, wiggling it from side to side before pulling it out. In these situations, especially the former, the prognosis was good, provided the practitioner could get all the pieces out.

Some practitioners, perhaps recognizing the risks associated with manual intervention, approached the issue obliquely: Hippocratic doctors apparently recommended holding the nose shut while sneezing to propel the placenta out through redirected force.[7] Others laid the newborn infant, still attached to the umbilical cord, between or below the mother's thighs and allowed the movements of the baby to tug it out.[8] The same "quick-birth" (*okytokion*) amulets that were tied around the laboring woman's thigh in order to speed up labor could also be used to draw out the placenta. Of course, as we saw in chapter 9, they needed to be removed at the right time so that they didn't pull the uterus out too.

In terms of herbal preparations, the midwife might have used unguent of marjoram.[9] This infusion was prepared by macerating in olive oil a mixture of marjoram, tufted thyme, cassia, wormwood, bergamot mint flowers, and myrtle leaves. The midwife manually applied this pungent, astringent oil to the cervix to draw down the placenta. Unguent of wormwood, another compound preparation, worked similarly.[10] Some of the most efficacious herbs were rare and costly, such as Mecca balsam, which only grew in a certain part of Judea.[11] Only a few gallons of its sap were harvested every year and sold for twice their weight in silver. The sap had many medicinal uses, including several gynecological and obstetrical ones. At a birth it could be used in a fumigation or sitz bath to dilate the cervix. After the birth it could be rubbed on the vagina or cervix to draw down the placenta.

If the cervix was already closed, the situation was trickier. Practitioners would inject oil douches into the vagina and try to manually dilate the cervix. If this did not work, they would need to use herbal sitz baths and vaginal fumigations—of pine bark, labdanum, the operculum (lid) of the murex sea snail, garlic leaves, or wormwood—to try to open the cervix before attempting manual extraction.[12] Drinks made with beaver testicles and pennyroyal, horehound, or dropwort might help as well.[13] Anxiety must certainly have been high for patients with retained placenta. Putrefaction set in quickly and without remedy, spelled certain death. A 5th-to-6th-century medical text attests to the unpleasant olfactory aspect of the experience: "The stench (of the retained placenta) fills and benumbs the head and upsets the stomach." The writer advises pumping strong fragrances into the room to counteract the stench: cardamon, frankincense, storax, aromatic onyx, and labdanum.[14]

Physicians advised gentle and attentive care for the postpartum woman. She was to rest on a soft bed in a dark room.[15] Her lochial flow could be caught with a soft sponge, a tuft of wool, or a piece of cloth, which was to be changed frequently. A diaper of clean wool was wrapped from her belly button in front up to the top of her buttocks in the back. In the first few days, her genitals were regularly treated with warmed olive oil and wine. As of the third day postpartum, she would take sitz baths in warm water or olive oil and apply herbal poultices to her vulva and perineum. The postpartum diet was mild: bread soaked in warm water, vegetable porridge, soft-boiled eggs.

This sort of care would likely have had good results. A clean wool diaper with a frequently-changed insert of sponge, cloth, or wool would have been antimicrobial; warmed olive oil and wine would have had a soothing and potentially antiseptic effect on lacerations; and sitz baths and poultices would have helped with the healing of bruised tissue and the reduction of hemorrhoids.

But as historian Misa Nguyen has pointed out, the medical prescriptions for postpartum care were focused only on the first few days after delivery and were, on the whole, interested in rehabilitating the woman's body for future reproduction.[16] They did not acknowledge the extent of what we now call the fourth trimester, and there is no mention of an extended confinement or recuperation period.

Furthermore, what women did or were supposed to be doing in the post-birth period was almost certainly determined by their social status. Wealthy free women had the assistance of slaves for their own care as well as the care and feeding of the infant. Enslaved women, conversely, were likely to have had even more work to do after giving birth. In addition to caring for their own infants, they were often compelled to act as wet nurses to other children born in the household. Certainly they would not have been afforded the same opportunities for rest and recovery as their enslavers. These social inequities accreted around cultural ideas about who could handle what in the postpartum period. Elite Roman men circulated the idea that elite Roman women spent too long resting in the postpartum period in contrast to foreign women, who gave birth quickly with little need for recuperation. One writer explained that women in Illyria (in the Roman province of Dalmatia) are pregnant often, give birth easily, and return to work promptly. "You would think," he quips, "they have not given birth to a child but found one!"[17]

This is an early expression of the racist idea of the noble savage that emerged in European ethnographies of Africa and the Americas starting in the 16th century. Generally speaking, the trope referred to the innate goodness and morality of indigenous people—those who were uncorrupted by "civilizing" influences. For women, it was used to characterize their reproductive practices. It goes like this: White women of European descent are weak and soft; they give birth with difficulty and need lots of (enslaved or hired) help in the postpartum period; they are prone to hysteria or attacks of the nerves. In contrast, native women and Black women are strong and hardy; they give birth easily and can get back to work right away; they don't need any help in the postpartum period and in fact have the reserves of strength to aid in the care of white women's children; they are not prone to hysteria.[18] Such assumptions created a physiological justification for the exploitation of native and Black women's reproductive labor and care work, first as slaves and then as hired laborers. It's not clear if and how the Romans exploited these tropes, but the framework is there. It could have been a way to denigrate elite Roman women and at the same time justify the exploitation of enslaved women who had been displaced from the edges of the empire to the city center of Rome.

FIRST BATH

Along with the birth of the placenta and the onset of the lochia, there was the immediate need to tend to the infant. The main sources for infant care were the writings of Soranus and later physicians who adopted, adapted, and translated his recommendations.[19] Consequently, the recommendations were geared toward upper-class families. These texts advised a number of dubious practices. It's not clear if people actually did the things that were recommended, but if they did, Roman infants would have been at significant risk for malnourishment, illness, and death.[20] First there was the newborn bath. According to Soranus, shortly after the birth, the midwife should rub the baby with ground salt and soda ash and rinse it off in a lukewarm bath.[21] Today, caretakers are discouraged from bathing an infant too soon after birth because it can dangerously lower the baby's body temperature, cause stress reactions, and deprive the infant of its protective coating of waxy vernix. Ground salt and soda ash, while having antiseptic cleaning properties, would have been quite caustic on delicate newborn skin.[22] Following the bath, the midwife was to dilate the infant's nostrils, mouth, and anus with her finger and pour olive oil into its eyes. The belief was that olive oil would clear out the eyes and prevent dim-sightedness later on.

SHAPING BODIES, SHAPING SEX

First the midwife and then the wet nurse were responsible for tending to the umbilical cord and swaddling and massaging the infant. In these tasks the stakes were high and any misstep could have severe consequences. As we have seen, the midwife was responsible for cutting the umbilical cord. The medical texts cautioned that if she cut it too soon or with the wrong implement, the mother could hemorrhage or the placenta could get sucked up into the body and putrefy. If she cut it too close to the belly, the infant could die. The midwife bound the cord stump with wool and covered it with linen soaked in olive oil.[23] She was supposed to press the stump gently into the baby's abdomen in order to promote a pleasingly concave shape for the belly button.

The midwife made a diaper from a clean wool cloth; then she wrapped the infant in wool or linen cloths, first swaddling individual limbs and then the entire body.[24] The use of wool, especially clean wool, would have mitigated somewhat the risks presented by bathing and sprinkling with salts. Wool—particularly wool that still has its lanolin—has naturally antimicrobial, moisture-wicking, and temperature-regulating properties.

But the swaddling wasn't just meant to keep the infant warm and soothed. It was supposed to mold the body of the infant into the ideal form, even shaping its sex/gender. Soranus advised the midwife to swaddle the bodies of male infants with consistent pressure all the way down, but for female infants to bind the chest tightly and the hips loosely, since "this form is more attractive in women."[25] If the midwife or wet nurse did not swaddle the infant properly, she could "cause to the limbs to become deformed."[26]

Massage, too, was important for molding the infant's body and its sex/gender.[27] Soranus explained that the first massage squeezed out any viscous and damaging material that was left in the infant's body from being in its mother's womb.[28] The midwife was supposed to press into the sides of the baby's buttocks, hollowing them out "for the sake of attractiveness." He instructed the midwife to pay special attention to the foreskin of male infants. The Greeks and Romans considered a long foreskin to be most attractive. The midwife could encourage this shape by drawing the foreskin down over the tip of the penis and even tying it there with a strand of wool.[29] Consistent drawing and stretching, it was thought, would cause the foreskin to take on a shape that would be most attractive in adulthood. For the Romans, the physical manifestation of sex/gender—especially masculinity—was something that needed molding from a young age. And this masculinity was easily endangered. Soranus wrote that the wet nurse had to be careful about how she carried baby boys around. If she lifted them up onto her shoulder and moved them around, she could bruise their testicles, causing them to retract or dissolve, leaving the boys with undescended testicles or even making them into eunuchs.[30]

FEEDING THE NEWBORN

Then there was the matter of feeding the infant. Opinions seem to have been strong and divided. A 1st- or 2nd-century-BCE physician, Damastes, advised bringing the baby to the breast immediately after birth.[31] He reasoned that nature put milk in the breasts of the birthing woman even before delivery so that the infant could eat right away. In the 2nd century CE his views were adopted by the physician Galen, who argued that "nature not only has prepared such nourishment [breast milk] for infants, but also provided them, right from the start, with innate capacities for the use of [it]."[32] He explained that if the nipple was placed in a newborn's mouth, the infant began suckling immediately and eagerly.

On the opposite side of the debate was Soranus, who advised waiting up to three days after birth to give the baby its first food.[33] This food, he said, should *not* be the milk of its mother. He cautioned that the thick yellow colostrum—what we now know to be the first nutrient-dense, antibacterial, and antimicrobial substance produced by the breasts—was unrefined and putrid milk, spoiled by the exertion and disturbance of the birth.[34] Instead, he advised that the newborn be fed warmed hydromel (honey water), which he thought was good for purging the stomach and bowels, followed by the milk of a wet nurse. If a wet nurse could not be found, then even honey mixed with goat's milk was preferable to the colostrum. The mother could nurse her own infant, but she had to wait for her actual milk to come in.

How many postpartum women were following the advice of Galen, Soranus, or, more likely, their midwives? What were those midwives actually saying? We don't know.[35] But within two centuries, Soranus's view had decidedly won out, at least in the medical writing. In the 4th century CE, the physician Oribasius recommended honey as the first food, followed by hydromel.[36] The mother was not to breastfeed the infant herself until at least the fourth day after birth. In 5th- or 6th-century-CE Roman Africa, the physician Muscio cautioned that the first milk (colostrum) was "not life-supporting," but "unwholesome, thick, and indigestible."[37]

The infant subjected to this feeding regimen would have faced a number of risks. Being given honey within its first year of life would have put it at slight risk for infant botulism and death. But more concerning was the danger posed by contaminated water.[38] There's a good chance that the water used to make the infant's hydromel would have contained bacteria from human or animal waste, particularly in urban centers like the city of Rome.[39] As historian and religious scholar Susan Holman has pointed out, what might have been a source of sickness—diarrhea, fever, dehydration, and electrolyte imbalance—for an older child or adult would have been fatal to a young infant.[40]

Delaying the first milk would have deprived the infant of an important source of early nutriment as well as the immune-boosting, antimicrobial protection of the colostrum. It also would have seriously compromised the mother's milk supply. After four days without breastfeeding, employing a wet nurse would have been almost inevitable. The birthing mother's body would have received the message that milk production wasn't necessary, decreasing or eliminating her supply.

All of these practices—bathing and cleaning the newborn, manually evacuating its orifices, and delaying milk—were aimed at the same thing: neutralizing the corrupting influences of the mother's body. The medical model of prenatal and postpartum care in ancient Rome was above all concerned with mitigating the risks posed to the fetus by its mother.[41] According to this model, those risks reached their peak at the moment of the birth, which was imagined as a violent struggle between the woman and child. After the child was successfully delivered, it could finally be rescued from the dangers of the womb. All of the first fluids and excretions of the newborn body—vernix, meconium, mucous—were seen as corrupt and harmful residues from the uterus. What was needed, then, was a significant break from the mother's body. Purged of its birth fluids through fingers, water, salt, soda ash, olive oil, and honey, and protected from the thick, corrupted first milk (colostrum) from its mother's breast, the baby was thought to have the best chance to survive and thrive. But the exact opposite was true. And so, this misogynistic belief—that the greatest threat to newborn life came from the residual fluids of the womb—led to a regimen that would have put the infant at grave risk of malnourishment, illness, and death.

The experience that Perpetua described in breastfeeding her son suggests that she followed different advice than the sort offered by Soranus or Muscio. The baby seems to have been relying on her for its sustenance and well-being. Perpetua's father lamented that the baby "will not be able to keep living after you die" and she described experiencing painful engorgement when she was separated from and not able to nurse him.[42] She seems to have had a robust and healthy milk supply. Perhaps, contrary to the prevailing medical advice, a midwife or her mother had advised her to put the baby to her breast early and often.

Outside of the medical texts, there was a strong "(mother's) breast is best" sentiment among Roman male elites, though unsurprisingly, these men were silent on how to support and facilitate maternal breastfeeding. Of course, Soranus's advice would have been expensive; the only alternatives to maternal breastfeeding were wet nursing or animal milk. Everyone seems to have agreed that animal milk—especially goat's milk—would work in a pinch, but was far inferior to human milk. So apart from the wealthiest Romans and from enslaved people, who often did not have control over their infants' feeding regimens, it's likely that the majority of Roman women actually did breastfeed their own children.[43] And they likely did so soon after birth. Absent bizarre medical advice, the combination of a crying infant and full, leaking breasts would have had one obvious solution.

NURSING AND WET NURSING

Sometime in the mid-2nd century CE (around the time that Cyrilla was fainting in the bath and a little after Petronilla was petitioning the magistrate) in the city of Rome, the wife of an elite man gave birth to a baby boy.[44] Her husband was part of the high-ranking senatorial class. He routinely hung around a Greek philosopher named Favorinus, who had attracted a large following of wealthy and politically influential Roman men. These men would spend their leisure time—of which they had much—eating, drinking, socializing, and debating philosophical ideas. One of the men, Aulus Gellius, wrote down some of Favorinus's ideas. When news came to the group of the birth of their friend's baby, Favorinus thought they should visit the new father. Aulus Gellius recorded the interaction, providing a rare glimpse inside the house of a newly postpartum woman.

When they arrived, the friends congratulated the happy new father. The birthing woman's mother was there and Favorinus asked her about the delivery: How long was the labor? How difficult? The group learned that the new mother was sleeping, tired out from the exertion and sleeplessness of birth. Favorinus exclaimed, "I have no doubt she will nurse the baby herself!" No, the grandmother countered, she would spare her daughter the "wearisome and difficult task of breastfeeding" after the "pains she has suffered in childbirth." Seizing the opening, Favorinus launched into a diatribe, at first against the grandmother and then, more broadly, against all Roman mothers who did not breastfeed their own children.

Favorinus argued that a woman who employed a wet nurse for her child participated in an "unnatural, imperfect, and half-motherhood." His concerns were twofold. The first was that women who did not nurse their own children compromised their maternal affection; their role was usurped by the nurse, generally a woman of inferior class.[45] The second and more dire concern involved the belief that breast milk conveyed elements of character directly from the breastfeeding woman's soul to the newborn infant. So, ignoble breast milk, as from an enslaved woman, would nurture ignobility in the child. Physiologically speaking, breast milk was understood to be a more concentrated or "cooked" form of menstrual blood, diverted after birth from the uterus to the breasts.[46] Just as the menstrual blood built up the body and soul of the fetus in utero, the breast milk built up the body and soul of the infant.[47]

His speech hit on some of the same misogynistic themes as the anti-abortion screeds we saw in chapter 5: Favorinus claimed that elite Roman women refused to nurse their babies because it "mars their beauty."[48] Such women, he scoffed, view their nipples as "beauty marks" meant not to feed their children but to adorn their breasts. We don't get to hear the grandmother's reply.

Other male writers praised elite Roman women who breastfed their own children. It was one of the prime characteristics of a good mother.[49] A typical description read: "She [the good mother] did not hand him over to wet nurses or attendants. She fed him with her own breasts, warmed him in her own embrace."[50] In another precursor to the noble savage trope, the late 1st- to early 2nd-century historian Tacitus contrasted negligent Roman mothers who handed their children over to enslaved Greek wet nurses with virtuous German women who breastfed their own children.[51]

It's difficult to know just how widespread a phenomenon these elite Roman men were lashing out against. As we've seen, medical opinion in the 2nd century was divided about whether and when a mother should breastfeed her own infant or use a wet nurse. Soranus's assumption was that his clientele, members of the upper crust of Roman society, were using wet nurses for their children. The opinion of the grandmother in the Favorinus episode corroborates this picture. In addition to allowing time for recovery, the use of a wet nurse also enabled the birthing woman to get pregnant again more quickly.[52] The medical writers recognized the link between lactation and infertility.[53] As long as a woman was lactating, they thought, the menstrual fluid was being diverted and converted into breast milk, leaving no excess nutriment for the conception and gestation of another child. Much of the postpartum advice of the medical writers concerned the intentional drying-up of the mother's milk with plasters of herbs and tight breast binding.[54] Despite the moralizing discourse from the elite male writers, it's likely that many if not most upper-class men supported and promoted the use of wet nurses. It may also be that there was tension between the birthing woman's family and her husband in this regard. In a 3rd-century-CE letter from Roman Egypt, a couple wrote to their son-in-law, chastising him for forcing their daughter to nurse her newborn baby.[55] They instructed him to hire a wet nurse.

Wet nursing was certainly necessary if the mother died. Perpetua's father was not being hyperbolic when he exclaimed that her child would not live after she died. Aside from wet nursing, the feeding methods available to a motherless infant were risky.[56] The Romans had breast pumps and feeding bottles (see fig. 19), and there may even have been a location for the sale of pumped milk in one of the public markets in Rome.[57] Goat or donkey milk could be substituted for human milk in

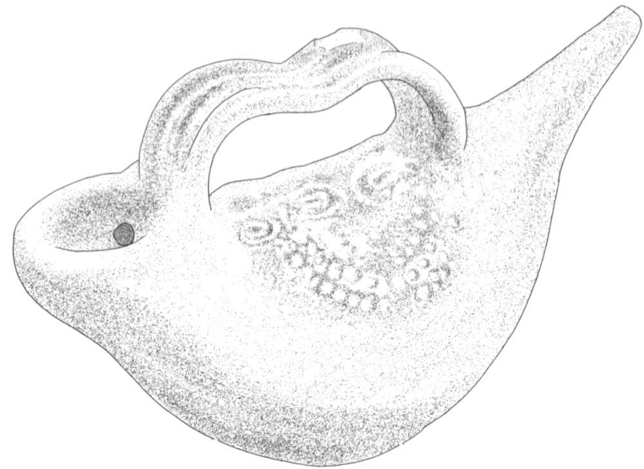

FIGURE 19. Roman pottery feeding bottle. A leather nipple may have been attached to the spout. Bottles like this could have been used to feed pumped breast milk, animal milk, or hydromel to infants and toddlers. Likely 1st century CE. Science Museum Group, Sir Henry Wellcome's Museum Collection A67762. Drawing by Hayley Monroe.

the bottles. Certainly, an infant who was not able to form a latch on the breast due to a cleft palate or other disability would have had to be fed in this way. But lack of refrigeration, along with inadequate cleaning practices, would have significantly compromised any milk delivered in a bottle. In these conditions, from the breast was almost certainly best.

It is likely that this care work often stayed in the family, with a sister, grandmother, or even a friend or neighbor taking on the breastfeeding of the motherless infant.[58] A tombstone inscription from Raetinium (the modern city of Bihác in Bosnia and Herzegovina) honors a sixty-two-year-old woman who is remembered as both the aunt and wet nurse of a man named Caius Julius Certus.[59] But when there was no family member to do the job, someone else was needed.

Like midwifery, wet nursing was a job performed by free, enslaved, and formerly enslaved women alike.[60] But much more so than midwifery, it put the workers in an intimate and protracted relationship with complex power dynamics.[61] In wealthy families with lots of slaves, wet nurses were typically women who were already part of the household. Having recently given birth themselves, they would have been responsible for breastfeeding their enslavers' children as well as other enslaved children born into the home.[62] Wealthy households without a suitable wet nurse on hand would have purchased a lactating slave or hired one from a neighbor. Other times a free or formally enslaved woman would hire herself out as a wet nurse for wages.

There is a tension in the historical record regarding wet nurses in ancient Rome. On the one hand, there are many loving funerary inscriptions and even beautiful artistic reliefs honoring wet nurses, tributes made by enslavers, patrons, former nurslings, and even the nurses themselves.[63] Wet nurses also set up gravestones for their nurslings, attesting to an affectionate and, at times, long relationship. In the late 2nd century CE in the city of Rome, a man named Marcus Aurelius Fortunatianus (his name tells us that he was likely a former slave of the emperor Marcus Aurelius) set up a grave monument for his family, including his wet nurse, an enslaved woman named Cyrene.[64]

Around the same time, in the city of Colonia (modern Cologne, Germany), somebody with a lot of money built a large grave monument depicting an enslaved wet nurse named Severina (see fig. 20).[65] We don't know who the dedicator or dedicatee were because the main part of the monument is missing. All that remains is a decorative altar on the top, about two and a half feet tall. The front contains a small portrait of a woman along with a scene of a shepherd tending to a flock of sheep. On the right and left sides of the structure, Severina is shown performing her duties: sitting in a high-backed wicker chair nursing an infant and laying a swaddled infant in a cradle. Above each scene is the inscription "Severina Nutrix," Severina the Wet Nurse. It could be a tombstone for Severina or her charge. Either way, it displays a deep bond between wet nurse and nursling.

Some wet nurses could reap great rewards for their labor. Pliny the Younger, the husband of the miscarrying Calpurnia from chapter 6, gifted his former wet nurse a farm when he became an adult.[66] And the

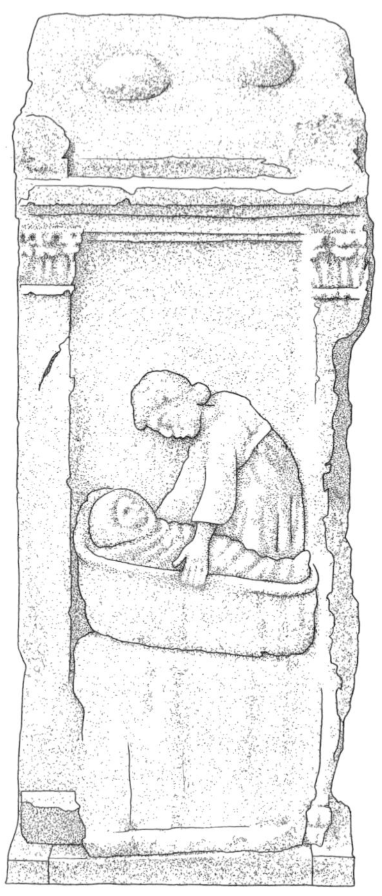
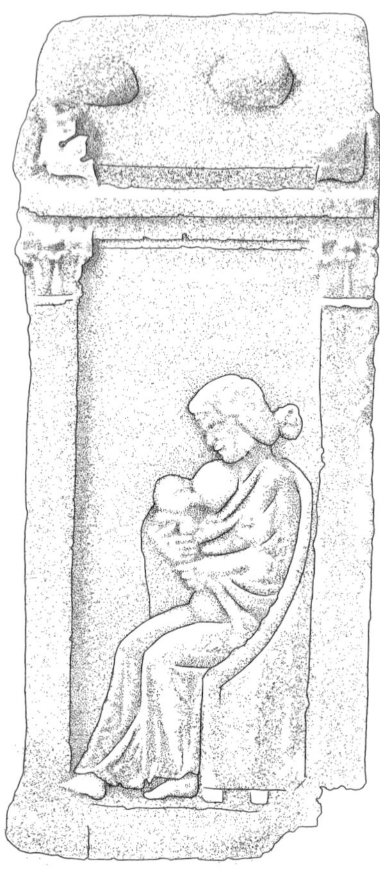

FIGURE 20. Tombstone depicting the wet nurse Severina tending to a swaddled infant in a cradle and breastfeeding the infant while sitting in a high-backed chair. 3rd century CE. Romano-German Museum, Cologne, Germany. Drawing by Hayley Monroe.

Roman legal texts recorded that an enslaved wet nurse could receive early manumission from her nursling. Generally, slaves could not be manumitted until they were thirty years old, and the enslavers who manumitted them had to be at least twenty. Exceptions to this rule included wet nurses and tutors, who by virtue of the great affection for them shown by their nurslings, could be manumitted early.[67]

On the other hand, in contrast to this façade of mutual affection, wet nursing was often a labor of necessity or compulsion that severely limited the wet nurse's own choices concerning her body, her life, and her family-building.[68] In Roman Egypt, the hiring of a wet nurse was a formal arrangement, initiated with a contract that detailed the extent and terms of service. Nearly fifty of these contracts or their receipts survive on papyri, ranging in date from the 1st century BCE to the 4th century CE.[69] These documents, of course, provide only a limited view into one small part of the vast Roman Empire, but they allow us to see some of the social and economic realities of the practice.[70]

The typical scenario in these contracts is that a freeborn wet nurse has been hired to care for an infant that has been abandoned.[71] When the birth parents were unable to care for their infants, for whatever reason, they left the babies on urban trash heaps.[72] The babies were picked up by other people, who then hired wet nurses. These wet nurses cared for the babies in their own homes until they were weaned, sometimes for up to two years. The infants returned to their adoptive families as slaves.

In a contract from 71 CE in the city of Alexandria, a man named Lucius Vetranius Philostratos agreed to pay a woman named Dionysia a monthly wage to care for and breastfeed in her own home a baby boy that he (or, more likely, someone enslaved by him) found on a trash heap.[73] At the end of the contract period, the boy would return to Lucius's household as a slave. If either Lucius or Dionysia violated the terms of the contract or terminated it early, they would owe a penalty to the other.

Sometimes the nurse that was hired was enslaved herself. In this case, her pay went to her enslaver. According to a receipt for wages paid on October 13, 187 CE, an enslaved wet nurse named Sarapias finished two years of breastfeeding and caring for a young girl named Helene.[74] Sarapias's work generated four hundred drachmas in revenue, all of which was paid to Sarapias's enslaver, Chosion. Although she is named as the nurse in the receipt, Sarapias had no monetary stake in the transaction. Because she was enslaved, all of her labor and its revenue belonged to her enslaver.

Evidence from later periods shows that the work of wet nursing often came at the expense of feeding and caring for one's own infant.[75] It was likely no different in the Roman world. In order to be a wet nurse, a woman had to have given birth to her own child. But would she have had enough time, energy, and milk to feed her own babies in addition to her nurslings? While some wet nurses, like those in the contracts from Roman Egypt, were working for pay and, to some extent, on terms they had agreed on, many others were enslaved women who were compelled to do this work for children in the enslaver's household.

In five wet nursing contracts from Alexandria, the terms of employment stipulate that the wet nurse breastfeed no infants other than the one entrusted to her care.[76] This stipulation came along with others that were meant to ensure the best chance of survival to the nursling: not "spoiling" her milk, not having sex with a man, and not becoming pregnant during the term of her employment.[77] But what did these restrictions mean for the nurse's own child? Four of these contracts involved enslavers hiring out enslaved women for wages that went directly to the enslavers. Even with the income from these arrangements, the enslavers probably wouldn't have wanted to compromise the care of the wet nurses' own children (the enslavers' property). In these cases, the enslaved women's children may have died or reached the age of weaning. But we can also imagine the case of a sickly infant whose care the enslaved woman was forced to abandon in order to take on the wet-nursing labor imposed on her by her enslaver. The brutal economic calculations of a slaver would have left little room for autonomous family-building among his or her slaves.

We can also imagine the economic pressures on free women to wean their own children early if it afforded them the opportunity to take on paid wet-nursing work. It may have looked like a good economic decision to start feeding one's own infant goat's milk in order to provide breast milk to a paying customer. But such a trade-off could have had drastic consequences for the infant weaned early.[78] In a world riddled with disease, long before the invention of formula, breast milk afforded children the best chance at survival for the first two years of their life. However, to look at it another way, historian Anna Sparreboom has suggested that the extended period of nursing provided by a wet-nursing job might have been welcome to some women as a means of spacing out their own pregnancies.[79] This is an intriguing idea for potential agency in a coercive situation.

There are a few instances of harmonious relationships between "milk-siblings"—children nursed by the same woman but not otherwise related.[80] In an inscription from Pisaurum on the northeastern coast of Italy, a soldier named Gaius Tadius Sabinus set up a tombstone for his wet nurse, Maria Marcellina, and his co-nursling or "milk-brother," Caedus Rufinus.[81] Such cases suggest that sometimes there was enough to go around, though these were probably the exception rather than the rule.

Like his enumeration of the qualities that made the best midwife, Soranus also formalized the profile of the best wet nurse.[82] As in the contracts from Roman Egypt, this best wet nurse was supposed to remain sober, abstain from sexual intercourse, avoid becoming pregnant, and stick to a particular dietary regimen to avoid "spoiling" her milk. He gave a detailed account of the size and quality of the best breasts for nursing: firm but not too firm, medium sized, without prominent veins, not "used up" by too many infants. This portrait reveals the stark brutality of enslavement or of having a body for hire. We can picture a Roman man examining the breasts of potential wet nurses, squeezing them like fruit, perhaps tasting the milk.

According to Soranus—and echoed in the writings of Rome's elite men—anything the wet nurse did could affect the physical and psychological development of the infant. Since she had even longer physical contact with the baby than its mother—up to two or three years in some cases—her actions had even more of an impact than the pregnant woman's.[83] According to Soranus, many things could "spoil" her breast milk: eating pungent foods, drinking alcohol, bathing, having sex, doing too little or too much exercise or not the doing the right kind of exercise.[84] The effects of spoiled milk were severe. Soranus stated that spoiled and sour milk could cause an infant's nervous system to suffer and bring on "epilepsy and apoplectic attacks."[85] If the wet nurse let her charge cry for too long without bringing him to the breast, his intestines could slip down into his scrotum, causing a hernia.[86] If she moved the baby around too much after nursing, she would make its body "moist and susceptible to disease."[87] If she was too loud or aggressive and frightened the child, she could "cause afflictions of the body and the soul."[88]

It was the potential effects of the nurse's milk on the infant's soul or psyche that caused the most hand-wringing. Whatever intrinsic character traits the nurse had she was thought to transfer to her nursling in her milk. Here, there was a fundamental conflict. Many of these women were enslaved—a state that was thought to indicate a fundamental inferiority of character. Did that mean that wet nurses transferred their slavishness to their nurslings? Of course the answer had to be no, because the elite classes of Rome relied so heavily on enslaved labor for their most intimate care work. But it did mean that wet nurses could be subject to intense scrutiny, control, and blame.[89]

RITUAL TRANSITIONS

Following the birth, the integration of the infant into the community was marked by assessments, celebrations, and rituals. According to Soranus, the midwife would examine the newborn and determine if it was "worth rearing."[90] Scholars have debated the meaning of this phrase.[91] Does it refer to the exposure of infants deemed unfit for rearing? Does it mean infants who were disabled or sickly or female? Infanticide—the direct killing of a child—seems to have been quite rare.[92] In some cases, parents did decide to expose their child, leaving it out, like the trash-heap children in Roman Egypt, to either die or be reared by someone else.[93] But whether or not this decision was based on the infant's physicality or sex is less clear. It was probably more a matter of economic or social pressures (for example, babies from illicit unions) rather than a judgment about the fitness of the child.

By examining the funerary remains of children (those older than newborns) from ancient Greece, archaeologist Debbie Sneed has shown that people cared diligently for babies born with various disabilities, including cleft palates and hydrocephaly, even if the prognosis for these babies was grim.[94] Caretakers used feeding bottles and tended to them for as long as they lived. The same may have been true in the Roman period as well.[95] Bioarchaeological evidence from skeletons indicates that individuals who were born with congenital abnormalities, such as a clubfoot, lived past infancy.[96] Additionally, artwork, including paintings and small sculptures, points to the presence of individuals with many different congenital conditions—Down's syndrome, cleft palate, dwarfism, intersex, short limbs, Klippel-Feil syndrome, polydactyly, microcephaly, and macrocephaly—living and being integrated into society.[97] While it's often repeated that disabled infants were disposed of, there is little evidence that points to this having been the case. And there doesn't seem to have been a preference for exposing female babies over male babies.

For parents, the birth of a new baby was generally a happy occasion. The house was decorated, birth announcements went around, and people sent presents for the new baby. Two joyful families in Pompeii chalked the news right onto the outside of their homes. One proclaimed, "Our daughter Juvenilla was born on Saturday, August 2nd at 8 p.m."; another simply read, "Cornelius Sabinus was born!"[98] The precise day and time given for Juvenilla's birth would have allowed for the reading of her horoscope—a projection of the course her life would take and the kind of person that she would be.

Parents gave thanks to the gods for a successful birth and healthy child. These could take the form of terracotta figurines dedicated at sanctuaries. In Roman Gaul (modern-day France), once the baby survived the first critical forty to sixty days of life, parents would dedicate life-sized swaddled terracotta infants to the gods as thanks (see fig. 21).[99] These figurines marked the transition out of the swaddle. In other parts of the Empire, people dedicated terracotta figurines of women or goddesses nursing infants.[100] Sometimes new parents set up reliefs with inscriptions. In the late 2nd century CE in Poetovio in Pannonia (modern Ptuj, Slovenia), Vitalis and Vintumila set up a votive relief—a rectangular piece of terracotta with an image and words inscribed on it—as

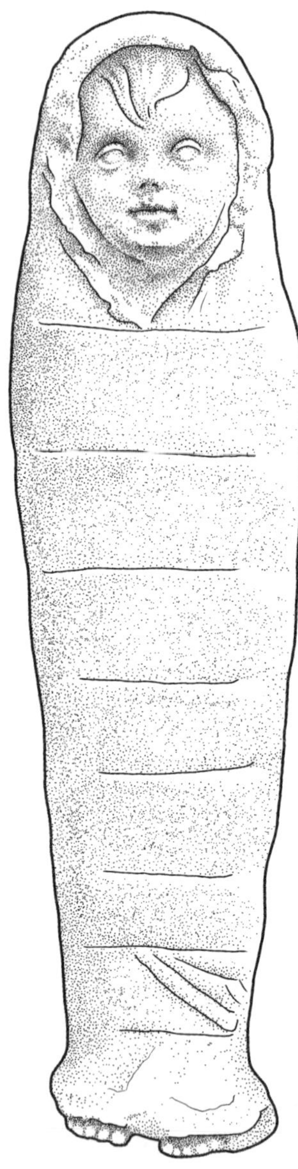

FIGURE 21. Terracotta votive of a swaddled infant. 4th–1st century BCE. Allard Pierson Museum, Amsterdam (inv. APM08900). Drawing by Hayley Monroe.

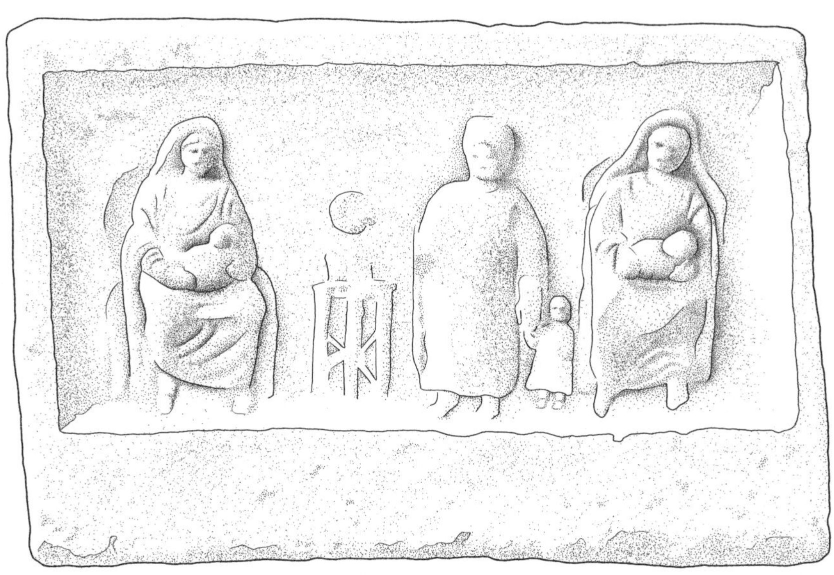

FIGURE 22. Terracotta votive relief dedicated by Vitalis and Vintumila to the nursing goddesses on behalf of their daughter, Maximilla. Poetovio (modern Ptuj, Slovenia), late 2nd century CE. Ptuj-Ormož Regional Museum, inv. RL 972. https://lupa.at/8762. Drawing by Hayley Monroe.

thanks for the well-being of their daughter, Maximilla (see fig. 22).[101] The image on the relief shows Vintumila holding the young Maximilla by the hand. On either side of them, goddesses sit nursing infants. It's not clear what age Maximilla was when this dedication was made, but it seems that she had come through the dangerous first years of infancy. Such dedications to nursing goddesses were popular in this community and may attest to a more robust practice of maternal breastfeeding than was typical in other parts of the empire.[102]

On the eighth day after birth (for girls) or the ninth day (for boys), Romans held a naming day celebration for the infant.[103] The details of the ceremony are sparse, but it seems that at this point the infant was introduced to and integrated into the wider community. Some historians have explained the interval between the biological birth and this "social birth" as a means of dealing with high infant mortality.[104] If a child died before their naming day, they hadn't actually been fully born yet. It also gave the parents time to decide whether to rear or expose the child.

But there may have been another reason for the delay. After the birth the mother had to rest and recover, and infant feeding had to be established. As we can see in the story of Favorinus and the protective grandmother, when the men arrived to see the new baby, the mother was sleeping. I imagine the grandmother wasn't too happy to have a bunch of men traipse into the house, disturbing her daughter and the new baby. Very young infants are incredibly susceptible to infection and disease. Waiting to bring outsiders around the child or to bring the child to the outside world would have helped mother and baby have the best chance of recovery and survival. Evidence in favor of this interpretation is that the Romans celebrated their birthdays on their actual day of birth, not on their naming day.[105]

DEALING WITH INFANT DEATH

What about when a baby didn't make it? As we saw in chapter 10, infant mortality was high. It's possible that 20 percent of infants who were born alive didn't make it to their first birthday.[106] Premature babies—those born before thirty-seven or thirty-eight weeks—didn't stand much of a chance due to immature lungs and other vulnerabilities. Many infants perished from nutritional deficiencies and infections.[107]

Sometimes ancient Romans explained the death of the very young as the malevolent action of a child-killing demon. From early Greek times, this demon was depicted as the ghost of a woman—any woman—who had died before she could get married and have children or who had lost her own children.[108] She enviously attacked pregnant women and newborn babies, causing miscarriage, stillbirth, and neonatal death.[109] This demonic ghost had many names, including Gello, Lamia, Mormo ("fearsome one"), Strix ("screech owl"), Megaira ("she who is envious"), and just *horrida mulier* ("horrible woman").[110] She was also connected to the evil eye—the embodiment of the envy of a god, demon, or mortal who turned their destructive gaze toward the happy and fortunate.[111] Sarah Iles Johnston, a scholar of ancient religions, has proposed that this demon was used to displace culpability from human actors.[112] If a baby died, it wasn't because of anything the mother or caregivers did; nor was it the result of a curse from an envious neighbor. Gello was to blame. She could be warded off, distracted, or thwarted with folktales—repelled by the use of her true name—or with spells, charms, and amulets.[113] In earlier periods in the Greek-speaking parts of the Mediterranean, she was stopped with the divine aid of Artemis. Under Christian influence it became King Solomon, Jesus, or other heavenly figures who interceded on the supplicant's behalf.[114]

Despite the high rate of infant mortality, the Romans cared and mourned deeply when their children died.[115] Graves for the very young attest to this affection. In Tavant in Gaul (modern-day France), a grave for a three-to-six-month-old baby boy contains a miniature sword, attesting to the dashed hopes of his parents, who perhaps dreamed that he might grow up to be a soldier like his father.[116] Very young infants were often buried near the home, sometimes in clay pots, which formed a kind of substitute womb.[117] In some locations, neonatal bones have been found grouped together in a designated location, such as a well or shrine.[118] Some of the archaeologists who initially discovered these group burials took them as evidence that infants were routinely discarded, but the scholarly consensus now is that this was not the case.[119] Rather, it was part of the ritual practice of ancient communities to bury their youngest members in these particular locations.

In the 2nd century CE, a Roman woman named Elpis set up a gravestone for her three children, sons Elpidius and Dalmatius, who both died at age seven, and an unnamed daughter who died at thirteen days old (see fig. 23).[120] She wrote that she was a "mother to worthy children." The inscription is rough, with uneven slanted letters that crowd into one another. Elpis's single name of Greek origin (meaning "hope"), as well as the single names of her two sons, suggest that she was enslaved. The lack of a named father indicates the same. What did it take for her to

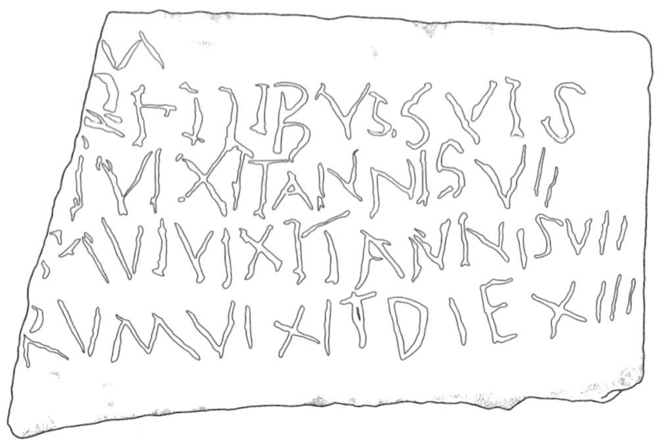

FIGURE 23. Fragment of a funerary plaque set up by Elpis for her three children. Rome, 2nd century CE. *CIL* 6.19227. Doria Pamphilj Gallery. Drawing by Hayley Monroe.

commission this gravestone? To what lengths did she go to be remembered as the mother of her children, even in what must have been her enormous grief? If she was enslaved, the fact that she identifies herself as the mother (*mater*) of her children is even more extraordinary.

WHO GETS TO BE A MOTHER?

Imprisoned alongside Perpetua in the Carthaginian prison was an enslaved woman named Felicity. She was not Perpetua's slave, but an enslaved woman in the community who had also taken up with the local Christian group. At the time of imprisonment, she was eight months pregnant. As she and her fellow Christians awaited their punishment, they prayed that she would give birth before the day appointed for their martyrdom. Otherwise, she would be held back in the prison until she had given birth. The law did not permit the execution of pregnant women until after they had delivered, in order to protect the rights of fathers and enslavers to their potential children.

The Christians' prayers were answered. Three days before the scheduled execution, Felicity went into labor. Despite the difficulties of an eight-month birth, and despite being mocked by the jailor while she labored—"If you're in so much pain now, what are you going to do when you're thrown to the beasts?"—she delivered a healthy baby girl.[121] Handing the infant off to a fellow Christian, she turned her attention to her imminent death.

Like Perpetua, Felicity perhaps seems callous. She left her newborn infant and gleefully entered the arena—"from the midwife to the gladiator"—breasts dripping with milk.[122] Both women abandoned their motherhood for their relationship with God. But what sort of motherhood would Felicity have had anyway? Children born to free or freed parents in legitimate marriages took their status from their father. But children born outside of legitimate marriage, to unwed and/or enslaved mothers, took their status from their mothers. Enslaved mothers gave birth to enslaved children. And these enslaved mothers did not get to be mothers in the same way that free women did.[123] To enslavers, enslaved women's reproductive labor was a commodity to manage and exploit.[124]

Enslaved women could have their children sold away from them or have their motherhood disrupted in other ways. One way enslavers controlled enslaved mothers was by consolidating the labor of breastfeeding.[125] All the enslaved children born in a household would be nursed by the same woman or group of women, freeing up the birthing mothers to be hired out as wet nurses or to quickly get pregnant again. Enslavers may have even sent all the infants and wet nurses to the country plantations, keeping the birthing mothers in their urban villas. The intention would have been to maximize reproductive output and weaken bonds between birthing mothers and their children.[126]

Sometimes enslavers offered enslaved women their freedom in exchange for childbearing. But there was a brutal catch. The children born while she was enslaved would themselves, of course, remain enslaved. An inscription from the 1st century CE in Delphi, Greece, records that a woman named Sostrata preemptively purchased her freedom.[127] The terms were severe. Despite having paid cash at the time of the inscription, Sostrata had to continue serving her enslavers, a married couple, until they died. She also had to birth and leave behind in slavery a child who was at least two years old—a future slave for the married couple's son. This contract was not unique. Enslaved women were often in the position of having to obtain their own freedom through the production of enslaved children.[128] As historian Kat Huemoeller has argued, enslavers tried to coerce reproduction from enslaved women with the promise of freedom, while at the same time offsetting "the reproductive loss associated with freeing women."[129]

The cruelties of a society saturated in slavery disrupted the mother-child bond in other ways. In some of the wet-nursing contracts from Roman Egypt, poor, free mothers put up their infants as collateral for debts, seemingly in order to obtain the resources necessary to raise them.[130] The creditor would pay the woman a sum of money up front, and the woman would breastfeed her own child for a stipulated period of time (two years, for instance), all the while (hopefully) repaying the loan. During that time, the child belonged to the creditor. In this way, some women were legally wet nurses to their own children. The emotional stakes of such an arrangement must have been high. On the surface it would have looked like a woman was breastfeeding her own baby. But legally speaking, she was nursing the slave of her creditor. We can only imagine the relief that a woman named Philotera felt when she was able to repay the debt that she owed to a man named Patrikos and regain her parental rights to her daughter, Mareas, whom she had been nursing as Patrikos's future slave.[131]

But there are glimpses of resistance amid the reproductive coercion. It seems that enslaved women sometimes used contraceptives and abortifacients to thwart the intentions of their enslavers. In a letter from 380 CE, one of the early Christan writers, Ambrose of Milan, referred obliquely to the case of an enslaved woman from Altinum (in northeastern Italy) who, at the request of her enslaver, was inspected by a midwife for signs of having been pregnant. The unnamed woman was "charged with wrong," meaning that the midwife determined that she had been pregnant and, it was assumed, had caused herself to abort.[132] Why would she have done this? She was likely attempting to thwart the enslaver's reproductive control of her body.

At other times, resistance looked like family-building even in the face of legal and social adversity. A funerary epitaph for an enslaved child named Threptus was set up jointly by his wet nurse, Oscia Sabina, and his mother, Lamyra.[133] Oscia Sabina and Lamyra may have been fellow slaves who both had affective ties to the young Threptus, Lamyra by birthing him and Oscia by nursing him. Perhaps they acted as his co-mothers, maybe even in an informal relationship with one another. At the risk of reading too much into this spare gravestone, this might have been an instance of queer family-making. It is, at least, evidence of resistive and cooperative childrearing under the harshest and most dehumanizing circumstances.

. . .

In the 2nd century CE, medical pediatric care was developing as a way to combat the risky business of caring for newborns. But often the "scientific" methods—which were based on theories—led to dangerous practices. They likely did more harm than many of the folk practices they were meant to replace. Attributing early infant sickness and death to the work of an envious demon and taking appropriate protective measures would have had a positive, community-building effect. Conversely, attributing early risk to the dangerous milk of the mother had real, dire consequences. Midwives and wet nurses were scapegoated as sources of potential harm to the newborn infant, when in fact it was their attentions that offered the best chances of survival. Doctors like Soranus and his successors worked to plug the labor of reproduction into the hierarchies of the empire, not necessarily to ensure the optimal survival of mother and baby. Further, these very hierarchies delineated who was allowed to be a mother. When Perpetua and Felicity died in the arena, one of them was abandoning her child, while the other was leaving behind her enslaver's property.

But glimmers of women's stories shine through with evidence of resistive practice. These glimmers are why it matters to try to reach back and tell the stories of people like Perpetua, Felicity, Serapias, Elpis, Oscia Sabina, and Lamyra. They existed within structures of patriarchy, misogyny, and slavery. They may have experienced the tensions between emergent theoretically based medical practice and traditional practice. But those structures and tensions did not wholly define them.

Afterword

I WAS INSPIRED to write this book in part as a response to a common refrain in the scholarship on Roman women. It generally goes something like, "Childbirth in ancient Rome was deadly and terrifying." Sometimes the scholar will elaborate, giving an estimate for maternal mortality as proof of the claim. I have approached these statements with curiosity. Surely there is more to it than that? That's like summing up the famous Battle of Cannae as "deadly and terrifying" with no mention of how Hannibal the Carthaginian tricked the Roman infantry—superior to his own in numbers and training—by drawing them in toward a shallow, buckling line of light-armed troops and outflanking them with his cavalry. Ancient Roman women, I think, deserve more than a line or two about fear and death.

When people write about their birth experiences today, they often describe feelings of splitting or shattering, of brushing up against death. In *The Argonauts,* Maggie Nelson writes, "To let the baby out you have to be willing to go to pieces."[1] But this shattering, this "touching death," as Nelson calls it, also brings expansion and transformation. In her writing on birth, childbirth educator Britta Bushnell focuses on this transformational aspect of the experience: "Birth is not just physical; it's emotional, mental and spiritual. It's breaking open, a transformative surrender that asks everything of us."[2] For this reason, she writes, "Storytelling and shared wisdom are vital in birth work. They illuminate the depth of what it means to give birth, not just physically, but as a process of profound transformation." What would an ancient Roman woman have written about her own experience of giving birth?

In a letter to his friend Lucilius, the Stoic philosopher Seneca (4 BCE–65 CE) wrote about his recent experience with an acute illness:

> My friends were essential to my recovery; I was comforted by their words of encouragement, by their attentiveness through the night, and by their conversation. Nothing . . . restores and helps a sick man as much as the affection of his friends; nothing snatches away the expectation and fear of death. . . . I was thinking that I would not continue to live with them, but through them. I imagined that I was not giving up but putting my strength in them. All these things gave me the will to help myself and to endure any torture.[3]

In Seneca's description, it is his friends who sustain his spirit, who pull him back from the brink of death with their affection and conversation. His reliance on them is an experience of extreme need, disembodiment, and resurrection—"I was thinking that I would not continue to live with them, but through them." It is their dedicated presence by his bed, their "words of encouragement" that give him "the will to help myself and to endure any torture." If these were the words available to Seneca, how might Cyrilla or Agrippina have described their experiences of birth? For Roman women, the inevitable intensity of birth was something to be faced in communities of women, working together to help each other prepare, labor, birth, and recover.

We can see this community at work in a birth scene on a small ivory plaque from Pompeii, part of a portable handloom (see fig. 24).[4] Here the laboring woman sits on a birth chair. She is supported from behind by an assistant, who holds her by the waist. The midwife kneels down in front of her on a low stool, holding a sponge in her right hand, gently parting the laboring woman's legs with her left. The figure behind the midwife is a goddess, probably Juno Lucina. This is almost certainly a mythological birth scene. The plaque forming the other side of the loom shows the death of the demigod Meleager, brought about by the actions of his mother, Althea. The two sides of the plaque display Althea's dual

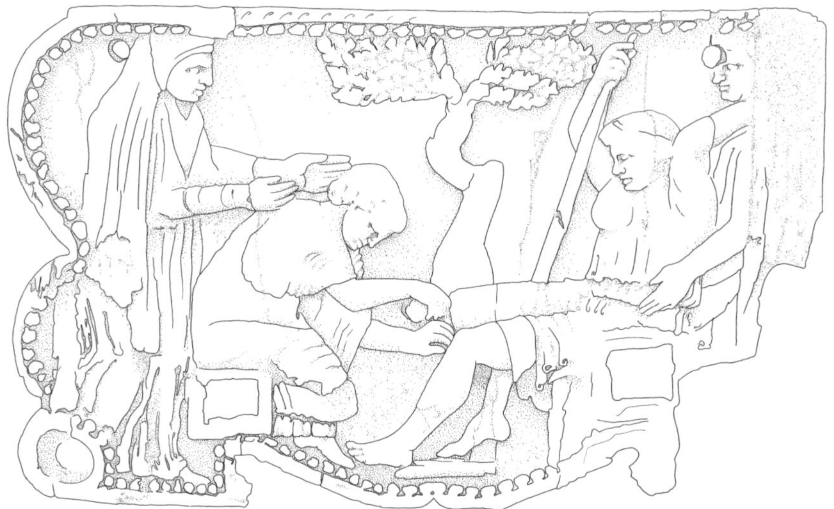

FIGURE 24. Ivory plaque from a handloom, depicting the mythological birth of the demigod Meleager to Althea. Pompeii, 1st century CE. National Archaeological Museum, Naples, Italy (109905A). Drawing by Hayley Monroe.

power over her son—her ability to bring him into existence through birth and her ability to extinguish him in death. It is a visualization of that most patriarchal and misogynistic of Roman fears—that a woman may have control over the life of a man. But in another way, it gives a glimpse of the idealized childbirth experience—women helping women, mortals and goddesses alike. If this ideal wasn't always realized—and almost certainly it was not—it was at least the model to which communities aspired.

Birth work—both the work of those who give birth and the work of those who support people through birth—has, for much of history, been invisible to or ignored by the writers of history. In ancient Rome, this invisibility led to the dismissal and disparagement of birth workers—midwives, attendants, wet nurses, and the mothers themselves. In excluding birth stories from the modern history of ancient Rome, we have repeated the epistemic violence.

If there is something inherently dangerous about birth—a contested claim—then it has always been communities of (mostly) women who have mitigated these dangers. But giving birth is so much more than fear and danger. Although I cannot discount that many Roman women must have been afraid, and some of them would have been in danger, nonetheless, I have to imagine that for some women in ancient Rome, birth was triumphant and transformative. In this book I have tried to access that perspective as much as I can, while paying heed to the cultural forces that shaped the experience of giving birth in the ancient Roman world.

ACKNOWLEDGMENTS

My mom started taking me to home births when I was seven, and my dad started taking me to academic libraries at about the same time. It was the combination of these two types of training—an embodied immersion in the world of midwifery and the academic study of ancient history—that led to the creation of this book. I am deeply grateful for the ways my parents have shaped me as a person and a scholar.

When I was struggling to begin writing, Kat Huemoeller said to me, why don't you tell a birth story? I credit her as the midwife of this book. She helped me conceive the project, read my book proposal and early chapters, got me unstuck and writing again so many times, discussed ideas with me, and read and gave me invaluable feedback on the final draft.

While writing this book I had to contend with large teaching loads, a pandemic, and multiple cross-country moves. But these obstacles made this book what it is. Because I was always teaching, I wrote this book with students in mind. Because I was always moving, I learned many different things from many different people. Much of this book was written in intervals of one hour a day.

There were many generous and loving individuals who helped me along the way. Heidi Marx, Kristi Upson-Saia, and Jared Secord were the first to believe in the project. Jared read early drafts of the first four chapters, and Heidi and Kristi read multiple versions of the first seven chapters. They also put in me in touch with my wonderful editor at UC Press, Eric Schmidt. Heidi organized a book workshop for me through the Working Group in Religion, Medicine, Disability, Health, and Healing in Late Antiquity (ReMeDHe). Respondents Susan Holman and Jane Draycott generously and carefully read the first seven chapters and provided feedback that dramatically reshaped the book. Claire

Burridge helpfully took notes during the workshop. ReMeDHe has been a warm, collegial, and endlessly supportive intellectual home for me.

When I was an adjunct at Wheaton College in Norton, Massachusetts, my involvement with *Eidolon* buoyed my spirit. Donna Zuckerberg, Yung In Chae, Sarah Scullin, and Tori Lee taught me to write things that people would want to read.

During the three years I spent as a visiting assistant professor at Vassar College, I benefited from the stimulating intellectual comradery and deep friendship of many brilliant people. I am especially grateful to Curtis Dozier, Barbara Olsen, Hamit Arvas, Christina Owens, Katie Gemmill, Pauline Goul, Katharine Hite, and Judy Dollenmayer. Kirstin Wesselhoeft and Klaus Yoder were friends and colleagues who let me attend the home birth of their child. I am grateful to the students in my Sex, Gender, and the History of Medicine and History of Midwifery courses for asking great questions and providing new insights. Around this time, I also posted on social media asking people what questions they had about childbirth in ancient Rome. I got dozens of responses, which shaped the book more than the respondents probably realize.

My colleagues (and their families) at the University of British Columbia Department of Ancient Mediterranean and Near Eastern Studies (AMNE) provided much friendship, writing companionship, and expertise. I'm grateful to the members of the ANME daily writing group, with whom I still frequently meet over Zoom. Tony Keddie read my book proposal. Flo Yoon read early drafts of the first four chapters. Matt McCarty answered questions about Roman epigraphy. Leanne Bablitz told me about Babatha. Isaac Soon is always sending promising sources my way. Rachel Philbrick has been a great friend since our grad school days. Hannah Roe has been a dear friend and writing partner. She read my book proposal and offered guidance on the publishing process. She and Phil Yoo allowed me the great joy of being their doula at the birth of their child. I'm also grateful to the UBC students who were in my Ancient Medicine in the Mediterranean and Near East course, who read drafts of the first two chapters of the book.

Since my recent move to the University of Wisconsin–Madison, my new colleagues have welcomed me warmly. I'm grateful to have started this job with Julia Horn, who read and gave me invaluable feedback on the sixth chapter.

I've learned so much from midwives, especially Kathi Mulder, Geradine Simkins, Patrice Bobier, Lynette Biery, and Melinda Parenteau. At Pomegranate

Community Midwifery in Vancouver, British Columbia, Kat Montgomery, Sophia Kraemer, Annie Passmore, Kerry Harris, and Katrina Blommaert guided me through my prenatal, birth, and postpartum journey. I thought I knew about birth, but I learned so much more from childbirth educator Stephanie Ondrak at the Childbearing Society. I see the true magic of midwifery in the work of Ninotte Lubin, founder, director, and lead midwife at Grace Community Birth Center in Grand Bassin, Haiti. I first met Ninotte when my mom and I traveled to Jacmel, Haiti, to volunteer at Mother Health International birth center after the devastating earthquake in 2010. Watching Ninotte and being a small part of her twelve-year journey to found and build Grace Community Birth Center and her ongoing efforts to fund it has been profound and life changing.

I happened to be pregnant and give birth around the same time as several dear old friends throughout North America. Phone calls with Anna Bonnell Freidin, Laura Hodges, Phoebe McGee, and Johanna Hanink helped me process my new parenthood journey and learn about all the different ways that people give birth. I'm also so grateful to the women in Vancouver whom I met through prenatal yoga and childbirth class and with whom I shared pregnancy and the early days of parenting.

Anna Bonnell Freidin read the final draft. This book has benefitted so much from her feedback, as well as from her research and writing on childbirth in ancient Rome. The three reviewers from the press gave excellent suggestions for ways to improve the final manuscript. Debbie Sneed and Julia Kelto Lillis answered questions over email. Caitlin Hines and Molly Jones-Lewis shared unpublished work. Chelsea Gardner and Melissa Funke had me as a guest on their *Peopling the Past* podcast to talk about midwifery in ancient Rome. Hayley Monroe created the beautiful illustrations. Isabel Cooperman has been the best research assistant. I first learned about herbalism more than a decade ago from Mary Blue and Denise DeSpirito. Jennifer Swalec and Abby Colodner have been close friends through many different stages of life. Ben Life always showed keen interest in my progress on the book. I'm grateful to Jyoti Arvey, who took over as my editor when Eric left UC Press for Basic Books and whose expert guidance has led me through the writing of the final chapters and the publication process. I'm also grateful for the editorial and production team at UC Press, including Stephanie Summerhays and Teresa Iafolla. Jan Spauschus provided meticulous copy editing.

My family has supported me so much. C Mulder inspires me with their writing practice and is a great untie to Teddy. Kathi and Craig Mulder, Terri and Leigh Bartlett, Hannah Mulder, Hazen Remus, Sam Bartlett, and Ellis Jordan all cooked meals, provided childcare, and put up with me being absent, either physically or mentally, while I wrote this book. Katie Strittmatter has always been an enthusiastic supporter. Gabi Mulder helped with some final tweaks. Both of my grandmothers died while I was writing this book; I have dedicated it to them because they were both enormously encouraging of me. Grandma Ann was only somewhat disappointed that I didn't go into politics, and Grandma Carolyn was so proud of my academic achievements. You could always find her wearing the sweatshirt of whatever college or university I was studying or teaching at.

The greatest appreciation goes to my husband, Stephen Bartlett, for innumerable acts of assistance, humor, and grace. He discussed every idea in this book with me probably more than he wanted to. I am thankful to Teddy for bringing so much joy and laughter to our lives. Finally, I'm also grateful for my cat, Maebe, who was my family before I ever knew Stephen and Teddy.

GLOSSARY OF HERBAL AND MEDICAL TERMS

I have described the following herbs based on how they were used in antiquity. For modern applications, reference should be made to contemporary sources on herbal medicine. Many of these plants had broad medicinal applications; I have focused on their role in reproductive health.

ABORTIFACIENT method or substance that induces an abortion

ALLHEAL any of several plants thought to have broad healing powers; varieties in the ancient Mediterranean probably included Asclepius's allheal (*Ferula nodosa* L. or *Echinophora tenuifolia* L.) and Chiron's allheal (*Helianthum ovatum* Dunal and *Helianthum vulgare* Gaertn.). See also "Hercules's woundwort"

AMENORRHEA absence of menstruation

AMNIOTIC FLUID fluid inside the amniotic sac

AMNIOTIC SAC translucent, fluid-filled sac that surrounds the fetus in the uterus

AROMATIC ONYX shell of the onyx cowrie (a type of sea snail, modern identification uncertain), which produces a pleasant-smelling smoke when burned

ASTRINGENTS drying herbs that contract tissue and stop fluid secretions

BAY (SWEET) *Laurus nobilis* L., astringent herb used in cooking and medicine; abortifacient

BELLOWS device with an air bag that emits a stream of air when squeezed by two handles; used for pumping air into the vagina and uterus

BIRTHWORT *Aristolochia rotunda*, *A. longa*, and *A. clematitis* L.; name means "best birth"; contains toxic aristolochic acid; emmenagogic, expulsive

BITUMEN also called asphalt or tar; a naturally occurring sticky, black, viscous byproduct of organic substances

BLOODLETTING also called venesection; therapeutic blood removal to balance the humors; done with surgical tools or leeches

CHOLERIC having too much black bile (a cold and dry bodily humor associated with autumn)

CLYSTER injection of liquid infused with herbs or other substances into the rectum or vagina for medicinal purposes or to cause evacuation; commonly called an enema today

COLOSTRUM thick yellow milk produced by the breasts immediately after the birth of a baby

COMMON CENTAURY *Centaurium erythraea* Rafn, flowering plant in the gentian family; emmenagogic, abortifacient

CRETAN THYME *Satureja thymbra* L., also called savory of Crete and Roman hyssop; expectorant, diuretic, expulsive

CUPPING process in which bulbous glass or ceramic cups are heated and applied to the body, creating suction and drawing fluids to the surface of the skin

DARNEL *Lolium temulentum* L., wheat-like grass used in vaginal fumigations to promote conception

DECOCTION concentrated medicinal liquid made by boiling or simmering dried or fresh plant matter in water or some other liquid for an extended time

DILATOR surgical instrument used to open or expand a tube or cavity in the body

DITTANY OF CRETE *Origanum dictamnus* L., acrid wooly herb native to Crete; expulsive

DIURETICS substances that increase the frequency and amount of urination

DOUCHE stream or spray of liquid used to clean a bodily orifice, particularly the vagina

DROPWORT *Spiraea filipendula* L., also *Filipendula vulgaris* Moench; its name comes from the tubers that hang in drops from the roots; used to expel the placenta

EGYPTIAN ALUM type of rock salt that contains aluminum; astringent

EMBRYOTOMY surgical operation in which a dead fetus is removed in pieces from the uterus or birth canal

EMETICS substances that cause vomiting

EMMENAGOGIC substance that stimulates menstruation

EMOLLIENTS substances that soften, soothe, and protect the skin and mucous membranes

EXPECTORANTS mucous-thinning and purging substances

EXPULSIVES herbs that expel matter from the uterus, including embryos/fetuses

FIELD BASIL *Ziziphora capitata* L.; pungent, diuretic herb used in plasters to glue wounds

FLUX pathological flow of fluid from the body, especially the vagina

FUMIGATION (VAGINAL) also called vaginal steaming or vapor bath; treatment in which steam from boiling water infused with herbs or other substances, or smoke from burning herbs or other substances, is directed into the vagina via a tube or straw

FUNDUS upper end (top) of the uterus

GARDEN CRESS *Lepidium sativum* L., peppery, warming herb; abortifacient, emmenagogic, aphrodisiac

HAZELWORT *Asarum europaeum* L., also called European wild ginger and wild spikenard; in the birthwort family (Aristolochiaceae); contains toxic aristolochic acid; warming, diuretic, emmenagogic

HELLEBORE (BLACK) *Helleborus cyclophyllus* Boiss, toxic plant distinguished by its black roots; purgative, emmenagogic, abortifacient

HELLEBORE (WHITE) *Veratrum album* L., also called false hellebore; poisonous, purgative plant; abortifacient

HERCULES'S WOUNDWORT *Opoponax hispidus* Friv., *Opoponax chironium* L., or *Opoponax persicus* Boiss & Heldr., also called Hercules's allheal, woundwort, or opoponax; resinous juice from the stalk of the plant has broad medicinal applications; emmenagogic, expulsive, abortifacient

HOREHOUND *Marrubium vulgare* L. or *Marrubium creticum* Miller, hairy, bitter plant in the mint family; expectorant, emmenagogic, expulsive

HULWORT *Teucrium pollium* L., small mountain shrub; antidote for poison and wild animal bites; laxative, emmenagogic

HUMORS fluids that were thought to compose the body in ancient medical thought: blood, phlegm, yellow bile, and black bile

HYDROMEL honey water

HYSTERICAL *PNIX* "uterine suffocation," a condition in which the uterus was thought to move around in the body and suffocate other organs

KISSA ancient Greek term for prenatal symptoms including nausea, exhaustion, and strange cravings

LABDANUM also called ladanum, sticky brown resin extracted from the rock-rose plant (*Cistus ladanifer* L. or *Cistus creticus* L.); used medicinally and in incense; used to expel the placenta

LACEDEMONIAN LEAP abortifacient method recommended in the Hippocratic text *Nature of the Child* that involved leaping and kicking the buttocks

LANOLIN yellow, waxy substance secreted by the sebaceous glands of wool-bearing animals, with waterproofing properties

LINSEED *Linum usitatissimum* L., also called flaxseed; used in a sitz bath for uterine inflammation; expectorant, aphrodisiac, purgative

LOCHIA normal discharge of blood, mucus, and uterine tissue following childbirth; lasts up to six weeks

LOVAGE *Levisticum officinale* W.D.J. Koch, pungent and aromatic culinary and medicinal herb; digestive, emmenagogic

LUPINE likely *Lupinus albus* L., a culinary and medicinal plant; seeds used to induce menstruation and urination

MACERATE to soften plant matter in a liquid such as olive oil, usually for the purpose of using the plant-infused liquid after straining out the solid matter

MAN ORCHID also called satyrion, a general name for aphrodisiacs from the orchid family; modern identification is unclear

MARSH MALLOW *Althaea officinalis* L., soothing, softening, mucilaginous (slippery, gel-producing) herb with broad healing properties

MECCA BALSAM *Commiphora opobalsamon* Engl., expensive herb that was grown only in Judea (Syria-Palaestina) and prone to adulteration; warming, expulsive, diuretic

MECONIUM first dark-green or black tar-like feces that an infant produces after birth

MYRRH *Commiphora myrrha* (T.Nees) Engl., tree native to Africa and the Arabian Peninsula that produces a fragrant, resinous sap; in ancient times, expensive and prone to adulteration; used cosmetically and medicinally; emmenagogic, expulsive

MYRTLE *Myrtus communis* L., evergreen shrub or small tree; astringent, diuretic

NARD also called spikenard; probably refers to *Nardostachys jatamansi* (D.Don) DC., native to the Himalayas; plant in the honeysuckle family that produces an aromatic, amber-colored oil; in ancient times, expensive and prone to adulteration; used cosmetically and medicinally; warming, drying, diuretic

NETTLE (STINGING) plants in the *Urtica* family; fresh leaves provoke a stinging feeling on contact; aphrodisiac, emmenagogic, diuretic

OAK GALLS also called oak apples; round, apple-like growths found on the leaves and branches of oak trees; astringent, styptic

ODOR THERAPY method of treating the wandering womb by using sweet-smelling substances to attract it or foul-smelling substances to repel it

OKYTOKION AMULETS "quick-birth" amulets; stones, plant matter, or other substances applied outside the body to promote the birth of the fetus and placenta

OPERCULUM OF MUREX *Murex* is a genus of sea snail and the operculum is the hard, lid-like structure attached to the foot of the snail that closes the hole to its shell

PENNYROYAL *Mentha pulegium* L., in the mint family (*Lamiaceae*); warming, emmenagogic, expulsive, abortifacient

PESSARY also called a vaginal suppository; pellet-shaped suppository inserted into the vagina, made from herbs combined with fat, wax, and/or wool

PHLEGMY having two much phlegm (a cold and wet bodily humor associated with winter)

PICA craving or consumption of non-food items such as clay or dirt

PITCH dark, sticky, semi-solid byproduct of burning wood for coal

PLASTER thick paste made from mashed or ground-up plant matter, minerals, or other substances (such as dung or charcoal) mixed with a liquid, spread on cloth, and applied to the skin

POLYHYDRAMNIOS a condition of having too much amniotic fluid

POULTICE moist, mashed-up plant matter applied to the skin directly or wrapped in cloth

PROBE blunt-ended surgical instrument used to explore inside a wound or cavity of the body

PURGATIVES also called cathartics; herbs causing evacuations of liquid and solid matter from the body, especially from the bowels

ROOT CUTTER knowledgeable procurer and distributer of medicinal plant matter

RUE *Ruta graveolens* L. and *Ruta chalepensis* L., common herb; warming, diuretic, emmenagogic, abortifacient

SACRUM triangular bone at the base of the spine

SAGAPENON juice from a plant in the giant fennel genus (*Ferula persica* Willd.); expectorant, emmenagogic, abortifacient

SCAMMONY *Convolvulus scammonia* L., twining plant with a thick, fleshy root that produces milky juice that when dried and ingested is a powerful purgative

SHEPHERD'S PURSE *Capsella bursa-pastoris* L., common herb; warming, purgative, emmenagogic, abortifacient

SHOULDER DYSTOCIA difficult vaginal birth in which one or more of the infant's shoulders gets stuck behind the pubic bone after its head has emerged

SILPHIUM also called silphion, laserwort, or laser; identification is uncertain; in the giant fennel genus; may be *Ferula drudeana* Korovin; has many culinary and medicinal uses; emmenagogic, expulsive

SITZ BATH warm, shallow bath with salts or herbs used to soothe the anus and genitals

SOAPWORT *Saponaria officinalis* L., common flowering plant whose leave and roots produce a soapy lather when boiled; used for stripping lanolin from wool and cleaning textiles; diuretic, purgative, emmenagogic, abortifacient

SOUND thin metal rod used to probe and expand orifices in the body, especially the urethra and cervix

SPIKENARD see "nard"

SQUIRTING CUCUMBER *Ecballium elaterium* (L.) A. Rich., plant with a small, round, cucumber-like body that rapidly expels a viscous, seedy liquid when touched; purgative, expulsive

STERNUTATIVES also called sternutatories; sneeze-inducing substances

STINKING BEAN TREFOIL *Anagyris foetida* L., pungent shrub; used as an *oxytokion* amulet; emmenagogic, expulsive

STORAX resinous, fragrant sap from a number of different trees; probably refers to *Storax officinalis* L.; in ancient times, expensive and prone to adulteration; emmenagogic

STYPTICS substances with blood-stanching properties

WALLFLOWER can refer to several plants in the genus *Erysimum* (formerly *Cheiranthus*); probably *Erysimum cheiri* (L.) Crantz; seeds have emmenagogic and expulsive properties

WASH see "douche"

WILD CARROT *Daucus carota* L., also called Queen Anne's lace; seeds are emmenagogic and aid in conception; root is diuretic, aphrodisiac, expulsive

WILD SPIKENARD see "nard"

WILLOW WEED *Polygonum persicaria* L., pungent, wheat-like, astringent plant

WORMWOOD refers to *Artemisia absinthum*, *A. arborescens,* or *A. campestris* L.; warming, purgative, diuretic, emmenagogic, expulsive

VERNIX also called vernix caseosa; waxy white substance that coats the skin of newborn infants

NOTES

INTRODUCTION

1. Banks, *Natality,* 3.
2. Birthtalk.org, "Laura Stavoe Speaks."
3. Birthtalk.org, "Laura Stavoe Speaks."
4. Filippini, *Pregnancy, Delivery, Childbirth,* 34.
5. Wick, *Sumud,* 2.
6. Wick, *Sumud.*
7. Somerstein, *Invisible Labor,* 223.
8. Simkins, *Into These Hands,* xxiv.
9. Gaskin, *Ina May's Guide to Childbirth,* 121–25.

1. CYRILLA FAINTS IN THE BATH

1. Galen, *Prognosis* 8. The titles of Galen's writings have been inconsistently translated from ancient Greek into English. For instance, the same treatise is sometimes called *Affected Places* and at other times *On the Affected Parts.* When I refer to Galen's writings, I use the titles provided in the appendix of Singer and Rosen, *Oxford Handbook of Galen.* On a separate note, I have given this woman the name Cyrilla, which I explain in greater detail ahead. Galen, as he does with all of his female patients, leaves her unnamed.

2. Unless otherwise indicated, translations from Ancient Greek and Latin are my own.

3. Cyrilla is in the care of midwives *(maiai),* as well as attendants (*hupēretousai* and *therapeuousai*), who could be enslaved women or hired nurses. The person who thinks Cyrilla is pregnant is "one of the women

watching over her" (*phullatousē*), which Vivian Nutton (Galen, *On Prognosis,* 113) translates as "chief nurse." On baths in private homes, see Draycott, *Roman Domestic Medical Practice,* 66.

4. The province was called Judaea from 6–135 CE, then became Syria-Palaestina in 136 CE.

5. On Galen's friendship with Boethus, see Flemming, "Demiurge and Emperor," 61–62; Tieleman, "Galen and the Stoics," 287–88, 294; Mattern, *Prince of Medicine,* 100, 163.

6. Galen, *Prognosis* 8.

7. Galen, *Prognosis* 7. Susan Mattern (*Prince of Medicine,* 163–64) raises the possibility that the mother of the boy, Cyrillus, is not Boethus's wife but another woman in his household. The boy, however, is identified as Boethus's son, and as Angela Hug (*Fertility, Ideology,* 12–13) points out, official Roman marriages were expected to produce children, while other unions were not. Boethus would have been more likely to claim as his son a child by his wife rather than one by another woman in his household.

8. On the life and work of Galen, see Mattern, *Rhetoric of Healing* and *Prince of Medicine*; on competition in Galen's writings, see Lloyd, "Galen's Un-Hippocratic Case Histories," 122–24. On the medical marketplace and diversity of practitioners, see Nutton, "Medical Market Place" and *Ancient Medicine,* 366–96; Israelowich, *Patients and Healers*; Flemming and Totelin, *Medicine and Markets*; Upson-Saia et al., *Medicine, Health, and Healing,* especially 289; Marx-Wolf, "Religion, Medicine, and Health," 514–16; Draycott, *Roman Domestic Medical Practice.*

9. King, *Hippocrates' Woman,* 176.

10. Galen was always adamant that he did not get paid for his medical care (Mattern, *Rhetoric of Healing,* 83); these 400 gold pieces, he tells us, were a gift. He may have been strident on this point because there was a widespread suspicion of doctors in Rome, particularly Greek doctors. Pliny the Elder (*Natural History* 29.7), writing a bit earlier than Galen, reports the belief that Greek doctors conspired to kill foreigners—a perversion of the much-storied Hippocratic Oath, which, of course, instructs physicians *not* to harm their patients. On pay for Roman soldiers, see Alston, "Roman Military Pay," 115—soldiers were paid about 300 *denarii* per year and there were 25 *denarii* to a gold *aureus,* so they received about 12 gold *aurei* per year.

11. In the Roman Republic, men had to be forty-two to be consul, but under the empire this rule was largely ignored, making it more difficult to estimate Boethus's age.

12. On the age of Roman girls at first marriage, see Caldwell, *Roman Girlhood,* 2–8.

13. Hug, *Fertility, Ideology,* 11.

14. Throughout this book, I generally use the terms "enslaver" and "enslaved" to refer to people who might otherwise be called "masters," "owners," and "slaves." This language follows the work of scholars who work on ancient and modern slavery and it aims to both humanize those who were (and are) enslaved and deny to enslavers their preferred terms of identification.

15. On these laws, which were part of a larger program of Augustan social legislation, see Milnor, *Gender, Domesticity,* 140–54. Angela Hug (*Fertility, Ideology,* 49–50) sees these laws as part of a moral panic that the free Roman population was not adequately reproducing itself.

16. McGinn, *Prostitution, Sexuality,* 76.

17. McGinn, *Prostitution, Sexuality,* 84.

18. Columella, *On Agriculture* 1.8.19–20.

19. Cao, *Alimenta,* 273; McGinn, "Roman Children," 346–47.

20. Hug, *Fertility, Ideology,* 25–29.

21. On the reproductive expectations for enslaved women, see Huemoeller, *Child Follows the Womb.*

22. Phang, *Marriage of Roman Soldiers,* 327.

23. On the expectation of producing children for the Roman state, see Hug, *Fertility, Ideology,* 8. Expectations did not always meet reality. Some very prominent women in ancient Rome, such as the first empress, Livia, had few or no children. Livia had two sons with her first husband, Tiberius, and no surviving children with her second husband, the emperor Augustus. But Augustus did not divorce her. Instead, he adopted her first son and made him his heir. Adoption would go on to become an important reproductive strategy among the upper classes in Rome.

24. Hug, *Fertility, Ideology,* 19.

25. Roman girls, on average, started menstruating later than people today, perhaps around age thirteen or fourteen (Hug, *Fertility, Ideology,* 33).

26. Caldwell, *Roman Girlhood,* 97.

27. Plutarch expresses a similar sentiment in his *Lives of Lycurgus and Numa* 4.1–2 (see Hug, *Fertility, Ideology,* 35). These writings display a significant departure from the Hippocratic recommendations used by midwives and doctors from the 5th century BCE onward, which viewed virginity, especially prolonged virginity, as essentially unhealthful. See Caldwell, *Roman Girlhood,* 83–84.

28. Soranus, *Gynecology* 1.34.

29. Soranus, *Gynecology* 1.30–32.

30. Soranus, *Gynecology* 1.34, "Women usually get married to have children and ensure succession . . . not for enjoyment."

31. Soranus, *Gynecology* 1.33.

32. Frier, "Marriage of Underage Girls" and "Normalizing Illegality?"; Freidin, *Birthing Romans,* 29–31. There is evidence of girls being married—and perhaps subjected to sexual intercourse—even younger than twelve. These would have been informal marriages until the girl reached twelve.

33. *AE* 1985, 355; translation is from Scarfo, "Pregnancy, Childbirth," 54.

34. Quintilian, *The Orator's Education* 6 pr. 4–16; Caldwell, *Roman Girlhood,* 4.

35. Caldwell, *Roman Girlhood,* 4–5; Bodel, "Minicia Marcella."

36. Hug, *Fertility, Ideology,* 36.

37. Caldwell, *Roman Girlhood,* 5.

38. Some historians estimate that upward of a third of children in ancient Rome died before the age of five (Parkin, "The Demography of Infancy"). On infant mortality in ancient Rome, see Hug, *Fertility, Ideology,* 17n30; Freidin, *Birthing Romans,* 33–34.

39. However, as Rebecca Flemming ("Gendering Medical Provision") has pointed out, Roman midwives provided healthcare to women and children outside of the context of pregnancy and childbirth. So the fact that Cyrilla has "usual midwives" doesn't necessarily mean that she has been pregnant before.

2. CYRILLA'S FLUX AND OTHER FLUIDS

1. The discussion that follows on medical understandings of the female body in antiquity and the role of menstruation in reproduction owes much to Dean-Jones, *Women's Bodies*; King, *Hippocrates' Woman*; Flemming, *Making of Roman Women*; and the many excellent articles by Ann Ellis Hanson.

2. This theory of four humors features in the Hippocratic text *Nature of Man.*

3. On the humors and health, see Upson-Saia et al., *Medicine, Health, and Healing,* 53–54, 98–99, 102–6. On humoral theory and other theories of health and disease, see Nutton, *Ancient Medicine,* throughout and especially 57–67.

4. Mulder, "Flabby Flesh," 146–50. Medical writers thought that these differences in male and female bodies were there from birth but became more

pronounced at puberty (Dean-Jones, "Cultural Construct of the Female Body," 187–88).

5. Hippocrates, *Diseases of Women* 1.1.

6. Lesley Dean-Jones ("Cultural Construct of the Female Body," 188) sums up the Hippocratic position on the female body thus: "The body of a mature woman was one big gland"—a spongy receptacle for excess fluid.

7. For an overview of the Greek and Roman obstetrical and gynecological texts, as well as their afterlives throughout the Mediterranean and Near East, see Lehmhaus, "Re-reading Gynaecology," 77–82.

8. Galen (*Prognosis* 14.649) says that it was Boethus and his other highly placed Roman friends who recommended him to the emperor Marcus Aurelius. Galen became the court physician in 168 CE. See Mattern, *Rhetoric of Healing* and *Prince of Medicine*, on Galen's relationship with Boethus and Marcus Aurelius.

9. Muir and Totelin, "Medicine and Disease," 86. On the legacy and use of Hippocratic texts in the Roman period, see Flemming, "Pathology of Pregnancy."

10. King, "Introduction." For a discussion of the Hippocratic gynecological texts and their philosophies of the female body, see Hanson, "'Diseases of Women,'" "Medical Writers' Woman," "Continuity and Change," and "Conception, Gestation"; Dean-Jones, *Women's Bodies*; King, *Hippocrates' Woman*; Flemming, *Making of Roman Women*; Totelin, *Hippocratic Recipes,* 197–224.

11. Hippocrates, *Nature of the Child* 3.

12. On the metaphor of bread-making, see Hippocrates, *Nature of the Child* 1; on the metaphorical significance of the womb as an oven and the fetus as a loaf of bread created by the baker/father, see duBois, *Sowing the Body,* 110–29. The metaphor of cheese-making comes from Aristotle (*Generation of Animals* 739b21–27), who expanded on the theories of generation found in the early Hippocratic writers; see also Totelin, "Eating of Curds" and "Breastmilk in the Cave," 244. In this analogy, the pregnant woman provides the milk (menstrual blood), the man provides the rennet (sperm), and the fetus is the cheese that results from the mixing of the two. Galen picks up this cheese-making analogy in *Semen* 2.5.30–31.

13. Hippocrates, *Nature of the Child* 9: at puberty, a passage forms in young women for the menses and the sperm; see also Hippocrates, *Generation* 2.

14. Scullin, "'She's Only a 4.'"

15. Martin, "Contradictions of Masculinity," 102–4.

16. Mattern (*Rhetoric of Healing,* 173–202) has a detailed chart of Galen's case histories.

17. Mattern, *Rhetoric of Healing,* 116–27.

18. Galen's writings about female bodies include texts dealing with some limited aspects of reproductive anatomy, conception, fetal development, and childbirth: *The Anatomy of the Uterus, The Shaping of the Embryo, Semen,* chapters 14 and 15 of *The Function of the Parts of the Human Body,* and his *Commentary on Hippocrates's Epidemics.*

19. About twenty-five of the patients in Galen's text are female, around fifteen of whom he represents as being his own patients (Mattern, *Rhetoric of Healing,* 112).

20. Von Staden, "Apud Nos," 273.

21. Celsus (*On Medicine* 4.27) recommends bloodletting for uterine complaints and Aretaeus (*On Cures for Acute Diseases* 2.10.3) recommends it for hysterical suffocation and the wandering womb. On bloodletting more generally, see the translation of Celsus, *On Medicine* 2.10–11, in Upson-Saia et al., *Medicine, Health, and Healing,* 231–34.

22. On blood collecting and putrefying in the uterus, see Hippocrates, *Nature of the Child* 4.

23. Soranus, *Gynecology* 4.1; Mulder, "Flabby Flesh," 153.

24. King, *Hippocrates' Woman,* 26; Hanson, "Hippocratic *Parthenos,*" 48.

25. King, *Hippocrates' Woman,* 23: "A major concern of the Hippocratic gynecology is the transformation of immature girls into reproductive women."

26. On the wandering womb, see Hanson, "Continuity and Change" and "Conception, Gestation"; Dean-Jones, *Women's Bodies*; Demand, *Birth, Death*; Adair, "Plato's View"; King, *Hippocrates' Woman*; Faraone, "Ancient Greek Exorcisms" and "Magical and Medical Approaches"; Dasen, "Healing Images"; Freidin, "Animal Wombs"; Wright, *Psychiatry.*

27. On uterine suffocation, see King, "Once Upon a Text"; Mattern, "Panic and Culture."

28. Hippocrates, *Diseases of Women* 2.14.

29. Hippocrates, *Diseases of Women* 1.2, 1.7, 2.15, 2.18, 2.20, 2.23–25, 2.35–36. On womb movements in Hippocratic writings, see Hanson, "Continuity and Change"; Dean-Jones, *Women's Bodies,* 69–77; and King, *Hippocrates' Woman,* 35–37.

30. Hippocrates, *Diseases of Women* 1.2, 1.7.

31. On the use of cupping vessels in antiquity, see Bliquez, *Tools of Asclepius,* 25–27, 56–72. On the widespread comparison of women's bodies and wombs to containers and vessels in the ancient world, see Lehmhaus, "Re-reading Gynaecology."

32. Bubb, "Ancient Conceptions."

33. On the uterus as octopus, see Freidin, "Animal Wombs." On the octopus metaphor in the ancient world more generally, see Coughlin et al, *Soul Is an Octopus.*

34. Plato, *Timaeus* 91a-d.

35. Dasen, *Sourire d'Omphale,* 57; Freidin, "Animal Wombs," 77n6. Other writers explained the wandering of the womb as a search for moisture: Hippocrates, *Diseases of Women* 1.7 and *Nature of Women* 3; Hanson, "Continuity and Change," 82–83; Dean-Jones, *Women's Bodies,* 71; Freidin, "Animal Wombs," 78.

36. Hanson, "Continuity and Change," 82.

37. Soranus, *Gynecology* 1.15.

38. On uterine prolapse in the ancient medical texts, see Hippocrates, *Diseases of Women* 1.2; Aretaeus, *On the Causes of Acute Diseases* 2.11.1; Aretaeus, *On the Causes of Chronic Diseases* 2.11.9–10; Soranus, *Gynecology* 4.35–39. For discussion of uterine prolapse and the wandering womb, see Dean-Jones, *Women's Bodies,* 71, 76–77; King, *Hippocrates' Woman,* 37; Dasen, "Métamorphoses de l'Utérus," 177, and *Sourire d'Omphale,* 74; Freidin, "Animal Wombs," 83.

39. Soranus, *Gynecology* 4.36; Freidin, "Animal Wombs," 83–84.

40. Hippocrates, *Generation* 9.

41. Von Staden, *Herophilus*; Bubb, *Dissection in Classical Antiquity,* 37–41.

42. Von Staden, *Herophilus,* 517–18; Bubb, *Dissection in Classical Antiquity.*

43. Bubb, *Dissection in Classical Antiquity.*

44. Aretaeus, *On the Causes of Chronic Diseases* 2.11.9.

45. Soranus, *Gynecology* 1.8.

46. Soranus, *Gynecology* 3.29.

47. Soranus, *Gynecology* 1.4 (the ideal midwife is "free from superstition"); 2.11 (midwives are superstitious and refuse to use iron blades to cut the umbilical cord); 2.19 (the ideal wet nurse "should not be superstitious").

48. Aretaeus, *On the Causes of Acute Diseases* 2.11.1–3, 5; *On the Causes of Chronic Diseases* 2.11.9–11; *On Cures for Acute Diseases* 2.10.1–3.

49. Hippocrates, *Diseases of Women* 2.14.

50. Hippocrates, *Diseases of Women* 2.24.

51. As part of a remedy for uterine prolapse, Soranus (*Gynecology* 4.38.3) writes, "Very hot cupping vessels should be applied near the navel on each side and sweet-smelling scents held continuously up to the nose."

52. Soranus, *Gynecology* 3.29; King, *Hippocrates' Woman,* 23.

53. Soranus, *Gynecology* 3.50.

54. A later Latin translation of Soranus's *Gynecology* (originally composed in Greek) by the North African physician Muscio (late 5th to early 6th century)

returns to a more traditional idea of the wandering womb. Departing from Soranus, Muscio explains that the womb can rise "up to the chest" (*Gynaecia* 130; translation is from Bolton, "Mustio's *Gynaecia*"). Similarly, another late Latin adaptation of Soranus by another North African physician, Theodorus Priscianus, advocates explicitly for odor therapy as a remedy for uterine suffocation (*Euporiston* 3.2.230.1–3). By the 11th century, the version of Soranus's *Gynecology* that trickled back to southern Italy (by way of Muscio's *Gynaecia*) had completely reincorporated odor therapy; it contains a detailed recipe for a uterine fumigation. See analysis in Hanson and Green, "Soranus of Ephesus," 1051–55.

55. Galen, *Affected Places* 6.5.

56. Galen, *Affected Places* 6.5. "Hysterical" in this context does not refer to a psychological condition as it does today, but to a physiological affliction of the uterus; see King, "Once Upon a Text."

57. Galen, *Affected Places* 6.5; translation is from Siegel, *Galen on the Affected Parts.*

58. For analysis of this passage and Galen's use of Hippocratic therapies, see Green, "Female Physiology and Disease," 46–53, and King, *Hippocrates' Woman,* 232–33.

59. Galen, *Affected Places* 6.5; for analysis of this passage, see King, "Galen and the Widow."

60. In this story the practitioner is a *maia,* "midwife."

61. For Galen's recommendation of odor therapy for a rising womb, see *The Therapeutic Method, to Glaucon* 1.15, and *The Composition of Drugs According to Places* K13.320. These passages are discussed in King, *Hippocrates' Woman,* 233, and Green, "Female Physiology and Disease," 50. Compare also to Galen, *Semen* 1.4.21: "The uterus, because of its desire for the . . . semen, goes to meet it, the whole uterus rushing toward the vagina and using its neck, like the esophagus, as a kind of hand that helps to propel the semen"; translation adapted from De Lacy's in Galen, *On Semen.*

62. On root cutters, see Lloyd, *Science, Folklore,* 119–35; Upson-Saia et al., *Medicine, Health, and Healing,* 238–39. On the variety of providers available, see Israelowich, *Patients and Healers*; Nutton, *Ancient Medicine.*

63. On the overlapping systems of healthcare and the medical marketplace, see Marx-Wolf, "Religion, Medicine, and Health," 514–16.

64. At the time of writing, there are 190 uterine amulets catalogued in the Campbell Bonner Magical Gems database: http://cbd.mfab.hu/visitatori_salutem.

65. On the manufacture of the uterine amulets, see Marino, "Setting the Womb," 284. On the carving methods used on these types of amulets and other

small carved objects in ancient Egypt, see Gwinnett and Gorelick, "Beads, Scarabs."

66. Soranus, *Gynecology* 1.63.

67. Galen, *Simple Drugs* K12.207; translation in Faraone, *Transformation of Greek Amulets,* 152. See also Bonner, *Studies in Magical Amulets,* 54; Gourevitch, "Popular Medicines," 265–66.

68. On the iconography of the uterine amulets, see Marino, "Setting the Womb"; Dasen, *Sourire d'Omphale*; Tsatsou, "Uterine Amulets" (who suggests that some of these amulets could have been used by men to erotically influence women); Freidin, "Animal Wombs."

69. Aubert, "Threatened Wombs," 449; Michel, *Die magischen Gemmen,* 75–88; Dasen, "Métamorphoses de l'Utérus," 173–75, "Femmes à tiroir," 134, "Représenter l'invisible," 46–47, "Healing Images," 181, and *Sourire d'Omphale,* 68–72; Faraone, *Vanishing Acts,* 46.

70. Bonner (*Studies in Magical Amulets,* 90–92) was the first to identify this symbol as an octopus-style uterus; see also Marino, "Setting the Womb," 152–58; Dasen, *Sourire d'Omphale,* 72–77; Freidin, "Animal Wombs," 79–83. The fact that these octopus-style uteruses do not actually have eight legs does not negate the identification. The word for octopus in ancient Greek was *poplypus,* simply meaning "many legs," and the animal was thought to have a variable number of tentacles, not strictly eight (Freidin, "Animal Wombs," 81).

71. On the meaning of Ororiouth, see Marino, "Setting the Womb," 95–97.

72. Bonner, *Studies in Magical Amulets,* 85; Marino, "Setting the Womb," 131–32, 120–25 (Isis); Dasen, *Sourire d'Omphale,* 64–65, 130–31 (Khnoum); Dasen, "Femmes à tiroir," 134, and "Représenter l'Invisible," 60 (baby Horus); Bonner, *Studies in Magical Amulets,* 9–60; Delatte and Derchain, *Intailles magiques,* 56 (Chnoubis).

73. Goff, *Symbols of Ancient Egypt,* 173; Dasen, "Femmes à tiroir," 134; Marino, "Setting the Womb," 139–44.

74. "Womb, retract!," CBd 225 and CBd 750; "Therapy for the womb," CBd 3410; compare to CBd 3430: "protect Selukia from the uterus." For discussion of these amulets, see Marino, "Setting the Womb," 100–101; Freidin, "Animal Wombs," 78–79.

75. On women and children as the primary users of amulets, see Faraone, *Transformation of Greek Amulets,* 27–28, 47–48, 78, 252–53.

76. Hanson, "Uterine Amulets," 287–90; Faraone, *Transformation of Greek Amulets,* 79–101, 253–54.

77. Galen, *Prognosis* 8.

78. In the Hippocratic *Diseases of Women* 1.65, the writer advises giving a woman suffering from the female flux a vaginal wash with acrid, emollient, and astringent substances. He provides a recipe for a vaginal ointment that includes willow weed, field basil, and honey, as well as a recipe for a drink that includes toasted linseed, sesame seed, butter, goat cheese, barley meal, and wine. See also *Diseases of Women* 1.49, 57, 58 on the advisement of astringent vaginal and uterine cleanses for fluxes and uterine ulcerations.

79. On the issues with retrospective diagnosis, see Graumann and Horstmanshoff, "'This I Suffered'"; Marx-Wolf, "Religion, Medicine, and Health," 512–13; Upson-Saia et al., *Medicine, Health, and Healing,* 12, 208. The chapters in Laes et al., *Disabilities in Roman Antiquity,* are also instructive on this matter, especially the introduction and those by Gevert and Laes, Goodey and Rose, and Graumann.

3. THE SELF-OBSERVANT WOMEN GET PREGNANT

1. Hippocrates, *Nature of the Child* 2.

2. Hippocrates was from the Aegean Island of Kos, near the coast of modern Türkiye (Turkey), and was active in the late 5th century, so I have set the episode here in 410 BCE. I have named her Demetria since this was a common name for women in ancient Greece and it is well-attested on Kos (Sherwin-White, *Ancient Kos*).

3. Galen, *Semen* 1.2.5–9.

4. The phrase that Galen uses here translates to something like "women of the sort who seemed to pay more attention to themselves." *Semen* 1.2.5.

5. Galen, *Semen* 1.4.28–33.

6. Hippocrates, *Nature of the Child* 2. The writer of the text says that this embryo came out after being "in the mother for six days." It would, however, be impossible to see a six-day-old embryo with the naked eye. Based on the description in the text, this embryo may have been between one and two months old and a quarter to one inch long. If this episode is real and not just a story, then it's likely that the enslaved singing girl got pregnant earlier than she thought she did or said that she was less far along than she was.

7. Galen, *Semen* 1.3.1–8; 1.3.13.

8. Galen (*Semen* 1.3.5) quotes Aristotle to agree with him that conception is like rennet or fig juice (semen) setting milk (menstrual fluid) into cheese (fetus).

9. Galen, *Semen* 1.5.1–7. The semen was also thought to form the bones and membranes—essentially it was responsible for anything white or translucent

in the body (*Semen* 1.10.1; also 1.11.1–2: "For all the fleshy parts were generated from blood; but all the membranous parts come from semen").

10. On female seed in ancient Greek medical texts, see Flemming, "One Seed, Two Seed," and Mulder, "Flabby Flesh." On Galen's theory of female seed, see Nickel, *Untersuchungen zur Embryologie Galens,* 29–49; De Lacy in Galen, *On Semen,* 47–51; Connell, "Sex Difference and Reproduction," 410–14.

11. Galen, *Semen* 1.2.1. Elsewhere, Galen writes about dissecting pregnant goats, sometimes while the goats were still living (Mattern, *Prince of Medicine,* 151–52).

12. Galen, *Semen* 1.2.10–11.

13. Galen, *Semen* 1.2.12.

14. Galen, *Semen* 1.7.8–12. Freidin ("Animal Wombs," 84–85) shows that the connection was not just metaphorical—the uterus was thought to have the same kind of suckers as an octopus, with which it held onto the semen and then the embryo.

15. Aristotle famously refers to the female as "a deformed male" (*Generation of Animals* 737a27–30); Connell, *Aristotle on Female Animals,* 118; Mulder, "Flabby Flesh," 150–51; Flemming, "One Seed, Two Seed," 164–65.

16. Galen (*Semen* 2.5.29–32) compares the forming embryo to curdling milk setting into cheese and to wet clay or wax being shaped by a molder.

17. On the themes of fluidity in fetal sex determination, see Mulder, "Flabby Flesh," 146–47, 150–51.

18. Galen, *The Function of the Parts of the Human Body* 14.6–7. He espouses a similar idea at *Semen* 2.5.41–52. Helen King (*One-Sex Body on Trial,* 35) calls this a "thought experiment," and Patricia Simons (*Sex of Men,* 147) refers to it as "an introductory teaching device." Thomas Laqueur ran with the idea of a pre-modern "one-sex" body that at some point in the early modern period become a "two-sex" body, but his hypothesis has been soundly challenged, comprehensively by Helen King (*One-Sex Body on Trial*) and recently by Brooke Holmes ("Let Go of Laqueur"), among others.

19. Vesalius, unlike most other anatomists of the early modern period, was unusually involved in crafting the images that accompanied his text, suggesting that he "believed in the power of images to create anatomical knowledge" (Kusukawa, *Anatomy and the World of Books,* 129).

20. Galen's anatomical ideas, based on animal dissections, persisted for centuries after the beginning of human dissection in the 14th century (Park, *Secrets of Women*).

21. My favorite essay on genital homology and evolution is Stephen J. Gould, "Male Nipples and Clitoral Ripples."

22. Galen (*Semen* 2.1.1–6) imagines that female semen, like male semen, collects in the testicles (the name that Galen gives to the ovaries as well as the male testicles) and is depleted during sex, as "the female discharges semen not externally, like the male, but into its own uterus." There is no understanding of the ova or the process of ovulation.

23. Galen (*Semen* 2.5.53–69) explains the underdevelopment of the female genitals through two analogies: the underdevelopment of teeth in newborn humans and the underdevelopment of eyes in moles. In both cases, there is not sufficient heat in the uterus to cause the teeth and eyes to "pop" out.

24. On nocturnal emissions of semen in women as in men, see Galen, *Semen* 2.1.25, 2.1.34.

25. The logic is circular. In *Semen* (2.4.13) Galen explains, "The female would not even desire sexual union apart from having testicles and semen." The existence of sexual pleasure in women proves the existence of their semen and testicles (cervical fluid and ovaries); the existence of their semen and testicles (by analogy with male bodies) proves the existence of sexual pleasure in women.

26. This translation is adapted from the one in Gellar-Goad, "Todd Akin."

27. Gellar-Goad, "Todd Akin."

28. This the *Laudatio Turiae* ("Praise of Turia") (Osgood, *Turia,* 156–69). Her name is missing from the inscription. She is commonly called Turia based on an initial identification of her with Turia, the wife of Quintus Lucretius Vespillo, some of whose biographical details fit those of the man who dedicated the inscription. But this identification has been discredited (Osgood, *Turia,* 117–24). However, "Turia" is how she is still widely known among scholars.

29. This and all translations hereafter are from Osgood, *Turia.*

30. (Pseudo) Aristotle, *History of Animals* 10.633b; Muscio, *Gynaecia* 2.16; Oribasius, *Medical Collections* 6.38. See discussion in Hug, *Fertility, Ideology,* 53–54.

31. Flemming, "Invention of Infertility," 571; Totelin, "Whose Fault," 57–58.

32. Hippocrates, *Superfetation* 30, with discussion in Totelin, *Hippocratic Recipes,* 198–99. Lucretius (*On the Nature of Things* 4.1233–47) gives a medical account of male infertility: sperm that is too thick or too runny and thin. Either way, it cannot properly reach the uterus and mingle with the female semen. Understanding of male infertility outside of the medical texts is confined to impotence, which was the subject of ridicule (Hug, *Fertility, Ideology,* 55–58).

33. Flemming, "Invention of Infertility," 571; also Hug (*Fertility, Ideology,* 55) on the remedies of Pliny the Elder.

34. Flemming, "Invention of Infertility," 573–74.

35. Hippocrates, *Diseases of Women* 1.10–24.

36. Hippocrates, *Diseases of Women* 1.2.

37. Hippocrates, *Diseases of Women* 1.17.

38. Hippocrates, *Diseases of Women* 1.2; compare to Hippocrates, *Barrenness* 1.

39. Hippocrates, *Diseases of Women* 1.10. On the phrases used to indicate sexual intercourse as a treatment for gynecological issues (for example, "let her go to her husband"), see Totelin, *Hippocratic Recipes,* 200n9. On intercourse as a treatment, see Dean-Jones, "Politics of Pleasure," 60–61; King, "Sowing the Field," 34–35.

40. For uterine suffocation, see Hippocrates, *Diseases of Women* 1.2, 7.

41. Hippocrates, *Girls* 468–70 (Potter edition); see also Flemming and Hanson, "Hippocrates' *Peri Parthenión*," 250.41–43, with discussion in Totelin, *Hippocratic Recipes,* 200. On the history of this disease of virgins from antiquity to the 20th century, see King, *The Disease of Virgins.*

42. Hippocrates, *Diseases of Women* 1.10; *Barrenness* 1.

43. Hippocrates, *Diseases of Women* 1.11.

44. Hippocrates, *Diseases of Women* 1.13.

45. Hippocrates, *Diseases of Women* 1.12; in *Barrenness* 1, the Hippocratic writer explains that smooth uterine walls can also be caused by ulcers—the prognosis for fertility is not good.

46. Hippocrates, *Diseases of Women* 1.9, 11.

47. Hippocrates, *Diseases of Women* 1.8.

48. Hippocrates, *Diseases of Women* 1.8; compare to Hippocrates, *Barrenness* 1: "If the woman receives treatment at the start of the illness, she will recover and become fertile. But if time has passed, she will remain barren."

49. Laurence Totelin (*Hippocratic Recipes,* 24) has pointed out that the treatments in the Hippocratic text *Barrenness* are "extremely long." They would have required dedicated medical attention over many months or even years. See also Totelin, "Whose Fault."

50. Hippocrates, *Barrenness* 243; see discussion in Flemming "Invention of Infertility," 574.

51. Hippocrates, *Superfetation* 29, with discussion in Totelin, *Hippocratic Recipes,* 198–99.

52. Flemming, "Invention of Infertility," 574.

53. There is some discussion in antiquity of certain stones, like the magnetite used in this fertility treatment, being alive—having breath and soul. See discussion and references in Dasen, *Sourire d'Omphale,* 37–38.

54. On sympathy, see Holmes, "Proto-Sympathy"; Freidin, *Birthing Romans,* 76–88.

55. On the different understandings of sympathy in medicine, philosophy, religion, and magic, see Freidin, *Birthing Romans,* 177, 182. As she explains (182), "Soranus uses sympathy to understand affections *within* the body (that is, among its parts), but expresses skepticism about sympathy and antipathy *between* bodies."

56. On magic in the ancient world, see Frankfurter, *Study of Ancient Magic.*

57. Olive oil as medicine: Dioscorides, *Medical Materials* 1.3; olive leaf as an amulet: *Greek Magical Papyri* 7.213–14.

58. In his *Natural History,* Pliny the Elder includes a mixture of remedies that might be defined—according to us as well as to ancient physicians like Galen and Soranus—as medical and magical. On Pliny's inclusion of magical practices, see Lloyd, *Science, Folklore,* 140.

59. *Greek Magical Papyri* 7.211–12. This translation is from Betz, *Greek Magical Papyri.*

60. This idea has also been called "persuasive analogy" (Freidin, *Birthing Romans,* 180n45). The breast milk of a nursing (that is, fertile) woman *persuades* the body of the infertile woman to become fertile. On the symbolism of ingredients used to treat infertility in the Hippocratic gynecology, see Totelin, *Hippocratic Recipes,* 197–224.

61. Similarly, an amniotic sac is used in a recipe for conception at Hippocrates, *Diseases of Women* 1.75: "Crush a woman's amniotic sac and the heads of worms, dilute Egyptian alum in goose fat; have her apply this mixture in wool to the mouth of her uterus." See discussion in Totelin, *Hippocratic Recipes,* 200. On the medical and magical uses of breast milk and menstrual blood, see Pedrucci, "Use of Breast Milk."

62. For more on squirting cucumber, see Freidin, *Birthing Romans,* 178–80. Fertile parts of animals were used similarly, for example, stag's penis (Hippocrates, *Barrenness* 224) and beaver testicles (Hippocrates, *Barrenness* 221). See discussion in Totelin, *Hippocratic Recipes,* 200–201n11.

63. These remedies were called the *Dreckapotheke,* literally "filthy pharmacy." On the *Dreckapotheke,* see Totelin, *Hippocratic Recipes,* 212–14.

64. Both of these recipes can be found in Hippocrates, *Diseases of Women* 1.89.

65. Totelin, *Hippocratic Recipes,* 213; Hanson ("Talking Recipes," 89) points out that recipes attributed to Cleopatra in Galen involve using dung to treat baldness—another instance of fertilizing. Instead of the "filthy pharmacy" cures having a fertilizing effect, Heinrich von Staden ("Women and Dirt") suggested that they may have been intended to have a purifying effect on female bodies, which were considered to be inherently filthy. In this case, like was intended to drive out like; the dung got rid of women's dirtiness and impurity.

66. On the question of where the recipes in the Hippocratic texts came from and whether they were authored by women or men, see Rousselle, "Observation féminine"; Muir and Totelin, "Medicine and Disease," 85–86.

67. Flemming, "Invention of Infertility," 574.

68. On the distinction drawn by ancient male medical writers between women who are experienced and women who are inexperienced, see Muir and Totelin, "Medicine and Disease," 84–85.

69. Juno Lucina means either "Juno of the light" or "Juno who brings to light." As to other gods that could be petitioned for help, Maureen Carroll (*Infancy and Earliest Childhood,* 18) explains, "It appears that just about any Etruscan, Italic or cross-cultural deity could cure a wide range of diseases or assist in bodily matters"; dedications related to fertility have been found at sanctuaries devoted to the male gods Apollo, Mars, and Hercules.

70. Dasen, "Femmes à tiroir," 129.

71. Ducaté-Paarmann, "Voyage à l'Intérieur," 71; Graham, "Making of Infants," 222.

72. Dioscorides, *Medical Materials* 2.100 (darnel); 3.52 (wild carrot).

73. Pliny the Elder, *Natural History* 28.253 (cow's milk); 30.43 (snails in saffron); Dioscorides, *Medical Materials* 3.56 (anise); 4.93 (stinging nettle seed); 3.128 (root of the man orchid)—here, too, the lines between medicine and magic are blurred, as Dioscorides writes, "The root [of the man orchid] is said to be aphrodisiac even when held in the hand but more so when drunk with wine" (translation adapted from Beck, *Dioscorides*).

74. Hug, *Fertility, Ideology,* 58–60.

75. Cicero (*On Divination* 2.145) records this anecdote to disparage the practice of dream interpretation. See the discussion in Hug, *Fertility, Ideology,* 59–60.

76. Pliny the Elder, *Natural History* 28.97. This remedy isn't much different than the herbal remedies supplied by the doctors and root cutters, except for the exotic ingredient of the hyena's eye. Hyenas were thought to be sexually virile and voracious creatures (as well as hermaphroditic; see Totelin, "Animal and Plant Generation," 58), so the inclusion of its eye in this remedy is intended to bring that quality to the infertile woman—a manipulation of sympathy. In a more clearly magical application of the hyena's power, a man who wears a hyena's anus on his left arm as an amulet can attract the erotic attention of any woman he looks at (Pliny the Elder, *Natural History* 28.106). On the magical uses of hyenas in Pliny the Elder, see Ogden, *Magic, Witchcraft,* 46–48.

77. It was magical spells in particular—spoken or written—that doctors like Galen and Soranus criticized as ineffective. For example, see Galen, *Simple*

Drugs K 12.251–52, with translation and discussion in Salvo, "Owners of Their Own Bodies."

78. *Digest* 48.8; *Opinions of Paulus* 5.23.

79. Salvo, "Owners of Their Own Bodies"; for an image of this curse tablet, see Nasrallah, *Ancient Christians,* 2, with further discussion at 192–98.

80. For full translations of the tablets, see Salvo, "Owners of Their Own Bodies," and Nasrallah, *Ancient Christians,* 193.

81. These magical elements would have been copied from a handbook (Salvo, "Owners of Their Own Bodies").

82. On possible interpretations of the story behind these tablets and the relationship between Karpimē Babbia and the writer of the tablets, see Salvo, "Owners of Their Own Bodies." Perhaps the writer was jealous of Karpimē Babbia's fertility, or maybe Karpimē Babbia had ridiculed her infertility. Maybe it was some kind of exchange, offering up another woman's fertility in exchange for her own. The logic of the curse fits the "envy" pattern identified by Ripat ("Roman Women") as being characteristic of women's "folk" healing practices—envy manifests as a physical, destructive force against the one who is envied.

83. These curse tablets are from a Greek-speaking part of the Roman Empire and date to about a century later than Turia lived, but they do show a kind of magical practice that was spreading throughout the Mediterranean.

84. Hippocrates, *Barrenness* 29.

85. Vaginal clyster: Hippocrates, *Barrenness* 10 (however, the author of the treatise recommends this especially for women who had previously gotten pregnant but were no longer able to, which does not seem to be Turia's situation); see Bliquez (*Tools of Asclepius,* 45–46, 208–13) on the various tubes used to treat gynecological conditions, including metal clysters, reeds, and long-necked gourds.

86. Hippocrates, *Barrenness* 9.

4. CONTROLLING CONCEPTION

1. There are a number of lost treatises on obstetrics, gynecology, and reproductive anatomy that were produced between the time of the Hippocratics and Soranus, including a treatise called *Midwifery* by Herophilus (4th to 3rd century BCE) that Soranus cites. It is possible that some of the shifts I am about to describe occurred earlier and we see them first in Soranus because his text is what survives. However, I do think the distinctly pronatalist context of

Rome is a good reason to suspect that what Soranus was doing was unique and unprecedented. On this point, see Freidin, *Birthing Romans,* chapter 3. On elite Roman men as the audience for Soranus's text, see Hanson and Green, "Soranus of Ephesus," 1027, and Flemming, *Making of Roman Women,* 232; on Soranus's optimal reproduction, see Freidin, "Well-Born."

2. Much has been written about the medicalization and pathologization of childbirth in the 19th to 21st centuries. The work of Jacqueline Wolf (*Deliver Me* and *Cesarean Section*) has particularly informed my thinking.

3. Hanson and Green, "Soranus of Ephesus."

4. For analysis of Soranus and his *Gynecology,* see Freidin, *Birthing Romans,* 123–65; on Soranus's works more broadly, as well as on his afterlife in late antiquity and the Middle Ages, see Hanson and Green, "Soranus of Ephesus"; Flemming, *Making of Roman Women,* 228–46.

5. Green, "'Cliff Notes.'"

6. King, "Motherhood and Health."

7. Soranus, *Gynecology* 1.42 (effects of pregnancy) and 1.30: "Pregnancy and birth exhaust the female body and make it waste away, while virginity, which protects women from such injuries, can be considered healthful." As Rebecca Flemming ("Pathology of Pregnancy," 106) has pointed out, Galen, too, highlighted the "pathological potential" of pregnancy, but he didn't take it as far as Soranus.

8. Soranus, *Gynecology* 1.42.

9. Freidin, *Birthing Romans,* 124.

10. Anna Bonnell Freidin (*Birthing Romans,* 124) explains, "The *Gynecology* promises to diminish the harm resulting from the 'natural' processes of pregnancy, birth, and nursing, advertising specific skills and expertise, *technê,* as an antidote to risk (or *tuchê*)."

11. Hippocrates, *Barrenness* 2; *Diseases of Women* 1.78; *Nature of Women* 96. For Soranus's critique of this method, see *Gynecology* 1.35.

12. Hippocrates, *Nature of Women* 99. This rather confusing passage in Hippocrates is explained by Aristotle, *Generation of Animals* 2.7 (747a7–14). See discussion in Totelin, *Hippocratic Recipes,* 103. Essentially, if the red from the stone transferred from eyes to saliva, it meant the passageways of the body were open, including the vagina and cervix.

13. Soranus, *Gynecology* 1.34.

14. Soranus, *Gynecology* 1.34.

15. Soranus, *Gynecology* 1.34.

16. Freidin (*Birthing Romans,* 140) writes, "Although unstated, Soranus' guidance suggests that a practitioner should not only question but physically

examine a prospective bride." Helen King ("Risky Business") is dubious that any physical examinations of the vagina or cervix would have taken place.

17. Soranus, *Gynecology* 1.34.

18. Soranus (*Gynecology* 1.41) disparages those who connect the waxing moon with growth and increased fertility and the waning moon with decreased fertility. He also criticizes the view that certain seasons are better for conceptions—for example, Hippocrates, *Superfetation* 30: "Spring is the best time for getting pregnant."

19. Soranus, *Gynecology* 1.36.

20. Soranus, *Gynecology* 1.37.

21. Soranus, *Gynecology* 1.38.

22. Soranus, *Gynecology* 1.40.

23. Soranus, *Gynecology* 1.40.

24. Soranus, *Gynecology* 1.40.

25. Soranus, *Gynecology* 1.38.

26. My thanks to Heidi Marx for this explanation of *pneuma*. For *pneuma* in Galen, see Rocca, "Pneuma as a Holistic Concept"; for *pneuma* in the embryology of the 3rd-century philosopher Porphyry, see Marx-Wolf, "Living Plants."

27. Soranus, *Gynecology* 1.39.

28. Soranus, *Gynecology* 1.39. Also called *ideoplasty* (Wilberding, "Porphyry and Plotinus," 421, and *Porphyry: To Gaurus,* 68).

29. Pliny the Elder (*Natural History* 7.52) explained that the effects of *ideoplasty* could be accidental, since the fetus could even be affected by a woman's recollection of sights and sounds, not just things she saw and felt at the moment of conception.

30. Soranus, *Gynecology* 2.9, 2.10.

31. Porphyry, *To Gaurus on How Embryos Are Ensouled* 10.5.1–6.9. See discussion in Wilberding, "Porphyry and Plotinus," and *Porphyry: To Gaurus.*

32. Cambron-Goulet and Côté-Remy, "Plotinus and Porphyry."

33. Porphyry addressed his treatise, *To Marcella*, to his wife. See the translation in Wicker, *Porphyry the Philosopher.*

34. Soranus, *Gynecology* 1.44.

35. These symptoms of early pregnancy are all listed in Pliny the Elder, *Natural History* 7.43. In Aristotle, the signs of conception are felt by the women themselves: "Women have evidence of conception when the place is dry after intercourse" (*History of Animals* 9 (7) 583a15–16), and "After conceiving, they have a feeling, especially in their flanks" (9 (7) 583a35); also, "After conception women feel weighed down throughout their whole body, and have clouded vision and headaches" (9 (7) 584a3–5).

36. Soranus, *Gynecology* 1.44.

37. Soranus, *Gynecology* 1.44.

38. Soranus, *Gynecology* 1.44; this translation is based on Temkin, *Soranus' Gynecology*. While the Hippocratic texts offered many remedies to cure infertility and promote conception, they did not enumerate the signs that conception had occurred. The one exception is Hippocrates, *Superfetation* 16, which I suspect may be a much later text than the majority of the Hippocratic writings, perhaps as late as the 2nd century CE. It reads, "That a woman is pregnant, if you do not recognize it otherwise: her eyes are compressed and become more hollow than usual, and their whites do not have the natural whiteness, but are more livid."

39. Soranus, *Gynecology* 1.44.

40. The *mole* is described in detail in Soranus, *Gynecology* 3.36–39.

41. Pliny the Elder, *Natural History* 7.63.

42. Soranus, *Gynecology* 3.37. However, according to Porphyry (*To Gaurus* 12.6) sometimes the *mole* could move, deceiving the midwives.

43. Soranus, *Gynecology* 3.37.

44. Soranus, *Gynecology* 3.38.

45. Galen, *Semen* 1.2.6. Translation is from De Lacy, *On Semen*.

46. Freidin, "Animal Wombs," 77.

47. Freidin, "Animal Wombs," 80–83.

48. Marino, "Setting the Womb," 157–58.

49. Freidin ("Animal Wombs," 82) points out that when the octopus-style uterus and the cupping-vessel–style uterus appear on an amulet together, there is a "parallel between the number of bits on the key and legs on the octopus symbol" that suggests "that the two symbols are connected."

50. Soranus, *Gynecology* 3.29.

51. On women's bodies as fields in ancient Greek thought, see duBois, *Sowing the Body,* 39–85; throughout the Mediterranean and Near East, see Lehmhaus, "Re-reading Gynaecology," 7–13.

52. Soranus, *Gynecology* 1.35.

53. Soranus, *Gynecology* 1.36.

54. As Laurence Totelin ("Whose Fault," 60) puts it, "There was no such thing as a passive field in the ancient world." The earth was a goddess whose fruits were the result of her own sexual desires and instigations.

55. Galen, *The Anatomy of the Uterus* 890; Bubb, *Dissection in Classical Antiquity,* 276–78.

56. Galen, *The Shaping of the Embryo* 661, 668.

57. Galen, *Semen* 2.4.34.

58. Wilberding, "Porphyry and Plotinus," 424.

59. Porphyry, *To Gaurus* 5.4.

60. Hanson and Green, "Soranus of Ephesus." Soranus's *Gynecology* was translated into Latin by two North African medical writers: Caelius Aurelianus (late 4th to early 5th century) and Muscio (late 5th to early 6th century). A third late-Latin text called "Book of Gynecology for the Midwife Soteris" is a fabricated dialogue between the midwife Soteris and Soranus. And, finally, some of the material from Soranus appears in the medical text of a fourth North African native, Theodorus Priscianus (4th century).

5. CORINNA HAS AN ABORTION

1. Corinna was a pseudonym given to her by her boyfriend, Ovid. We don't know who the real Corinna was, though she was likely a prominent, well-known upper-class woman in Rome. Some scholars have taken her to be entirely fictitious, fabricated by Ovid so he could riff on contemporary concerns and play around with different genres and themes of Roman poetry—a stance that Ovid himself even seems to adopt in some of his poems (for discussion see Wyke, "Mistress and Metaphor in Augustan Elegy"; Sharrock, "Ovid and the Discourses of Love"; Heath, "Why Corinna?").

2. Ovid, *Amores* 2.13 and 2.14. On the military language of poem 2.14, see Hines, *Rome's Visceral Reactions*—mothers attack their wombs and fetuses with weapons, just like warriors attacking enemies on a battlefield.

3. Juvenal, *Satires* 6.592–601.

4. Tacitus, *Annals* 14.63.

5. Tacitus, *Germania* 19.5.

6. *Sibylline Oracles* 2.279–86; translation is from Lightfoot, *Sibylline Oracles.* This text is thought to have been revised by Christians sometime between 30 BCE and 250 CE. For discussion, see Mistry, *Abortion,* 23–24.

7. *Didache* 2.2.A8 (translation is by Milavec, *Didache*); Nifosi, *Becoming a Woman,* 142.

8. Tertullian, *Apology* 9.8; translation and discussion in Mistry, *Abortion,* 38–39.

9. *Digest* 48.8.8; this and all translations of the *Digest* in this chapter's notes are Watson's from *The Digest of Justinian.*

10. *Digest* 48.19.38.5; Nardi, *Procurato aborto,* 433–37.

11. On the law against aphrodisiacs, see *Digest* 48.19.38. On punishment for fertility drugs (in the case that the woman dies), see *Digest* 48.8.3; Gardiner, *Women in Roman Law,* 158–59; Richlin, *Arguments with Silence,* 258–59.

12. *Digest* 48.19.39.

13. Cicero, *In Defense of Cluentius* 32.

14. Hirt, "La législation romaine," 284.

15. *Digest* 25.4.1.1. For discussion, see Hirt, "La législation romaine," 281.

16. *Digest* 27.1.2.6; 5.4.3; 29.

17. *Digest* 1.5.7; see also 2.30.1, where the unborn heir is treated as already born and delays the inheritance claims of the heirs that come after him in line of succession.

18. *Digest* 25.4.1.1.

19. There are many sources in the law code for this; for example, *Digest* 28.2.4; 28.2.25.1; 28.2.27; 29.2.30.1; 29.5.4.

20. *Digest* 1.5.18; also 48.19.3, x14; *Opinions of Paulus* 1.13.5; see discussion in Hirt, "La législation romaine," 282.

21. This right is the *vitae necisque potestas* (literally "right of life and death"). See Westbrook, "Vitae Necisque Potestas."

22. *Digest* 5.3.27.pr.

23. *Digest* 44.2.7.1–3. However, the jurists also drew some distinctions between the children of enslaved women and other "fruits" *(fructus)*. See Huemoeller, *Child Follows the Womb.*

24. Dixon, *Roman Mother,* 17; Rawson, "Family Life."

25. On the drive of the Roman state to reproduce its free population, see Hug, *Fertility, Ideology.*

26. Theodorus Priscianus, *Euporiston* 3.6.23.

27. Soranus, *Gynecology* 1.60.

28. Soranus, *Gynecology* 1.61–65.

29. Soranus, *Gynecology* 1.36. Flemming ("Fertility Control," 899) suggests that Soranus's advice on the most fertile period is not as problematic as it seems given recent research on the variability of menstrual and ovulatory cycles.

30. Soranus, *Gynecology* 1.61.

31. Soranus, *Gynecology* 1.61.

32. Soranus, *Gynecology* 1.62–63.

33. On contraceptive amulets, see Dasen, *Sourire d'Omphale,* 42–44.

34. *Greek Magical Papyri* 63.26–28; translation is from Betz, *Greek Magical Papyri.* The bean was supposed to take the place of a potential fetus.

35. *Greek Magical Papyri* 22a 11–14; Soranus, *Gynecology* 1.63.

36. On abortifacient methods in the ancient world, see Riddle, *Contraception and Abortion* and *Eve's Herbs*; Kapparis, *Abortion.* Abortifacients can be found in the works of most ancient Greco-Roman medical writers, including the Hippocratics, Aristotle, Dioscorides, Pliny the Elder, Soranus, Galen, Theodorus Priscianus, and Aetius of Amida.

37. Demand, *Birth, Death,* 60; Richlin, *Arguments with Silence,* 258.

38. Riddle, *Contraception and Abortion,* 81; Hippocrates, *Fleshes* 19; Pliny the Elder, *Natural History* 28.81.

39. Dioscorides, *Medical Materials* 4.148 (white hellebore); 4.162 (black hellebore); 4.70 (scammony); 1.6 (cardamom); 2.155 (garden cress); 2.156 (shepherd's purse); 2.163 (soapwort). All of the translation of Dioscorides in this chapter are adapted from Beck, *Dioscorides.*

40. Soranus, *Gynecology* 1.64–65.

41. This argument about silphium's contraceptive and abortifacient properties (and its extinction) originates with Riddle, *Eve's Herbs.* Popular media ran with it. A recent example is from the dubious website Ancient Origins (Clemens, "Silphium").

42. Pollaro and Robertson, "Extinction of Silphium."

43. McDaniel, "Ancient Romans Didn't Overharvest."

44. Dioscorides, *Medical Materials* 3.80 (under the entry for "laserwort").

45. Hippocrates, *Superfetation* 27; see also *Diseases of Women* 1.46, where silphium is used to expel a retained placenta after childbirth.

46. Hippocrates, *Superfetation* 27.

47. Dioscorides, *Medical Materials* 3.45 (rue); 3.31 (pennyroyal); 3.39 (marjoram); 1.11 (Cretan spikenard); 3.36 (Cretan thyme); 3.35 (catmint); 4.93 (stinging nettle); 4.150 (squirting cucumber); 3.51 (lovage); 3.7 (common centaury; called "feverfew" by Beck, *Dioscorides*); 1.10 (hazelwort).

48. Dioscorides, *Medical Materials* 2.149 (leek); 2.151 (onion); 2.152 (garlic); 2.155 (garden cress); 2.112 (radish); 2.120 (cabbage); 1.28 (fig).

49. Dioscorides, *Medical Materials* 2.74 (lanolin, here called "fat from greasy wool"); 2.163 (soapwort).

50. Dioscorides, *Medical Materials* 1.64 (myrrh); 1.66 (storax).

51. Dioscorides, *Medical Materials* 2.136; also listed as both emmenagogues and abortifacients are garden cress (2.155), shepherd's purse (2.156), Hercules's woundwort (3.48), sagapenon (sagapenum) (3.81), white hellebore (4.148), black hellebore (4.162), common centaury (3.7).

52. Soranus, *Gynecology* 1.64 (as abortifacients); 3.32 (for treatment of air in the uterus).

53. Dioscorides, *Medical Materials* 1.105 (wild olive); 5.62 (wine flavored with allheal); 1.14 (cinnamon); 1.64 (myrrh); 1.1 (iris).

54. Dioscorides, *Medical Materials* 3.32.

55. Dioscorides, *Medical Materials* 1.19; unguent of marjoram "draws down the menses and the afterbirth" (1.48), as does unguent of wormwood (1.50).

56. Hippocrates, *Diseases of Women* 1.78.

57. Demand (*Birth, Death,* 58–59) distinguishes between therapeutic and elective abortions in the Hippocratic corpus. Therapeutic expulsives are used when the fetus has died, while abortifacients are meant to destroy the fetus.

58. Pliny the Elder, *Natural History* 34.165; Dasen, *Sourire d'Omphale,* 26.

59. The word that Pliny uses in this passage is *abortus,* which was ambiguous. It could mean abortion or miscarriage, though it likely means miscarriage in this context, since it is talking about a clearing-out, not a destroying.

60. Hippocrates, *Nature of Women* 94.

61. Dioscorides, *Medical Materials* 3.4.

62. This remedy for conception appears in manuscript *H* of Muscio's *Gynaecia.* The translation is adapted from Bolton, "Mustio's *Gynaecia,*" 421.

63. There are other herbs that Dioscorides identifies as being expulsive, emmenagogic, and aphrodisiac. That is, he makes explicit the connection between drawing down menses or fetuses and promoting conception—for example, 3.36 (leeks); 2.155 (garden cress); 3.52 (wild and cultivated carrot); 4.93 (stinging nettle); 2.109 (lupine).

64. Soranus, *Gynecology* 1.63.

65. Soranus, *Gynecology* 1.60.

66. Some herbs were explicitly listed as being emmenagogic, abortifacient, and expulsive. The entry in Dioscorides for Hercules's woundwort (3.48) explains that it "draws down the menses," "destroys fetuses," and "draws fetuses"; the fact that it lists all three of these actions suggests that they were understood to be different from one another. Nancy Demand (*Birth, Death,* 58–59) corroborates my skepticism about subterfuge; Monica Green (*The Trotula,* 222n144) makes the same argument about emmenagogues and fetal expulsives in the Trotula (a medieval collection of gynecological writings).

67. See, for example, King, *Hippocrates' Woman,* 132–56.

68. Sage-Femme Collective, *Natural Liberty.*

69. Totelin (*Hippocratic Recipes,* 223–24) points out that "efficacy" itself is a cultural construct. What does it mean for something to work? We cannot retroject our modern definitions—or expectations—onto antiquity.

70. Flemming ("Fertility Control," 897, 900–901) corroborates my analysis of efficacy.

71. Hippocrates, *Diseases of Women* 1.72.

72. Hippocrates, *Epidemics* 5.53. This same case is recorded also at *Epidemics* 7.74. The physician writes that the abortion happened "either from something she drank or spontaneously." See discussion in Demand, *Birth, Death,* 57–58.

73. Macrobius, *Saturnalia* 2.5.9; translation is from Richlin, *Arguments with Silence,* 261.

74. Velleius Paterculus, *History* 2.100; Seneca, *On Benefits* 6.32.

75. Soranus, *Gynecology* 1.60.

76. Mistry (*Abortion,* 34n53) collects the work of those scholars who posit an "abortion epidemic" among the Romans, including Nardi, *Procurato aborto.*

77. See, for example, Dixon, *Roman Mother,* 61–62.

78. See especially Frier, "Natural Fertility."

79. Mistry, *Abortion,* 33–34.

80. Ovid, *Amores* 3.14.27–28: "Women, why do you stab yourselves with sharp instruments and give poisons to your unborn children?"

81. Pliny the Elder, *Natural History* 10.172, with discussion in Mistry, *Abortion,* 32–33. For further discussion of abortion in Pliny, see Beagon, *Roman Nature,* 216–20; Flemming, *Making of Roman Women,* 161–69; Richlin, *Arguments with Silence,* 256–59. Like the medical writers, Pliny disapproves of abortion ("I do not discuss abortifacients," 25.25) but lists many abortifacient methods and recipes under the guise of warning against them.

82. Flemming ("Fertility Control," 901) argues that Soranus wanted to make methods of contraception and abortion "available to wives, under the pro-natalist banner." In this case, available to wives would have meant knowable to husbands, since husbands were the audience of Soranus's *Gynecology.*

83. As Flemming ("Fertility Control," 901) puts it, wives were expected to produce legitimate children, while sex workers were expected to "legitimate male sexual pleasure, a legitimacy that was predicated on the separation of the transaction from procreation." On the expectation (of elite men) that certain women were supposed to use contraceptives and abortifacients in order to maintain their appearance, see Hines, *Rome's Visceral Reactions.*

84. Flemming, "Fertility Control," 906: husbands determined whether to expose children or to take in exposed children—another form of fertility control.

6. PREGNANCY PROBLEMS AND PRENATAL CARE

1. Kristina Killgrove ("Pregnant Women"), one of the leaders of this excavation, wrote about the preliminary findings for *Forbes.*

2. Henneberg and Henneberg, "Skeletal Material"; Carroll, *Infancy and Earliest Childhood,* 61.

3. On the work of bioarchaeologists, see Killgrove, "Bioarchaeology."

4. Malaria, when present in pregnant people, can cause anemia in the fetus and the related issue of *cribra orbitalia*—porous bone in the upper part of the eye socket. This condition has been found in infant skeletal remains in Roman Britain and in Roman-era Ravenna and Rimini, on the northeast coast of Italy (Lewis, "Disease and Trauma"). *Cribra orbitalia* has also been linked to weaning practices, when iron-deficient and absorption-inhibiting cereals replaced breastmilk (Carroll, *Infancy and Earliest Childhood,* 66–67).

5. On what has been learned from bioarchaeology about the prenatal and early lives of Roman infants, see Carroll, *Infancy and Earliest Childhood,* 66–70.

6. Pliny the Younger, *Letters* 8.10.

7. Pliny the Younger, *Letters* 8.11.

8. Pliny the Elder, *Natural History* 7.42 (sneeze); 7.43 (blown-out lamp); 30.128 (viper); 30.130 (raven's egg); 28.80 (menstrual blood); 32.8 (sea hare); discussion in Richlin, *Arguments with Silence,* 261–63.

9. Pliny the Elder, *Natural History* 21.147.

10. Hippocrates, *Diseases of Women* 1.25; Soranus, *Gynecology* 1.46.

11. Hanson, "Medical Writers' Woman"; Dean-Jones, "Autopsia, Historia" and "Hippocratic Physician"; Demand, *Birth, Death,* 64–65.

12. Connell, "Women's Medical Knowledge."

13. For example, Hippocrates, *Fleshes* 19: "It is . . . obvious to women of experience when a woman becomes pregnant: she immediately feels a chill, then heat, shivering, and a tension, and she feels sluggish in her joints, throughout her whole body, and in her uterus."

14. See Totelin, *Hippocratic Recipes,* on the polyvalent properties of medicinal substances.

15. Richlin, *Arguments with Silence,* 242.

16. Dasen, *Sourire d'Omphale,* 45–47.

17. Pseudo-Plutarch (*On Rivers* 20.2) writes, "In this river [the Euphrates] grows a stone called *aëtites* [eagle stone], which, when midwives apply it to the navels of women who are in hard labor, causes them to give birth with little pain"; Dasen, *Sourire d'Omphale,* 45.

18. For discussion of this myth, see Bettini, *Women and Weasels,* 27–44.

19. Ovid, *Metamorphoses* 9.281–323.

20. Antoninus Liberalis, *Metamorphoses* 29.

21. Bettini, *Women and Weasels,* 69–82.

22. Theodorus Priscianus, *Euporiston* 3.350–51. Translation is from Bettini, *Women and Weasels*, 269n67.

23. Pliny the Elder, *Natural History* 30.125.

24. Pliny the Elder, *Natural History* 28.42; see discussion in Richlin, *Arguments with Silence*, 263.

25. Bettini, *Women and Weasels*, 81–82.

26. Sutton and Scott, *Optimal Foetal Positioning*. Their observations and recommendations have been expanded upon by Gail Tully with her Spinning Babies® method (https://www.spinningbabies.com/). A recent nursing dissertation (Sears, "Impact of the Spinning Babies") that studied the effects of the method showed that it reduced the cesarean section rate among first-time birthers. Tully has come under some criticism for promoting pseudoscientific methods such as homeopathy, but many providers take the moves and leave the woo-woo.

27. Witkiewicz et al., "Perinatal Outcomes."

28. Demand, *Birth, Death*, 88–91; Baumbach, "Speak, Votives."

29. Kanta et al., *Honors to Eileithyia*; Demand, *Birth, Death*, 91–94.

30. Feucht, "Motherhood in Pharaonic Egypt"; Nifosi, *Becoming a Woman*.

31. Dasen, *Sourire d'Omphale*, 62–63; Spieser, "Meskhenet et les sept Hathors," 69–73.

32. Dasen, *Sourire d'Omphale*, 64.

33. Schultz, *Women's Religious Activity*, 52, 55–57, 69; on Mater Matuta, see Carroll, *Infancy and Earliest Childhood*, 71–72, and "Mater Matuta." On native Italian and Etruscan goddesses and gods related to fertility, pregnancy, and childbirth, see Glinister, "Ritual and Meaning."

34. Flemming ("Wombs for the Gods," 116) argues that a "focused indeterminacy" of meaning in the body part votives is part of their strength. The fact that they don't identify precisely what they are for means that they could be used for multiple purposes, including promoting childbirth and healing pathologies.

35. Dasen, *Sourire d'Omphale*, 40–1, 87–108.

36. CBd 760. See discussion in Dasen (*Sourire d'Omphale*, 87–108)—these amulets tended to be multipurpose.

37. Several amulets make use of this imagery of Hercules wrestling the lion and/or a pregnant Omphale brandishing a club: CBd 455, 761, 762, 763, 764, 765, 1047, 1170, 1336, 1454, 1591, 1632, 1706 (Hercules wrestling lion); 1703, 2338, 3033, 3658 (pregnant Omphale). One amulet (CBd 1631) shows Hercules wrestling the Nemean lion on top of a cupping-vessel uterus that is surrounded by the ouroboros snake.

38. Dasen (*Sourire d'Omphale*, 94–7) argues that these Hercules amulets were for problems with organs of the abdomen generally and could be used for problems with the uterus or the stomach. As therapy for the stomach, they

tapped into Hercules's reputation as a glutton, giving the wearer relief from indigestion and biliary colic. The KKK symbol that appears on these amulets is best understood as an anti-colic formula.

39. On the imagery of the pregnant, club-brandishing Omphale more broadly, see Dasen, *Sourire d'Omphale,* 87–108.

40. Dasen, *Sourire d'Omphale,* 42.

41. Dasen, *Sourire d'Omphale,* 107–8.

42. See CBd 1356 for a comparable amulet featuring Khnoum and Isis as well as baby Horus; see discussion in Mastrocinque, *Intailles magiques,* 57.

43. CBd 1055; with discussion in Dasen, "Femmes à tiroir" and "Représenter l'invisible."

44. *IG* IV^2 121; see discussions in Demand, *Birth, Death,* 93–94; Scott, "Gender in the Temple."

45. On incubation healing in ancient Greece, see Oberhelman, *Dreams, Healing*; Renberg, *Where Dreams May Come.*

46. It was important that Kleo had left the boundary of the sanctuary before giving birth, since birth and death were forbidden on sacred ground (Scott, "Gender in the Temple," 325–26).

47. *IG* IV^2 121.

48. Demand, *Birth, Death,* 94.

49. For sources on the myths of King Midas and Eos, see theoi.com.

50. *IG* IV^2 121–24. Scott, "Gender in the Temple"; many of the other miracle cures of women inscribed on these stones relate to infertility or false pregnancies.

51. Scott, "Gender in the Temple," 325.

52. Matthew 8.1–4; Mark 1.40–42 (leprosy); Mark 5.25–29 (bloody flux).

53. Hippocrates, *Nature of the Child* 19, with discussion in Demand, *Birth, Death,* 94.

54. Hippocrates, *Fleshes* 19.

55. An exception is Metrodora's *On the Conditions of the Womb* (ca. 3rd–6th century CE), though this text contains no instructions on prenatal care. The first nineteen chapters of Metrodora's text are translated in Upson-Saia et al., *Medicine, Health, and Healing,* 142–48.

56. On women's contributions to and citations in male-authored medical texts, see Flemming, "Women, Writing."

57. See chapter 4.

58. On the proto-eugenics of Soranus's *Gynecology,* see Freidin, "Well-Born."

59. Hanson and Green, "Soranus of Ephesus"; Bolton, "Mustio's *Gynaecia.*"

60. See, for example, Blumenfeld-Kosinski, *Not of Woman Born*; King, *Midwifery, Obstetrics*; Green, *Making Women's Medicine Masculine.*

61. Soranus, *Gynecology* 1.46.

62. Duden, *Disembodying Women.*

63. Mulder, "Hippocratic Oath."

64. Soranus, *Gynecology* 1.46–47.

65. Soranus, *Gynecology* 1.48–53; Muscio, *Gynaecia* 30–33.

66. Soranus, *Gynecology* 1.54–56; Muscio, *Gynaecia* 34.

67. Hanson, "Eight Months' Child."

68. Hanson, "Eight Months' Child"; for the reckoning of philosophical time more generally, see Freidin, "The Birthday Present."

69. Hanson, "Eight Months' Child."

70. Soranus, *Gynecology* 1.56; Muscio, *Gynaecia* 36.

71. Freidin, *Birthing Romans.*

72. Morgan and Michaels, *Fetal Subjects,* 8.

73. Yurie Hong ("Collaboration and Conflict") has pointed out that this maternal-fetal antagonism can be seen as early as the Hippocratic texts.

74. Soranus, *Gynecology* 1.46.

75. Soranus, *Gynecology* 1.49, 51.

76. Soranus, *Gynecology* 1.51.

77. Soranus, *Gynecology* 1.54, 56.

78. Draycott, *Roman Domestic Medical Practice,* 38–39 (health regimens only available to the elite), 118–20 (the various enslaved people who cared for the health of the elite).

79. In the city of Rome, an estimated 98 percent of the one million inhabitants were non-elite (Draycott, *Roman Domestic Medical Practice,* 39).

80. Garnsey, *Food and Society,* chapter 1; Bourbou, "Bioarchaeology of Roman Diet," 82

81. Garnsey, *Cities, Peasants,* 48; Bourbou, "Bioarchaeology of Roman Diet," 82.

82. Draycott, *Roman Domestic Medical Practice,* 39.

83. Bourbou, "Bioarchaeology of Roman Diet," 81–82.

84. Bourbou, "Bioarchaeology of Roman Diet," 87, citing Prowse et al., "Age-Related Variation," on the Isola Sacra; Craig et al., "Coastal Site of Velia," on Velia. Other studies (Keenleyside et al., "Population from Leptiminus"; Killgrove and Tykot, "Food for Rome," on Casal Bertone and Castellaccio Europarco) have not found sex-based variation in diet. In agreement with Craig et al. ("Coastal Site of Velia"), Bourbou ("Bioarchaeology of Roman Diet, 85) argues that where sex-based variation is present, it is

likely based on occupational access to "high trophic level foods like meat and fish."

85. Bourbou, "Bioarchaeology of Roman Diet."

86. Draycott, *Roman Domestic Medical Practice,* 40.

87. Draycott (*Roman Domestic Medical Practice,* 61–64) is somewhat optimistic on this front, noting the many different forms that gardens could take. Laes ("Women, Children," 181) is more pessimistic, arguing that "few families would have had the luxury of possessing a small city garden where they could raise some crop."

88. Laes, "Women, Children," 180–81.

89. Bourbou, "Life and Death"; on the widespread evidence of scurvy and rickets in the Roman Empire, see Laes, "Women, Children," 178–79; on vitamin C deficiencies and scurvy in Roman children, see Carroll, *Infancy and Earliest Childhood,* 67.

90. Soranus, *Gynecology* 2.44. On the visible manifestations of rickets in the bioarcheological record, see Carroll, *Infancy and Earliest Childhood,* 68 (bowing of the leg bones, or the arm bones if the rickets were active while the child was crawling).

91. Galen (*Venesection, Against Erasistratus* K11.164) mentions the issue of "women, namely mothers" remaining indoors and not "exposing themselves to direct sunlight" (translation is from Brain, *Galen on Bloodletting*). This passage was identified by Bagley, "Roman Children," 110, who discusses the possible causes of vitamin D deficiency in Rome (102–13).

92. Soranus, *Gynecology* 2.44.

93. Soranus, *Gynecology* 1.49, 54.

94. On working women as mothers in ancient Rome, see Finnigan, "Working Moms."

95. On the sexual availability of enslaved women to free men, see Perry, *Gender, Manumission,* 8–42; Finnigan, "Working Moms," 122–35.

96. Plutarch, *Advice to Bride and Groom* 140B.

97. Drexler et al., "Intimate Partner Violence"; Agarwal et al., "Comprehensive Review of Intimate Partner Violence."

98. Pomeroy, *The Murder of Regilla*; Witzke, "Violence Against Women," 258–59.

99. Freidin (*Birthing Romans,* 150) corroborates my interpretation of Soranus's recommendations as contributing to maternal-fetal conflict. For a different view, see Porter ("Compassion in Soranus' *Gynecology*"), who sees Soranus's prenatal guidelines as "compassionate." At best, I think, we could term his approach paternalistic.

100. Daniels, "Fathers, Mothers," 83–84.

7. PETRONILLA PETITIONS THE MAGISTRATES

1. *P.Gen.* 2.103, 2.104.

2. *P.Gen.* 2.103. Translation is from Rowlandson, *Women and Society,* 290-91. The letter was written by a professional scribe, but the "farewell" is written in a second hand that was likely Petronilla's.

3. Rowlandson, *Women and Society,* 290–91.

4. *P.Gen.* 2.104. On the appointment of guardians to fatherless children, see Evans Grubbs, *Women and the Law,* 236–54.

5. McGinn, "Roman Children."

6. *Digest* 37.9.1.3–13. All translations of the *Digest* in this chapter are from Watson, *Digest of Justinian.*

7. *Digest* 25.4.1.pr. On related cases of divorce and disputed pregnancy, see Evans Grubbs, *Women and the Law,* 198-202. Procedures for disputed pregnancy were used in cases where the spouses had divorced or where one spouse had died. The law does not discuss a married couple's disagreements over pregnancy, likely because the husband would have held the power in such situations.

8. *Digest* 25.4.1.pr.

9. *Digest* 25.4.1.13.

10. The Roman jurists decided that up to three shares of an inheritance could be held back in the case of a pregnancy following the father's death, since they considered it reasonable for up to three children to be born at once (*Digest* 5.4.3). On the legal concerns surrounding suppositious children and inheritance, see Evans Grubbs, *Women and the Law,* 264–69.

11. *Digest* 25.4.1.10. See discussions in Hanson, "Division of Labor," 176; Evans Grubbs, *Women and the Law,* 261-64.

12. *Digest* 9.22.10; Evans Grubbs, *Women and the Law,* 266.

13. Plautus, *Truculentus;* Mulder, "Female Trouble," 39–40.

14. *P.Fam.Tebt.* 20, with discussion in Rowlandson, *Women and the Law,* 269.

15. *Digest* 25.4.1; Evans Grubbs, *Women and the Law,* 200–201.

16. *Digest* 25.4.1.3.

17. *Digest* 3.2.15–19, 25.6; Evans Grubbs, *Women and the Law,* 265.

18. In the medical texts there are tests for fertility, virginity, and fetal sex, but not simply for pregnancy. On tests for virginity in the ancient medical texts, see Lillis, *Virgin Territory,* 33. It's possible that there were similarities between tests for pregnancy and virginity, but this is speculation on my part. Julia Kelto Lillis ("Late Ancient Christians") has argued, however, that vaginal inspections were not central to virginity tests.

19. *Digest* 3.2.19.

20. *BGU* 4.1104; Rowlandson, *Women and Society,* 171–72; Evans Grubbs, *Women and the Law,* 268.

21. Rowlandson, *Women and Society*; Bagnall and Cribiore, *Women's Letters.*

22. See chapter 11.

23. On the Babatha archive, see Evans Grubbs, *Women and the Law*, 131-133; Oudshoorn, *Roman and Local Law,* 5–12.

8. THE REAL MIDWIVES OF ANCIENT ROME

1. There are resonances here with Adrienne Rich's "hands of flesh, hands of iron" (*Of Woman Born*)—her description of the different approaches to birth throughout Western history, from female midwives, who used their hands, to male doctors, who used obstetrical tools such as forceps.

2. He may be in the act of bloodletting (Flemming, "Gendering Medical Provision," 285).

3. It was common practice at this time in Ostia (and elsewhere in the Roman world) for people to display an image of their work on their tombstone: cobblers making shoes, ropemakers making ropes, smiths forging iron, etc. (Larsson Lovén, "People at Work in Ostia").

4. *CIL* 6.6647 (Hygeia); *CIL* 11.3391 (Volusia); *CIL* 10.3972 (Maria Peregrina); *IGUR* 3.1240 (Julia Primigeneia); *CIL* 6.8207 (Sallustia Imerita); *CIL* 6.8947 (Antonia Thallusa); *CIL* 8.4896 (Irene). These inscriptions are all in Laes, "The Educated Midwife" and "Midwives in Greek Inscriptions."

5. On inscriptions for midwives see Laes, "The Educated Midwife" and "Midwives in Greek Inscriptions"; Alonso Alonso, "Medicae y Obstetrices"; Scarfo, "Pregnancy, Childbirth."

6. There are more free midwives commemorated in the Greek than the Latin tombstone inscriptions (Laes, "Midwives in Greek Inscriptions," 156–57).

7. *CIL* 6.6647; Laes, "The Educated Midwife," 280.

8. There is another tombstone for another midwife named Hygia (*CIL* 6.4458).

9. Writing about the ancient Greek world, Helen King (*Hippocrates' Woman,* 174) points out that our understanding of midwives in the past continues to be heavily influenced by present debates about midwives, doctors, and their roles in normal and abnormal childbirth.

10. On the different types of midwives in the United States, see Simkins, *Into These Hands,* xxxvii–xli; Davis-Floyd and Johnson, *Mainstreaming Midwives.*

11. US Government Accountability Office, "Midwives."

12. On midwifery in the medieval and early modern periods, see Ehrenreich and English, *Witches, Midwives*; Donnison, *Midwives and Medical Men*; Blumenfeld-Kosinski, *Not of Woman Born*; Wilson, *Making of Man-Midwifery*; Federici, *Caliban and the Witch*; King, *Midwifery, Obstetrics*; Green, *Making Women's Medicine Masculine*; Giladi, *Muslim Midwives*; Park, "Managing Childbirth"; Fox and Brazier, "Regulation of Midwives."

13. On midwifery in 19th- and 20th-century America, see McGregor, *Midwives to Medicine*; Fraser, *African American Midwifery*; Lay, *Rhetoric of Midwifery*; Bridges, *Reproducing Race*; Owens, *Medical Bondage.*

14. Upson-Saia et al., *Medicine, Health, and Healing,* 283.

15. Just 5 percent of physicians in inscriptions from the western part of the Roman Empire were women (Hemelrijk, *Women and Society,* 125).

16. *IG* II² 6873; Demand, *Birth, Death,* 132–33; Totelin, "Do No Harm."

17. Laurence Totelin ("Do No Harm") notes that "scholars tend to consider Phanostrate's title of *iatros* superior to that of *maia,*" but, she argues, "That is a little dismissive of the considerable skills involves in managing pregnancy and childbirth, and at times abortion."

18. *CIL* 6.9478; Tatarkiewicz, *"Cursus Laborum,"* 69.

19. *AE* 2018, 541; Tatarkiewicz, *"Cursus Laborum,"* 78.

20. On inscriptions for female doctors and midwives, see Alonso Alonso, "Medicae y Obstetrices"; Tatarkiewicz, *"Cursus Laborum,"* 68–69, 73–74, 77–78.

21. Tatarkiewicz, *"Cursus Laborum,"* 77–78.

22. Alonso Alonso, "Medicae y Obstetrices."

23. Alonso Alonso, "Medicae y Obstetrices"; Tatarkiewicz, *"Cursus Laborum,"* 78.

24. *AE* 2001, 263; Alonso Alonso, "Medicae y Obstetrices," 283, 289.

25. *CIL* 10.3980; Alonso Alonso, "Medicae y Obstetrices," 283, 290.

26. Hemelrijk, *Women and Society,* 125.

27. *IG* XIV.1751; *IGUR* II.675; Irving, "Restituta"; Tatarkiewicz, *"Cursus Laborum,"* 69.

28. Some scholars think that midwives like Scribonia learned and even took direction from male doctors—for example, Demand, *Birth, Death,* 66; Bettini, *Women and Weasels,* 177. But this assumption may come from the model of

modern nurse midwifery and may not accurately reflect the situation in the ancient world.

29. Mattern, *Prince of Medicine,* chapter 2; Upson-Saia et al., *Medicine, Health, and Healing,* 29, 283–84; Nutton, *Ancient Medicine,* 55, 68.

30. Upson-Saia et al., *Medicine, Health, and Healing,* 283–84, 289.

31. Upson-Saia et al., *Medicine, Health, and Healing,* 286.

32. Martial, *Epigrams* 1.47, 8.74, 10.77. On Pliny the Elder's disdain for doctors, see Richlin, *Arguments with Silence,* 246.

33. Upson-Saia et al., *Medicine, Health, and Healing,* 285.

34. The gifts and honors were awarded to both male and female physicians (Upson-Saia et al., *Medicine, Health, and Healing,* 286–88).

35. On women's medical writing in the ancient world, see Flemming, "Women, Writing" and "Gendering Medical Provision," 277.

36. King, "Motherhood and Health."

37. Hippocrates, *Fleshes* 19 (*akestrides*); *Diseases of Women* 1.46 (*omphalētomos*); *Diseases of Women* 1.68 (*iētreuousa*). See King ("Motherhood and Health") on the lack of midwives in the Hippocratic texts; see Connell, "Women's Medical Knowledge," on the women with medical expertise in the Hippocratic texts.

38. Demand, *Birth, Death*; King, "Motherhood and Health."

39. On the deliberate marginalizing and silencing of female experts in ancient male-authored medical texts, see Lehmhaus, "Re-reading Gynaecology," especially 70–75.

40. Soranus, *Gynecology* 1.3–4: the best midwives were "unperturbed, unafraid in danger, . . . sympathetic, . . . robust, . . . well-disciplined and always sober, . . . discreet, . . . not greedy for money, . . . free from superstition, . . . [with] soft hands" (translation is adapted from Temkin, *Soranus' Gynecology*).

41. Ecca, "Fixing Ethical Rules."

42. Galen, *Recognizing the Best Physician*; translation in Upson-Saia et al., *Medicine, Health, and Healing,* 289–94.

43. *Digest* 50.13.1. Translations of the *Digest* in this chapter are from Watson, *Digest of Justinian*. Rebecca Flemming ("Gendering Medical Provision," 272–73) takes this decree as solid evidence that midwives were counted among medical practitioners in the urban centers of the empire.

44. Soranus, *Gynecology* 1.3–4.

45. Soranus, *Gynecology* 1.4.

46. Eunapius, *Lives of the Philosophers and Sophists* 6.21–25.

47. See, for example, Giulia Ecca's ("Fixing Ethical Rules") description of illiterate midwives as "simply craftswomen, who probably used rudimentary

methods." On this point, see Connell ("Women's Medical Knowledge," 64), who, in assessing women's medical knowledge in antiquity, argues, "It ought to be accepted that theories and practices do not have to be written down in order to be philosophical." On the logic of women's "folk" healing practices, see Ripat, "Roman Women."

48. On ancient Rome as a slave society, see Hopkins, *Conquerors and Slaves*; Bradley, *Slavery and Society*; duBois, *Slaves and Other Objects*; Joshel, *Slavery in the Roman World.*

49. On enslaved scribes in ancient Rome, see Moss, *God's Ghost Writers.*

50. Bradley, *Slavery and Society,* 159–60.

51. Fett, "Consciousness and Calling."

52. *CIL* 6.6325.

53. Soranus, *Gynecology* 1.3–4.

54. Fett, "Consciousness and Calling," 72.

55. Fett, "Consciousness and Calling," 74.

56. Molly Jones-Lewis made this proposal about Panaratus and Prosdocia in a talk at the 2024 meeting of the Classical Association of Atlantic States: "Except for Panaratus and Prosdocia: Workplace Law in the Funerary Inscription of Scribonia Attike and Ulpius Amerimnus." She develops this idea further in a forthcoming book about doctors in Roman law and society.

57. On the negative depictions of old women and female healers generally, see Ripat, "Roman Women," 105.

58. Terence, *The Woman of Andros* 229–30.

59. Plautus, *The Braggart Soldier* 697.

60. Bettini, *Women and Weasels,* 178–87; Felton, "Witches, Disgust"; King, *Hippocrates' Woman,* chapter 9.

61. Felton, "Witches, Disgust," 191–93.

62. Ripat, "Roman Women," 124; Felton, "Witches, Disgust," 196–97. In a poem about the civil wars of the late 1st century BCE (Lucan, *The Civil War* 6.558–59), a witch named Erictho takes advantage of the devastation and chaos. She cuts a fetus from its dead mother's womb to use in a magic rite. Later in the poem (6.710–11), she places the dismembered parts of the infant on an altar.

63. Felton, "Witches, Disgust," 195–200.

64. Ammianus Marcellinus, *History* 16.10.19.

65. *Historia Augusta, 16: Antoninus Diadumenus* 4.

66. Pliny the Elder, *Natural History* 28.70; Bettini, *Women and Weasels,* 179.

67. Pliny, the Elder *Natural History* 28.67.

68. Pliny the Elder, *Natural History* 28.66.

69. Pliny the Elder discusses hair, breast milk, saliva, and menstrual fluid (*Natural History* 28.70–86).

70. Pliny the Elder, *Natural History* 28.83.

71. Pliny the Elder, *Natural History* 28.82–83.

72. Pliny the Elder, *Natural History* 28. 80–81; Ripat, "Roman Women," 109–11.

73. Pliny the Elder, *Natural History* 28.261–62.

74. Pliny the Elder, *Natural History* 28.253; Flemming ("Women, Writing," 271–76; "Gendering Medical Provision," 277n34) argues that "Olympias of Thebes" is probably a pseudonym.

75. Pliny the Elder, *Natural History* 28.249.

76. Pliny the Elder, *Natural History* 28.255.

77. Pliny the Elder, *Natural History* 28.257.

78. Park, *Secrets of Women*; Rebecca Flemming ("Women, Writing," 271–76) views this association between midwives and sex workers pessimistically. According to Pliny the Elder, she explains (274), both are "experts in a type of innate female knowledge that is essentially about being a woman, rather than being based in any kind of training." Amy Richlin (*Arguments with Silence,* 244) tempers this pessimism: "We might doubt that midwives looked as unimportant to women generally as they did to medical writers generally."

79. Soranus, *Gynecology* 1.4.

80. Soranus, *Gynecology* 2.11.

81. For example, Ecca, "Fixing Ethical Rules," 137–38.

82. For example, in *The Protevangelium of James.* Anna Tatarkiewicz discusses these texts in the forthcoming "Spaces and Practitioners."

83. *Digest* 50.13.1.

84. *Code of Justinian* 6.43.3.1.

85. Galen, *Prognosis* 8.

86. Soranus, *Gynecology* 3.3.

87. Hyginus, *Myths* 274; King, *Hippocrates' Woman,* 181–87, and *One-Sex Body on Trial.*

88. *CIL* 8.15593; Laes, "The Educated Midwife," 282.

89. In the vignette that follows, I take the details about Ostia from the chapters in Karivieri, *Multicultural Harbour City,* especially the chapters by Janet Delaine on apartment living, Arja Karivieri on lighting in homes and public spaces, Ray Laurence on streets, and Marja-Leena Hänninen on bathing.

9. AT THE BIRTH

1. Plutarch, *Dialogue on Love* 771B.

2. Pliny the Elder, *Natural History* 30.129–31, 28.102.

3. Soranus, *Gynecology* 2.2.

4. Nifosi, *Becoming a Woman,* 67n95; Soranus (*Gynecology* 2.5) points out that having the midwife stand in a pit in the ground doesn't work in second-floor rooms.

5. On the roles for men at births, see Hanson, "Division of Labor."

6. *O.Florida* 14; translation is from Nifosi, *Becoming a Woman,* 55.

7. Dioscorides, *Medical Materials* 2.109.

8. *P.Mich.* inv. 188; translation is from Rowlandson, *Women and Society,* 284–86.

9. *CIL* 6.8947; Scarfo, "Pregnancy, Childbirth," 242–43.

10. Treggiari, "Jobs for Women," 87; Kampen, *Image and Status,* 116; Scarfo, "Pregnancy, Childbirth" 122–23.

11. On these birth scenes, see Kampen, *Image and Status,* 38–39; Huskinson, *Roman Children's Sarcophagi,* 10–12; Jaeggi-Richoz, *Fabrique des bébés,* 239–53; Freidin, *Birthing Romans,* 231n66.

12. Kampen, *Image and Status,* 35–36; Kleiner, "Family Ties," 56. The woman bathing the child in these types of scenes has been interpreted as a midwife (Dasen, *Sourire d'Omphale,* 229; Jaeggi-Richoz, *Fabrique des bébés,* 244–45) or a nurse (Freidin, *Birthing Romans,* 230n65). It's possible that the image was meant to be ambiguous. Midwives would have provided immediate after-birth care, while nurses would have taken over on the second or third day.

13. Freidin (*Birthing Romans,* 233) points out that these scenes do not strictly represent the exact moment following the birth but participate in a fluid postpartum temporality of perhaps several days.

14. Kampen, *Image and Status,* 36; Wood, "Mortals, Empresses," 86. On the role of the Fates in these biographical sarcophagus scenes, see Freidin, *Birthing Romans,* 228–34.

15. Freidin, *Birthing Romans,* 231.

16. Nifosi, *Becoming a Woman,* 60–61.

17. Hanson, "Division of Labor"; King, *Hippocrates' Woman,* 177, 180.

18. Galen, *The Substance of the Natural Capacities* 152.

19. Demand, *Birth, Death,* 68; King, *Hippocrates' Woman,* 178–79; Flemming, "Women, Writing," 257–59; Tatarkiewicz, *"Cursus Laborum,"* 68. For a survey of female practitioners throughout the Mediterranean and Near East, see Lehmhaus, "Re-reading Gynaecology," 61–75.

20. Blumenfeld-Kosinski, *Not of Woman Born.*

21. *P.Oxy.* 51.3642.

22. Blumenfeld-Kosinski, *Not of Woman Born*; Park, *Secrets of Women.*

23. Seneca, *Epistles* 117.30; Tatarkiewicz, *"Cursus Laborum,"* 9.

24. *IGUR* 4.1702. For an analysis of this long inscription, see Graumann and Horstmanshoff ("'This I Suffered'"), who propose that the elder Lucius was probably a physician, which would explain why there is so much detail about the younger Lucius's medical conditions.

25. This translation is from Upson-Saia et al., *Medicine, Health, and Healing,* 324–25.

26. Graumann and Horstmanshoff, "'This I Suffered,'" 41.

27. On the ancient sources for Juno Lucina, see Tatarkiewicz, *"Cursus Laborum,"* 133–35.

28. Plautus, *The Pot of Gold* 692; Terence, *The Brothers* 487–88; Tatarkiewicz, *"Cursus Laborum,"* 134–35.

29. Hippocrates, *Diseases of Women* 1.77.

30. Hanson, "Long-Lived 'Quick Birther.'"

31. These homeopathic amulets are found in Pliny the Elder, *Natural History* 30.123–26.

32. Dioscorides, *Medical Materials* 5.142, 5.154.

33. CBd 759.

34. On these pagan and Christian birth amulets, see Hanson, "Long-Lived 'Quick Birther.'"

35. Simkin and Cheney, *The Birth Partner.*

36. Soranus, *Gynecology* 3.42.

37. Translation from Tomlin, "Special Delivery." This amulet can be viewed online at the British Museum: https://www.britishmuseum.org/collection/object/H_2009-8042-1

38. Hanson, "Gradualist View," 106.

39. Freidin, *Birthing Romans,* 167.

40. Freidin, *Birthing Romans,* 185–90. See the description in Dioscorides (*Medical Materials* 3.150) of stinking bean trefoil, a flowering shrub native to the Mediterranean, which could be used as a quick-birthing amulet but had to be thrown away immediately after the birth. The same herb when drunk could also help to dislodge a retained placenta.

41. For more on the use of amulets, see chapter 2.

42. Anna Bonnell Freidin (*Birthing Romans*) articulated this idea of a "community of care" made up of human and nonhuman actors that are called into the birth space by the amulets.

43. On the role of Fates and Fortuna/Tyche in Roman birth, see Freidin, *Birthing Romans,* 228; she describes the presence of the Fates in birth scenes as "a haunting nonhuman foil to the community assisting and caring for mother and child."

44. A description of the midwife's stool can be found in Soranus, *Gynecology* 2.3.

45. *P.Oxy.* 49.3491, 8; see discussion in Nifosi, *Becoming a Woman,* 57.

46. This image suggests that the typical untying of knots at a birth scene did not necessarily include necklaces (or, perhaps, *okytokion* amulets).

47. Soranus, *Gynecology* 2.2, 2.4, 2.5.

48. Soranus, *Gynecology* 2.6.

49. Hippocrates, *Superfetation* 8.

50. Soranus, *Gynecology* 2.11.

51. Hippocrates, *Diseases of Women* 1.77.

52. Hippocrates, *Diseases of Women* 1.34.

53. Hippocrates, *Barrenness* 224.

54. Hippocrates, *Diseases of Women* 1.34.

55. Pliny the Elder, *Natural History* 28.102.

56. Soranus, *Gynecology* 2.3.

57. Soranus, *Gynecology* 2.5.

58. *Homeric Hymn* 3*: To Apollo* 115–19.

59. Soranus, *Gynecology* 4.7.

60. Soranus, *Gynecology* 2.4.

61. Soranus, *Gynecology* 4.7

62. Soranus, *Gynecoloy* 2.5.

63. Soranus, *Gynecology* 4.6.

64. Soranus, *Gynecology* 4.7.

65. Soranus, *Gynecology* 2.5. Compare to 4.7, where he explains that the midwife should tell the laboring woman that "she is in no danger and should take courage."

66. Wolf, *Deliver Me.*

67. De Luca, "'God Was the First Anesthetist.'"

68. De Luca, "'God Was the First Anesthetist.'"

69. Wolf, *Cesarean Section,* 84–85, 99.

70. Soranus, *Gynecology* 2.4.

71. Muscio, *Gynaecia* 53.

72. Soranus, *Gynecology* 2.4, 2.14, 2.15, 2.49, 3.10, 3.23, 3.28.

73. Galen, *The Function of the Parts of the Human Body* 15.7.

74. Galen, *The Function of the Parts of the Human Body* 15.7.

10. DIFFICULT BIRTH

1. Pliny the Elder, *Natural History* 7.46; Tacitus, *Annals* 4.53.

2. Cleveland Clinic, "Breech Baby."

3. The swift and dramatic shift to cesarean sections for breech births was the result of a study known as the "Term Breech Trial," published in 2000 (Hannah et al., "Planned Caesarean Section"), which indicated worse fetal outcomes for vaginal as compared to cesarean section deliveries for breech births. The conclusions of this study—and the sweeping changes that resulted from it—were challenged by subsequent research (for example, Goffinet et al., "Planned Vaginal Delivery"; Daviss et al., "Evolving Evidence"; Vistad et al., "Vaginal Breech Delivery"), though with no effect on the recommendation of c-section for breech births.

4. Wolf, *Cesarean Section,* 171–73; Fischbein and Freeze, "Breech Birth at Home."

5. Efforts to turn a breech fetus can include acupuncture with moxibustion (Neri et al., "Acupuncture Plus Moxibustion"), a chiropractic maneuver known as the Webster technique, the Miles Circuit (Muza, "The Miles Circuit"), and external cephalic version.

6. Pliny the Elder, *Natural History* 7.45. Pliny explains that breech birth is a bad omen for the one who is born this way.

7. Pliny the Elder, *Natural History* 7.46.

8. Hippocrates, *Diseases of Women* 1.33.

9. Hippocrates, *Diseases of Women* 1.69.

10. Hanson, "Uterine Amulets," 183–90.

11. Soranus, *Gynecology* 4.8. If the fetus is coming buttocks first, Soranus even advises manually pushing it up the birth canal and straightening the legs so that it comes out feet first. This would not be the preferred method today.

12. Hippocrates, *Superfetation* 4.1–2.

13. Hippocrates, *Superfetation* 5.1.

14. Hippocrates, *Superfetation* 6.1.

15. Hippocrates, *Superfetation* 4.1–2, 5.1, 6.1, 6.74.

16. Cronk, "Hands off."

17. The causes of difficult labor that follow appear in Soranus, *Gynecology* 4.1–5. A similar description (probably based on Soranus's text) of the causes of difficult labor appears in Paul of Aegina 3.76.

18. See also Hippocrates, *Diseases of Women* 1.33.

19. Soranus, *Gynecology* 4.1.

20. Soranus, *Gynecology* 4.2.

21. Incollingo Rodriguez, "Women's Experiences of Weight Stigma."

22. Soranus, *Gynecology* 4.5.

23. Wolf, *Cesarean Section,* 3, who takes these numbers from midwife Martha Ballard's 18th-century birth records.

24. Laes, "Women, Children," 178.

25. Wolf, *Cesarean Section,* 27–28, 55.

26. On the much-debated question of whether male physicians attended normal births, see Dean-Jones, *Women's Bodies,* 1994; Hanson, "Division of Labor"; King, *Hippocrates' Woman,* 179–80, and "Motherhood and Health." As we saw in chapter 9, there were likely some births that were attended or managed by a solo male practitioner or a male family member, but these situations were probably not the norm.

27. Connell, "Women's Medical Knowledge," 67–68.

28. Soranus, *Gynecology* 4.1–5.

29. Soranus, *Gynecology* 2.11, 2.6.

30. Soranus, *Gynecology* 4.14.

31. Flemming, "Women, Writing."

32. Soranus, *Gynecology* 4.6: "Extreme grief, which makes the body loose, and other emotional issues, which can be learned about by asking [the patient], are not conducive to easy labor."

33. Soranus, *Gynecology* 4.6: "We ascertain that the fetus is transverse or has its hand thrust forward . . . by inserting the fingers."

34. Soranus, *Gynecology* 4.6: "The pulse and breathing of the laboring woman can let us know if she is in danger."

35. Soranus, *Gynecology* 4.7.

36. The methods given here appear in Soranus, *Gynecology* 4.7.

37. Soranus, *Gynecology* 4.7.

38. Soranus, *Gynecology* 4.7.

39. Hippocrates, *Excision of the Fetus* 4.

40. Hippocrates, *Diseases of Women* 1.68; Scullin, "'She's Only a 4.'"

41. Soranus, *Gynecology* 4.7.

42. Soranus, *Gynecology* 4.7.

43. Hippocrates, *Diseases of Women* 1.68.

44. Soranus, *Gynecology* 1.7.

45. Dupras et al., "Birth in Ancient Egypt," 61–64; Carroll, *Infancy and Earliest Childhood,* 53.

46. Soranus, *Gynecology* 4.3.

47. For example, Celsus, *On Medicine* 7.29; Paul of Aegina 3.76 (difficult labor), 6.74 (embryotomy).

48. Soranus, *Gynecology* 4.7.

49. Soranus, *Gynecology* 4.3.

50. Hippocrates, *Excision of the Fetus* 1; Hippocrates, *Diseases of Women* 1.70; Celsus, *On Medicine* 7.29; Hippocrates, *Superfetation* 7; Soranus, *Gynecology* 4.9–13; Tertullian, *On the Soul* 25.4. See also Gourevitch, "Chirugie obstétricale."

51. Hippocrates, *Excision of the Fetus* 1.

52. Hippocrates, *Superfetation* 7; Tertullian, *On the Soul* 25.4–6; Bliquez, *Tools of Asclepius,* 30, 43n74, 44, 255.

53. Baker, "Soranus and the Pompeii Speculum"; Bliquez, *Tools of Asclepius,* 251–55 (Bliquez calls this a "uterine speculum," but I think "vaginal" is more appropriate since it was inserted into the vagina, not the uterus).

54. On the rectal speculum, see Bliquez, *Tools of Asclepius,* 249–51. Jackson, "Roman Bivalve Dilators," suggests that the rectal speculum, at least the models that survive from antiquity, may have been developed in the 1st century CE. But there was some kind of smaller rectal speculum being used in the Hippocratic texts—perhaps, Bliquez (*Tools of Asclepius,* 251) posits, just two spoons being operated like a speculum.

55. Bliquez, *Tools of Asclepius,* 253. A total of eleven Roman vaginal speculums have been found.

56. Muscio, *Gynaecia* 186; Bliquez, *Tools of Asclepius,* 252.

57. Aetius, *Medical Collection* 16.23; Tertullian, *On the Soul* 25.4–5; Bliquez, *Tools of Asclepius,* 255.

58. Bliquez, *Tools of Asclepius,* 43, 257–59.

59. Bliquez, *Tools of Asclepius,* 255–57, 260. There is one mention of a hook (Celsus, *On Medicine* 7.29) that was sharp along the inner curve, which might have been used to remove the head of the fetus.

60. Bliquez, *Tools of Asclepius,* 40–43, 242, 257, 259.

61. Soranus, *Gynecology* 2.3.

62. Soranus, *Gynecology* 4.11. Compare to Aetius, *Medical Collection* 16.23 and Paul of Aegina 6.74, who both recommend the polyp knife, as well as the common scalpel; Bliquez, *Tools of Asclepius,* 256–57.

63. Soranus, *Gynecology* 4.10.

64. Tertullian, *On the Soul* 25.4. Translation is from Holmes, "A Treatise on the Soul."

65. Parkin, "The Demography of Infancy"; Carroll, *Infancy and Earliest Childhood,* 147.

66. Carroll, *Infancy and Earliest Childhood,* 54, 149–50.

67. Soranus, *Gynecology* 4.9.

68. Celsus, *On Medicine* prooem. 49–50.

69. Galen wrote about the surgery on this enslaved boy twice, in *The Doctrines of Hippocrates and Plato,* Testimonies and Fragments 7; and in *Anatomical Procedures* 7.12–13. For an animated description of the episode, see Mattern, *Prince of Medicine,* 173–75.

70. Owens, *Medical Bondage.* These enslaved women are known as the "Mothers of Gynecology" and there is a monument to them in Memorial Park in Montgomery, Alabama.

71. Wolf, *Cesarean Section,* 23–24, 169.

72. Park, *Secrets of Women*; Tatarkiewicz, *"Cursus Laborum,"* 128–30.

73. Pliny the Elder, *Natural History* 7.47; Kottek, "Caesarean Section," 435.

74. Blumenfeld-Kosinski, *Not of Woman Born,* 41, 45–46.

75. Blumenfeld-Kosinski, *Not of Woman Born,* 48–90.

76. Some people think that c-sections were performed in ancient Rome because a 6th-century-CE legal text mentions an early law (supposedly from the 8th century BCE) that held that a dead pregnant woman could not be buried without cutting the fetus out of her (Lex Caesarea in the *Digest*). But there is no mention of c-section in the ancient Greco-Roman medical texts. Apparently, c-section formed part of the practice of the Indian doctor Susruta, who was active sometime between the 5th century BCE and the 2nd century CE; c-section also appears in Rabbinic texts composed between the 2nd century BCE and 6th century CE (Blumenfeld-Kosinski, *Not of Woman Born,* 22–23; Kottek, "Caesarean Section").

77. Bliquez, *Tools of Asclepius,* 259–60.

78. Baskett, "Operative Vaginal Delivery," 4–5 (forceps), 7 (vacuum extraction); Wolf, *Cesarean Section,* 71–72 (c-sections); Bernstine and Callagan, "Ultrasonic Doppler." The fetal Doppler is different from continuous electronic fetal monitoring (EFM). Today, handheld Dopplers are used intermittently to take fetal heart tones during labor as an alternative to continuous EFM.

79. Wolf, *Cesarean Section,* 45-46, 76.

80. See chapter 8.

81. Wolf, *Cesarean Section,* 35.

82. Wolf, *Cesarean Section,* 84-85, 97, 98.

83. Muraca et al., "Maternal and Neonatal Trauma."

84. CDC, "Births—Method of Delivery"; Government of Canada, "Perinatal Health Indicators."

85. World Health Organization, "Caesarean Section Rates."

86. Patey et al., "Intermittent Auscultation."

87. *CIL* 3.2267; translation is from Hug, *Fertility, Ideology,* 252.

88. *CIL* 14.2737; translation is from Hug, *Fertility, Ideology,* 251.

89. Hug (*Fertility, Ideology,* 249–54) translates seventeen Latin inscriptions for women who died in childbirth, ranging in date from the 1st century BCE to the 4th century CE.

90. *AE* 1991.1076; translation is from Hug, *Fertility and Ideology,* 250.

91. *CIL* 3.9632; translation is from Hug, *Fertility, Ideology,* 252.

92. Kaibel, *Epigrammata Graeca,* 218; translation is adapted from Carroll, *Infancy and Earliest Childhood,* 61.

93. Parkin, *Demography and Roman Society,* 104.

94. Pliny the Elder, *Natural History* 7.47.

95. Hanson, "Gradualist View," 98; Hanson, "Hair on Her Liver," 245–54; Hong, "Collaboration and Conflict"; Hippocrates, *Nature of the Child* 19; Aristotle, *History of Animals* 9(7).584a.27–32.

96. It was believed that male fetuses started moving earlier in the uterus than female fetuses because of their superior strength: Hippocrates, *Nature of the Child,* 10; Aristotle, *History of Animals,* 9(7).583b3; Pliny the Elder, *Natural History,* 7.41–42.

97. Southon, *Agrippina.*

98. Pliny the Elder, *Natural History* 7.45.

99. Freidin, *Birthing Romans,* 55.

100. World Health Organization, "Maternal Mortality."

101. Schofield, "Did the Mothers," 258–59; cited in Freidin, *Birthing Romans,* 56.

102. Freidin, "Carrying Risk." On maternal mortality and its social impact in ancient Rome, see Freidin, *Birthing Romans,* 54–57.

103. Hug, *Fertility, Ideology,* 17–18.

104. On birth as a transition from wet to dry, see Freidin, *Birthing Romans,* 89–106.

105. *P.Münch.* 3.57.

106. Freidin, *Birthing Romans,* 55.

107. On tuberculosis in antiquity, see Simons, "Tuberculosis." Freidin (*Birthing Romans,* 55) gives statistics for England and Wales in 1890, in which year childbirth accounted for 8.8 percent of the deaths of women aged fifteen to forty-four, while tuberculosis counted for almost 32 percent of these deaths.

108. Wolf, *Deliver Me* and *Cesarean Section.*

109. Wolf, *Deliver Me* and *Cesarean Section*; see also Somerstein, *Invisible Labor.*

110. Wolf, *Cesarean Section,* 3.

111. Wolf, *Cesarean Section*; Somerstein, *Invisible Labor.*

11. AFTER BIRTH

1. *The Passion of Perpetua and Felicity.* The account in this chapter is based on the Latin text and translation in Heffernan, *Passion of Perpetua.* On the different versions of this text in Latin and Greek, see also Cobb, *Passion of Perpetua*; Constantinou and Skouroumouni-Stavrinou, "Lactating Woman," 6–7n22.

2. On the issues with dating this text, see Muehlberger ("Perpetual Adjustment"), who argues for a later date of composition by someone other than Perpetua, and Cobb (*Passion of Perpetua,* 6–8), who argues for an earlier date.

3. For discussions of lactation in this story, see Dova, "Lactation Cessation"; Totelin, "Breastmilk in the Cave"; Constantinou and Skouroumouni-Stavrinou, "Lactating Woman."

4. On women dying in the postpartum period, see Tatarkiewicz, *"Cursus Laborum,"* 139–42.

5. *P.Fouad* 1.75; translation is from Rowlandson, *Women and Society,* 293–94.

6. Soranus, *Gynecology* 4.16; Aetius, *Medical Collection* 16.24. On the risks of a retained placenta and methods for extraction, see Tatarkiewicz, *"Cursus Laborum,"* 110–11.

7. This is the practice of the Hippocratics as reported by Soranus (*Gynecology* 4.14). In the surviving Hippocratic texts, sternutatives (sneeze-inducing substances) are only prescribed for expulsion of stillborn infants, not the placenta.

8. Hippocrates, *Superfetation* 8.

9. Dioscorides, *Medical Materials* 1.48.

10. Dioscorides, *Medical Materials* 1.50.

11. Dioscorides, *Medical Materials* 1.19.

12. Dioscorides, *Medical Materials* 1.69 (pine); 1.97 (labdanum from rockrose); 2.7 (opercula of murex); 2.152 (garlic); 3.113 (wormwood).

13. Dioscorides, *Medical Materials* 2.24 (beaver's testicles); 3.31 (pennyroyal); 3.105 (horehound); 3.120 (dropwort).

14. Aetius, *Medical Collection* 16.24; translation is from Ricci, *Aetios of Amida.*

15. Caelius Aurelianus, *Gynaecia* 1.107; Tatarkiewicz, *"Cursus Laborum,"* 139–42.

16. Misa Nguyen discusses postpartum care in her forthcoming "Science and Medicine."

17. Varro, *On Agriculture* 2.10.9; Tatarkiewicz, *"Cursus Laborum,"* 142n15.

18. On racist stereotypes around birth and hysteria in the 19th century, see Briggs, "Race of Hysteria." On similar racist ideas about the relationship between childbirth pain and the "level of civilization," see De Luca, "'God Was the First Anesthetist,'" 635.

19. Soranus seems to have been the first medical writer in the Greco-Roman tradition to write extensively on the care of the newborn and young child (Bolton, "Patience for the Little Patient").

20. Holman, "Molded as Wax."

21. Soranus, *Gynecology* 2.13. Galen (*Health*, K6.33) also advised sprinkling the newborn with salts "so that its skin will be firmer and denser than the internal parts" (translation from Singer, *Galen: Writings on Health*).

22. The point about the antiseptic properties of the salt comes from Holman, "Molded as Wax," 82.

23. Soranus, *Gynecology* 2.14.

24. Soranus, *Gynecology* 2.15; Muscio, *Gynaecia* 67–68.

25. Sornaus, *Gynecology* 2.15.

26. Soranus, *Gynecology* 2.35.

27. On shaping the body of the infant, see Dasen, "'All Children Are Dwarfs'" and "Roman Birth Rites," especially 204–6; also Graham, "Infant Votives."

28. Soranus, *Gynecology* 2.32.

29. Soranus, *Gynecology* 2.34.

30. Soranus, *Gynecology* 2.40.

31. Damastes's views are reported (and criticized) by Soranus, *Gynecology* 2.18. There is also an extant fragmentary manuscript from Damastes called "On the Care of Pregnant Women."

32. Galen, *Health* K6.36. Translation is from Singer, *Galen: Writings on Health*.

33. Soranus, *Gynecology* 2.17.

34. Soranus, *Gynecology* 2.18; aversion to colostrum is an anthropologically widespread phenomenon and not unique to ancient Greece and Rome (Totelin, "Breastmilk in the Cave," 243). In antiquity colostrum was thought to be contaminated by the lochia that flowed in greatest quantities in the days immediately following birth (Totelin, "Breastmilk in the Cave," 240–45). See also Lawrence, "Breastmilk, Breastfeeding," 230; Constantinou and Skouroumouni-Stavrinou, "Lactating Woman," 29–30; Totelin, "Weaning and Lactation Cessation," 145.

35. Infant feeding and care practices probably varied quite a bit throughout the empire, following local knowledge and customs (Powell et al., "Infant Feeding Practices," 92–93).

36. Oribasius, *Medical Collections* 12.17; Holman, "Molded as Wax," 87. On Oribasius's medical writings and his approach to women see Musgrove, "Oribasius' Woman."

37. Muscio, *Gynaecia* 74; translation is from Bolton, "Mustio's *Gynaecia*."

38. Holman, "Molded as Wax."

39. On the conditions of urban living in the Roman Empire, see Mattern, *Rhetoric of Healing,* 4–6; Carroll, *Infancy and Earliest Childhood,* 69; Upson-Saia et al., *Medicine, Health, and Healing,* 37–51.

40. Holman, "Molded as Wax," 89.

41. The term "medical model" is taken from writing on modern midwifery, which contrasts a medical model with a midwifery model of care (Rothman, *In Labor*; Simkins, *Into These Hands,* Introduction) or a technocratic with a holistic model of birth (Davis-Floyd, *Birth as an American Rite*).

42. *The Passion of Perpetua and Felicity* 2, 6.

43. Constantinou and Skouroumouni-Stavrinou ("Lactating Woman," 13) point out that in the Greek parts of the Roman Empire, the women in our sources who breastfeed their own children tend to be of lower social status; it was elite women who were expected to employ wet nurses.

44. Aulus Gellius, *Attic Nights* 12.1. Translations in this chapter are adapted from Rolfe, *Gellius. Attic Nights.* On attitudes toward breastfeeding in this episode, see Dasen, *Sourire d'Omphale,* 260–62; Lawrence, "Breastmilk, Breastfeeding," 231–34; Totelin, "Breastmilk in the Cave," 240.

45. Compare to Plutarch, *The Education of Children* 5; Soranus, *Gynecology* 2.18.

46. Galen, *Health* K6.36; see discussion of this theory in Mulder, "Adult Breastfeeding"; Lawrence, "Breastmilk, Breastfeeding"; Constantinou and Skouroumouni-Stavrinou, "Lactating Woman," 14–15; Lehmhaus, "Re-reading Gynaecology," 56.

47. Mulder, "Adult Breastfeeding"; see also Penniman, *Raised on Christian Milk.*

48. Aulus Gellius, *Attic Nights* 12.1.8.

49. For a comparison of the discourse around the "perfect breastfeeding mother" in the ancient world and today, see Groff and Steger, "Ethics of Ancient Lactation."

50. Pseudo-Quintilian, *Major Declamations* 18.3.

51. Tacitus, *Germania* 20; Mulder, "Adult Breastfeeding," 233–34.

52. Soranus, *Gynecology* 2.18; Muscio, *Gynaecia* 725–27; Plutarch, *The Education of Children* 5; Bolton, "Mustio's *Gynaecia*," 41.

53. Totelin, "Breastmilk in the Cave," 241–42.

54. Totelin ("Weaning and Lactation Cessation," 142–46) describes some of the medicaments used to dry up the milk.

55. *P.Lond.* 3.951; translation in Bagnall and Cribiore, *Women's Letters,* 213.

56. On the substitutes for maternal milk, see Centlivres Challet, "Feeding the Roman Nursling."

57. Hundreds of these feeding bottles have been found, made from ceramic or glass; residue analysis has been performed on some of them, showing that they contained milk, though it's not clear whether it was human or animal milk (Carroll, *Infancy and Earliest Childhood,* 82–85). Carroll is skeptical about the identification of the "breast pump" objects, but I do not share her pessimism. It's likely that breastmilk was expressed many different ways throughout the vast Roman Empire, including by hand and via passive or active pumps. See also Constantinou and Skouroumouni-Stavrinou ("Lactating Woman," 10). For many excellent images of these objects, including the different shapes they took around the Mediterranean, see Jaeggi-Richoz (*Fabrique des bébés*); on p. 483 she shows a modern woman pumping milk with a replica of one of the breast pumps and feeding her six-month-old baby with a replica of one of the feeding bottles. On a possible marketplace for pumped milk, see Mulder, "Adult Breastfeeding."

58. Constantinou and Skouroumouni-Stavrinou ("Lactating Woman," 18–19) describe how networks of lactating women likely supported each other.

59. *CIL* 3.10038; Sparreboom, "Wet-Nursing," 147n15. Certus may be commemorating his aunt as his own wet nurse or simply for her profession as a wet nurse (Laes, "Amitae and Materterae," 151–52).

60. Bradley, "Wet-Nursing at Rome," 202–3.

61. Joshel, "Nurturing the Master's Child."

62. Keith Bradley ("Wet-Nursing at Rome," 212–13) proposes that there were probably a few enslaved wet nurses who were responsible for nursing all of the children born into a household, rather than each enslaved mother nursing her own child.

63. Bradley ("Wet-Nursing at Rome," 204–6) provides a table of sixty-nine funerary inscriptions involving Roman *nutrices,* (wet) nurses.

64. *CIL* 6.37753; Laes, *Children in the Roman Empire,* 77.

65. Ursula Rothe ("Der Grabstein der Severina Nutrix") thinks that the monument is for Severina; Sandra Jaeggi-Richoz (*Fabrique des bébés,* 231), following Nicolas Mathieu (*L'Epitaphe*) is more skeptical, arguing that the monument is likely for the nursling and was perhaps commissioned by the wet nurse.

66. Pliny the Younger, *Letters* 6.3.1; Bradley, "Wet-Nursing at Rome," 201–2, and *Discovering the Roman* Family, 13–14; Laes, *Children in the Roman Empire,* 69; Scarfo, "Pregnancy, Childbirth," 128.

67. *Digest* 40.2.13; Joshel, "Nurturing the Master's Child," 6: Sparreboom, "Wet-Nursing," 150–51.

68. Joshel, "Nurturing the Master's Child," 5–6; Pedrucci, "Mothers for Sale."

69. Parca, "Wet Nurses"; Ricciardetto and Gourevitch "Cost of a Baby."

70. There may have been more wet nurses hired in Roman Egypt than in the other provinces of the Roman Empire. For instance, in Pannonia (covering parts of modern-day Eastern Europe, including Croatia and Hungary), maternal breastfeeding was valorized and may have been more prevalent than in other parts of the empire (Freidin, *Birthing Romans*, 37).

71. Parca, "Wet Nurses."

72. Ricciardetto and Gourevitch, "Cost of a Baby," 41–42.

73. *CPG* 1.22; translation in Van Minnen, "Alexandrian Documents."

74. *P.Oxy.* 1.91; translation at https://papyri.info/ddbdp/p.oxy;1;91.

75. Wolfarth, *Milk*; Banks, *Natality*.

76. *BGU* 4.1058; *BGU* 4.1107; *BGU* 4.1109; *CPG* 1.13; *CPG* 1.22; translations in Van Minnen, "Alexandrian Documents." Pedrucci ("Mothers for Sale") points out that in later periods, wet nursing could spread disease (usually syphilis) from the nursling to the nurse and then to the nurse's own children and partner (or vice versa). This may have been true for the Roman period as well and could be one reason behind the contractual stipulation to nurse only one infant at a time.

77. Parca, "Wet Nurses," 211.

78. Totelin ("Weaning and Lactation Cessation," 136–38) points out that weaning at any age posed dangers for the infant as it transitioned from the safety of breast milk to food and water with new bacteria and parasites.

79. Sparreboom, "Wet-Nursing," 148.

80. On the *conlactanei* "milk-brother" inscriptions, see Gianni, *All in the Family*, 52–95; Treggiari, "Jobs for Women," 86; Joshel, "Nurturing the Master's Child," 22n52; Sparreboom, "Wet-Nursing," 148n16; Dasen, *Sourire d'Omphale*, 270–73.

81. *CIL* 11.6345. See translation and discussion in Gianni, *All in the Family* 83-84.

82. Soranus, *Gynecology* 2.19–27; Lawrence, "Breastmilk, Breastfeeding," 228–30. Constantinou and Skouroumouni-Stavrinou ("Breast Rules") show how Soranus was participating in a wider medical and philosophical discourse about the profile of the best wet nurse.

83. Soranus, *Gynecology* 2.27. Analysis of children's bones from the Kellis 2 cemetery in Egypt and from Leptiminus in Tunisia show that they were

breastfed for about three years, while children in Roman London nursed for up to four years (Carroll, *Infancy and Earliest Childhood,* 65); see also Totelin ("Weaning and Lactation Cessation") for a discussion of the ancient evidence for length of breastfeeding and the weaning timeline, including a useful chart synthesizing recent bioarchaeological studies.

84. On the connection between sex and alcohol in Soranus, see Lawrence, "Breastmilk, Breastfeeding," 230–31. Sex during breastfeeding was thought to spoil the milk, restart menstruation, and, if the nurse got pregnant, deprive the nursling of nutriment "by redirecting it to the foetus" (Totelin, "Weaning and Lactation Cessation," 145).

85. Soranus, *Gynecology* 2.38.

86. Soranus, *Gynecology* 2.39.

87. Soranus, *Gynecology* 2.40.

88. Soranus, *Gynecology* 2.40.

89. Constantinou and Skouroumouni-Stavrinou ("Breast Rules," 86): "The only way to reduce [the wet nurse's] power over the nursling was to place her body and paid work under continuous surveillance and control."

90. Soranus, *Gynecology* 2.6.

91. Christian Laes ("Infants Between," 372) thinks there was a week-long period of decision-making in which the parents, in consultation with the midwife, determined what they were going to do with the child. But given the little evidence for this practice outside of Soranus, I wonder if Soranus may have created a life-or-death ritual out of the midwives' routine assessment practices on newborns.

92. Evans Grubbs, "Dynamics of Infant Abandonment."

93. On the number of exposed and abandoned children, see Laes, "Women, Children," 24.

94. Sneed, "Disability and Infanticide."

95. On the care necessary for the survival of disabled individuals, see Southwell-Wright, "Perceptions of Infant Disability," 126–27. On the care given to infants generally, see Carroll, *Infancy and Earliest Childhood,* 149–50.

96. Laurence, *Roman Archaeology,* 115–16; Southwell-Wright, "Perceptions of Infant Disability," 118–20.

97. Laes, "Women, Children," 27–28.

98. *CIL* 4.8149 and *CIL* 4.294; Laes, "Infant Between," 371n40. In the first announcement (for Juvenilla), the inscription literally reads "in the second hour of the evening," which would have differed depending on the time of year. The Romans divided the daylight into twelve equal portions that they called "hours," so, summer hours were longer than winter hours. I've estimated that

the time of her birth was 8:00 p.m. based on my guess of what the "second hour of the evening" would have been on August 2. My point is that for the Romans, this birth announcement gives a specific time, even if it's not entirely legible for us. On time and timekeeping in ancient Rome, see Miller, *Time and Ancient Medicine,* and Ker, *The Ordered Day.*

99. Carroll, *Infancy and Earliest Childhood,* 72–76. This practice in Roman Gaul (modern-day France) in the first few centuries CE continued an earlier practice from Roman Italy that seems to have stopped in the 1st century BCE.

100. Carroll, *Infancy and Earliest Childhood,* 71, 77–81.

101. *AE* 1986, 564; Šašel Kos, *Pre-Roman Divinities,* 174 (no. 35, fig. 21). See Hemelrijk, *Women and Society* 255–56 (no. 76, fig. 52) for a translation of the inscription.

102. Forty of these votive reliefs, dedicated to the Nutrices Augustae (sacred nurses) and dated to the 2nd and 3rd centuries CE, have been found in Poetovio (Carroll, *Infancy and Earliest Childhood,* 77–79).

103. The naming day was called the Dies Lustricus, which translates to something like "the day of purifying/cleansing." On the Dies Lustricus, see Hänninen, "From Womb to Family"; Dasen, "Roman Birth Rites," 207–8; Laes, *Children in the Roman Empire,* 66–67; Carroll, *Infancy and Earliest Childhood,* 152. Ancient writers explained the difference in time for girls and boys as a function of girls' earlier maturation.

104. Laes, "Infants Between"; Romero and López, "Pueri Nascentes."

105. On Roman birthdays, see Laes, "Conception, Birth," 34. A few infants who died before their naming day were commemorated with tombstones bearing their names (Laes, "Infants Between," 135–36).

106. Parkin, "Demography of Infancy."

107. Carroll, *Infancy and Earliest Childhood,* 148.

108. Johnston, *Restless Dead,* 161–200. On the very early origins of these demons in Mesopotamia, see Lehmhaus, "Re-reading Gynaecology," 18.

109. See Johnston, *Restless Dead,* 161–200, who notes the issues with calling this entity a "demon" since she started her life as a mortal woman. She is more appropriately called a ghost.

110. Johnston (*Restless Dead,* 161–200) refers to these vengeful ghosts collectively as *aōrai,* "women who died before their time."

111. Johnston, *Restless Dead,* 195; on the effects of the evil eye on children, see Plutarch, *Table-Talk* 5 (680c-f); Aulus Gellius, *Attic Nights* 9.4.7–8. In ancient Rome, vision was explained as the sending forth of physical particles through the eyes, particles that could hit upon and infect the person or object

that was seen. Apotropaic ("turning aside") charms, such as Gorgon heads, penises, and eyeballs, were thought to attract the envious gaze and bear the brunt of its physical effects. On the effects of envy as a malevolent and manipulatable force, see Johnston, *Restless Dead,* 190–92, 196–98, as well as 189n81, for instances when a person was thought to have initiated a reproductive attack on another person; see also Ripat, "Roman Women."

112. Johnston, *Restless Dead,* 161–200.

113. Johnston, *Restless Dead,* 166–67; Björklund, "Protecting Against Child-Killing Demons."

114. Björklund, "Protecting Against Child-Killing Demons," 19, 41.

115. Golden, "Did the Ancients Care" and "Other People's Children." On mourning and burial practices for infants, see Carroll, *Infancy and Earliest Childhood,* 147–237; Laes, "Conception, Birth," 24–25. On grief over child death in the Roman literary sources, see Hug, *Fertility, Ideology,* 17–18.

116. Carroll, *Infancy and Earliest Childhood,* 149.

117. On the burial of infants near the home, see Moore, "Hearth and Home"; Carroll, "Infant Death and Burial"; Laurence, *Roman Archaeology,* 111–15. Archaeological evidence shows that children up to two and a half years old could be buried in or near the home, a practice called *suggrundaria* (Laes, "Infants Between," 131–32). *Suggrunda* are the eaves of the roof, so *suggrundaria* refers to burial in a wall niche underneath the roof, though it is applied generally to infants buried anywhere around the house. These home burials are similar to what some people report doing with miscarried or stillborn infants today.

118. Laes, "Infants Between," 131.

119. Laurence (*Roman Archaeology,* 111–15) calls the scholarly obsession with infanticide a "distraction" from other more plausible explanations, such as natural high infant mortality.

120. *CIL* 6.19227; Laes ("Infants Between") records twenty-eight inscriptions for infants who died within forty days of birth.

121. *The Passion of Perpetua and Felicity* 15.

122. *The Passion of Perpetua and Felicity* 18. On Felicity's dripping breasts, see Totelin, "Breastmilk in the Cave."

123. On the legal principle *partus sequitur ventrem* ("the offspring follows the womb"), which made the children of enslaved women slaves, see Huemoeller, *Child Follows the Womb.*

124. See Turner, "Invisible Threads," on the enslaved woman's body as a "legally codified . . . site where more slaves were produced"; see also Huemoeller, *Child Follows the Womb.*

125. Huemoeller, *Child Follows the Womb.*

126. This strategy could only be employed in large household with many slaves. As Huemoeller (*Child Follows the Womb*) points out, enslavement in the Roman world was widespread but mostly small scale, with only one or a few slaves per household. In these situations, enslaved women probably breastfed their own children.

127. *FD* 3.6.39; see discussion in Huemoeller, *Child Follows the Womb.*

128. Huemoeller, *Child Follows the Womb.*

129. Huemoeller, *Child Follows the Womb.*

130. Parca, "Wet Nurses," 216–17.

131. *CPG* 1.8; translation in Van Minnen, "Alexandrian Documents."

132. Ambrose, *Letter* 5.

133. *CIL* 6.23589; see discussion in Sparreboom, "Wet-Nursing," 154–55. Based on her double name, Oscia Sabina may have been a manumitted former slave at the time that this tombstone was erected.

AFTERWORD

1. Nelson, *The Argonauts,* 124.

2. These quotes are from a post on Bushnell's Instagram account (@brittabushnellphd) on January 7, 2025. See also Bushnell, *Transformed by Birth.*

3. Seneca, *Epistles* 78.

4. Michael Koortbojian (*Myth, Meaning, and Memory*) has argued that this plaque depicts a male warrior getting a knee injury dressed rather than a birth scene, but this very much goes against the scholarly consensus on the object, which clearly depicts a group of women: Kampen, *Image and Status*; Wood, "Literacy and Luxury," who initially identified it as the end of a papyrus-roll winder but revised the identification to a handloom in "Women's Work"; Tatarkiewicz, "*Cursus Laborum*"; Freidin, *Birthing Romans.*

BIBLIOGRAPHY

ANCIENT SOURCES

Where available, I have included English translations of the ancient sources. Otherwise, references are to the sources in their original language (Ancient Greek or Latin).

Aetius of Amida
Medical Collection
Olivieri, A., ed. *Aetii Amideni Libri Medicinales.* 2 vols. Teubner, 1935–1950.
Ricci, James V., trans. *Aetios of Amida: The Gynecology and Obstetrics of the IVth Century, A.D.* Blakiston, 1950.

Ambrose, Bishop of Milan
Members of the English Church, trans. *The Letters of S. Ambrose, Bishop of Milan.* Oxford, 1881. https://www.gutenberg.org/files/58783/58783-h/58783-h.htm

Ammianus Marcellinus
History Rolfe, J. C., trans. *Ammianus Marcellinus. History, Volume I: Books 14–19.* Loeb Classical Library, Harvard University Press, 1950.

Antoninus Liberalis
Metamorphoses Celoria, Francis, trans. *The Metamorphoses of Antoninus Liberalis: A Translation with a Commentary.* Routledge, 1992.

Aretaeus

On Cures for Acute Diseases; On the Causes of Acute Diseases; On the Causes of Chronic Diseases Adams, Francis, ed. and trans. *The Extant Works of Aretaeus, the Cappadocian.* Printed for the Sydenham Society, 1856.

Aristotle and Pseudo-Aristotle

Generation of Animals Peck, A. L., trans. *Aristotle. Generation of Animals.* Loeb Classical Library, Harvard University Press, 1942.

History of Animals Balme, D. M, ed. and trans. *Aristotle. History of Animals, Volume III: Books* 7–10. Loeb Classical Library, Harvard University Press, 1991.

Aulus Gellius

Attic Nights Rolfe, J. C., trans. *Gellius. Attic Nights, Volume II: Books* 6–13. Loeb Classical Library, Harvard University Press, 1927.

Caelius Aurelianus

Gynaecia Drabkin, Miriam F., and Israel E. Drabkin, ed. *Caelius Aurelianus, Gynaecia: Fragments of a Latin Version of Soranus' Gynaecia from a Thirteenth Century Manuscript.* Johns Hopkins University Press, 1951.

Celsus

On Medicine Spencer, W. G., trans. *Celsus. On Medicine, Volume* 1 *Books* 1–4. Loeb Classical Library, Harvard University Press, 1935.

Cicero

In Defense of Cluentius Hodge, H. Grose, trans. *Cicero. Pro Lege Manilia. Pro Caecina. Pro Cluentio. Pro Rabirio Perduellionis Reo.* Loeb Classical Library, Harvard University Press, 1927.

On Divination Falconer, W. A. *Cicero. On Old Age. On Friendship. On Divination.* Loeb Classical Library, Harvard University Press, 1923.

Code of Justinian

Krueger, P., ed. *Corpus Iuris Civilis, Vol.* 2. *Codex Iustinianus.* 14th ed. Weidmann, 1967.

Columella

On Agriculture Ash, Harrison Boyd, trans. *Columella. On Agriculture, Volume I: Books* 1–4. Loeb Classical Library, Harvard University Press, 1941.

Didache

Milavec, Aaron, ed. and trans. *The Didache: Text, Translation, Analysis, and Commentary.* Liturgical Press, 2004.

Digest

Watson, Alan, ed. and trans. *The Digest of Justinian, Volumes* 1–4. University of Pennsylvania Press, 2009.

Dioscorides

Medical Materials

Beck, Lily Y., ed. and trans. *Dioscorides. De Materia Medica,* 4th ed. Georg Olms Verlag, 2020.

Wellman, M., ed. *Pedanii Dioscuridis Anazarbei De materia medica libri quinque,* 3 vols. Weidmann, 1907-1914.

Eunapius

Lives of the Philosophers and Sophists Miles, Graeme, and Han Baltussen, ed. and trans. *Philostratus, Eunapius. Lives of the Sophists. Lives of the Philosophers and Sophists.* Loeb Classical Library, Harvard University Press, 2023.

Galen

Affected Places Siegel, Rudolph E., trans. *Galen on the Affected Parts: Translation from the Greek with Explanatory Notes.* S. Karger AG, 1976.

Anatomical Procedures Singer, C. *Galen: On Anatomical Procedures; De anatomicis administrationibus. Translation of Surviving Books with Introduction and Notes.* Oxford University Press, 1956.

The Anatomy of the Uterus Goss, C. M., trans. "On the Anatomy of the Uterus." *The Anatomical Record* 144: 77–84 (1962).

Commentary on Hippocrates's Epidemics

Vagelpohl, Uwe, ed. and trans. *Galen: Commentary on Hippocrates Epidemics Book I. Parts I–III.* De Gruyter, 2014.

Vagelpohl, Uwe, ed. and trans. *Galen: Commentary on Hippocrates Epidemics Book II. Parts I–VI.* De Gruyter, 2016.

Vagelpohl, Uwe, ed. and trans. *Galen: Commentary on Hippocrates Epidemics Book IV. Parts I–VIII.* De Gruyter, 2022.

The Composition of Drugs According to Places Kühn, K. G. *Claudii Galeni Opera Omnia.* 22 vols. Knobloch, 1821–1833.

The Doctrines of Hippocrates and Plato De Lacy, Phillip, ed. and trans. *Galen. On the Doctrines of Hippocrates and Plato.* 2 vols. 3rd ed. Akademie-Verlag, 1984.

The Function of the Parts of the Human Body May, Margaret Tallmadge, trans. *Galen. On the Usefulness of the Parts of the Body (Peri Chreias Moriōn De Usu Partium).* Cornell University Press, 1968.

Health Singer, P. N., trans. *Galen: Writings on Health: Thrasybulus and Health (De sanitate tuenda).* Cambridge University Press, 2023.

Prognosis Nutton, Vivian, ed. and trans. *Galen. On Prognosis.* Akademie-Verlag, 1979.

Semen De Lacy, Phillip, trans. *Galen. On Semen.* Akademie-Verlag, 1992.

The Shaping of the Embryo Singer, P. N. *Galen: An Anthology.* Oxford University Press, 2024.

Simple Drugs Kühn, K. G. *Claudii Galeni Opera Omnia.* 22 vols. Knobloch, 1821–1833.

The Substance of the Natural Capacities Brock, A. J., trans. *Galen, On the Natural Faculties.* Loeb Classical Library. Harvard University Press, 1916.

The Therapeutic Method, to Glaucon Dickson, K. *Stephanus the Philosopher and Physician: Commentary on Galen's Therapeutics to Glaucon.* Brill, 1998.

Venesection, Against Erasistratus Brain, Peter. *Galen on Bloodletting: A Study of the Origins, Development and Validity of His Opinions, with a Translation of the Three Works.* Cambridge University Press, 1986.

Greek Magical Papyri

Betz, Hans Dieter, ed. *The Greek Magical Papyri in Translation, Including the Demotic Spells.* 2nd ed. University of Chicago Press, 1992.

Hippocratic Corpus

These works are all attributed to the physician Hippocrates, but they were likely written by a number of people over several centuries. These people are referred to as "The Hippocratics" and their writings are called "The Hippocratic Corpus."

Barrenness Potter, Paul, ed. and trans. *Hippocrates. Generation. Nature of the Child. Diseases 4. Nature of Women and Barrenness.* Loeb Classical Library, Harvard University Press, 2012.

Diseases of Women Potter, Paul, ed. and trans. *Hippocrates. Diseases of Women 1–2.* Loeb Classical Library, Harvard University Press, 2018.

Epidemics Smith, Wesley D., ed. and trans. *Hippocrates. Epidemics 2, 4–7.* Loeb Classical Library, Harvard University Press, 1994.

Excision of the Fetus Potter, Paul, ed. and trans. *Hippocrates. Coan Prenotions. Anatomical and Minor Clinical Writings.* Loeb Classical Library, Harvard University Press, 2010.

Fleshes Potter, Paul, ed. and trans. *Hippocrates. Places in Man. Glands. Fleshes. Prorrhetic 1–2. Physician. Use of Liquids. Ulcers. Haemorrhoids and Fistulas.* Loeb Classical Library, Harvard University Press, 1995.

Generation Potter, Paul, ed. and trans. *Hippocrates. Generation. Nature of the Child. Diseases 4. Nature of Women and Barrenness.* Loeb Classical Library, Harvard University Press, 2012.

Girls

Flemming, Rebecca, and Ann Ellis Hanson, eds. and trans. "Hippocrates' *Peri Partheniôn* ('Diseases of Young Girls'): Text and Translation." *Early Science and Medicine* 3, no. 3 (1998): 241–52.

Potter, Paul, ed. and trans. *Hippocrates. Coan Prenotions. Anatomical and Minor Clinical Writings.* Loeb Classical Library, Harvard University Press, 2010.

Nature of Man Jones, W. H. S., trans. *Hippocrates. Heracleitus. Nature of Man. Regimen in Health. Humours. Aphorisms. Regimen 1–3. Dreams. Heracleitus: On the Universe.* Loeb Classical Library, Harvard University Press, 1931.

Nature of Women Potter, Paul, ed. and trans. *Hippocrates. Generation. Nature of the Child. Diseases 4. Nature of Women and Barrenness.* Loeb Classical Library, Harvard University Press, 2012.

Nature of the Child Potter, Paul, ed. and trans. *Hippocrates. Generation. Nature of the Child. Diseases 4. Nature of Women and Barrenness.* Loeb Classical Library, Harvard University Press, 2012.

Superfetation Potter, Paul, ed. and trans. *Hippocrates. Coan Prenotions. Anatomical and Minor Clinical Writings.* Loeb Classical Library, Harvard University Press, 2010.

Historia Augusta

Antoninus Diadumenus Magie, David, trans. *Historia Augusta, Volume II.* Rev. David Rohrbacher. Loeb Classical Library, Harvard University Press, 2022.

Homeric Hymn 3: To Apollo

West, Martin L., ed. and trans. *Homeric Hymns. Homeric Apocrypha. Lives of Homer.* Loeb Classical Library, Harvard University Press, 2003.

Hyginus

Myths Grant, Mary, ed. and trans. *The Myths of Hyginus.* University of Kansas Publications in Humanistic Studies, no. 34. University of Kansas Press, 1960.

Juvenal
Satires Braund, Susanna Morton, ed. and trans. *Juvenal. Persius. Juvenal and Persius*. Loeb Classical Library, Harvard University Press, 2004.

Lucan
The Civil War Duff, J. D., trans. *Lucan. The Civil War (Pharsalia)*. Loeb Classical Library, Harvard University Press, 1928.

Lucretius
On the Nature of Things Rouse, W. H. D., trans. *Lucretius. On the Nature of Things*. Rev. Martin F. Smith. Loeb Classical Library, Harvard University Press, 1924.

Macrobius
Saturnalia Kaster, Robert A., ed. and trans. *Macrobius. Saturnalia, Volume I: Books* 1–2. Loeb Classical Library, Harvard University Press, 2011.

Martial
Epigrams
Bailey, D. R. Shackleton, ed. and trans. *Martial. Epigrams, Volume I: Spectacles, Books* 1–5. Loeb Classical Library, Harvard University Press, 1993.
Bailey, D. R. Shackleton, ed. and trans. *Martial. Epigrams, Volume II: Books* 6–10. Loeb Classical Library, Harvard University Press, 1993.

Muscio/Mustio
Gynaecia Bolton, Lesley. "An Edition, Translation and Commentary of Mustio's *Gynaecia*." PhD diss., University of Calgary, 2015.

Opinions of Paulus
Scott, S. P., trans. *The Civil Law*. Vol. I. Central Trust Company, 1932.

Oribasius
Medical Collections Raeder, J., ed. *Oribasii Collectionum Medicarum Reliquiae*. 4 vols. Teubner, 1928–1933.

Ovid
Amores Showerman, Grant, trans. *Ovid. Heroides. Amores*. Rev. G. P. Goold. Loeb Classical Library, Harvard University Press, 1914.

Metamorphoses Miller, Frank Justus, trans. *Ovid. Metamorphoses, Volume II: Books* 9–15. Rev. G. P. Goold. Loeb Classical Library, Harvard University Press, 1916.

The Passion of Perpetua and Felicity

Heffernan, Thomas J. *The Passion of Perpetua and Felicity.* Oxford University Press, 2012.

Paul of Aegina

Heiberg, J. L., ed. *Paulus Aegineta.* 2 vols. Teubner, 1921–1924.

Adams, Francis, trans. *The Seven Books of Paulus Aegineta.* 3 vols. Sydenham Society, 1844–1847.

Plato

Timaeus Bury, R. G., trans. *Plato. Timaeus. Critias. Cleitophon. Menexenus. Epistles.* Loeb Classical Library, Harvard University Press, 1929.

Plautus

The Braggart Soldier de Melo, Wolfgang, ed. and trans. *Plautus. The Merchant. The Braggart Soldier. The Ghost. The Persian.* Loeb Classical Library, Harvard University Press, 2011.

The Pot of Gold de Melo, Wolfgang, ed. and trans. *Plautus. Amphytrion. The Comedy of Asses. The Pot of Gold. The Two Bacchises. The Captives.* Loeb Classical Library, Harvard University Press, 2011.

Truculentus de Melo, Wolfgang, ed. and trans. *Plautus. Stichus. Trinummus. Truculentus. Tale of a Traveling Bag. Fragments.* Loeb Classical Library, Harvard University Press, 2013.

Pliny the Elder

Natural History

Jones, W. H. S., trans. *Pliny. Natural History, Volume VI: Books* 20–23. Loeb Classical Library, Harvard University Press, 1951.

Jones, W. H. S., trans. *Pliny. Natural History, Volume VIII: Books* 28–32. Loeb Classical Library, Harvard University Press, 1963.

Rackham, H., trans. *Pliny. Natural History, Volume II: Books* 3–7. Loeb Classical Library, Harvard University Press, 1942.

Pliny the Younger

Letters Radice, Betty, trans. *Pliny the Younger. Letters, Volume II: Books 8–10. Panegyricus.* Loeb Classical Library, Harvard University Press, 1969.

Plutarch and Pseudo-Plutarch

Advice to Bride and Groom Babbitt, Frank Cole, trans. *Plutarch. Moralia, Volume II: How to Profit by One's Enemies. On Having Many Friends. Chance. Virtue and Vice. Letter of Condolence to Apollonius. Advice About Keeping Well. Advice to Bride and Groom. The Dinner of Seven Wise Men. Superstition.* Loeb Classical Library, Harvard University Press, 1928.

Dialogue on Love Minar, Edwin L., F. H. Sandbach, and W. C. Helmbold., trans. *Plutarch. Moralia, Volume IX: Table-Talk, Books 7–9. Dialogue on Love.* Loeb Classical Library, Harvard University Press, 1961.

The Education of Children Babbitt, Frank Cole, trans. *Plutarch. Moralia, Volume I: The Education of Children. How the Young Man Should Study Poetry. On Listening to Lectures. How to Tell a Flatterer from a Friend. How a Man May Become Aware of His Progress in Virtue.* Loeb Classical Library, Harvard University Press, 1927.

Lives of Lycurgus and Numa Perrin, Bernadotte, trans. *Plutarch. Lives, Volume I: Theseus and Romulus. Lycurgus and Numa. Solon and Publicola.* Loeb Classical Library, Harvard University Press, 1914.

On Rivers Banchich, Thomas M., trans. *Pseudo-Plutarch. About Rivers and Mountains and Things Found in Them.* Canisius College Translated Texts, 2010. https://roman-emperors.sites.luc.edu/Pseudo-P%20Revised.pdf

Table-Talk Clement, P. A., and H. B. Hoffleit, trans. *Plutarch. Moralia, Volume VIII: Table-Talk, Books* 1-6. Loeb Classical Library, Harvard University Press, 1969.

Porphyry

To Gaurus on How Embryos Are Ensouled

Brisson, L., et al. *Porphyre: Sur la manière dont l'embryon reçoit l'âme.* In *Histoire des doctrines de l'antiquité classique* 43. J. Vrin, 2012.

Wilberding, James, trans. *Porphyry: To Gaurus on How Embryos Are Ensouled and On What Is in Our Power.* Bloomsbury, 2011.

To Marcella Wicker, Kathleen O'Brien, ed. and trans. *Porphyry the Philosopher: To Marcella; Text and Translation.* Scholars Press, 1987.

Protevangelium of James

Elliot, J. K., ed. and trans. *The Protevangelium of James.* Brepolis, 2022.

Quintilian and Pseudo-Quintilian

The Major Declamations Stramaglia, Antonio, ed., and Michael Winterbottom, trans. *Quintilian. The Major Declamations, Volume I.* Loeb Classical Library, Harvard University Press, 2021.

The Orator's Education Russell, Donald A., ed. and trans. *Quintilian. The Orator's Education, Volume III: Books* 6–8. Loeb Classical Library, Harvard University Press, 2002.

Seneca

Epistles Gummere, Richard M., trans. *Seneca. Epistles, Volume III: Epistles* 93–124. Loeb Classical Library, Harvard University Press, 1925.

On Benefits Basore, John W., trans. *Seneca. Moral Essays, Volume III: De Beneficiis.* Loeb Classical Library, Harvard University Press, 1935.

Sibylline Oracles

Lightfoot, J. L., ed. and trans. *The Sibylline Oracles: With Introduction, Translation, and Commentary on the First and Second Books.* Oxford University Press, 2007.

Soranus

Gynecology

Ilberg, Johannes, ed. *Sorani Gynaeciorum libri IV. De signis fractuarum. De fasciis. Vita Hippocratis secundum Soranum.* Teubner, 1927.

Temkin, Owsei, trans. *Soranus' Gynecology.* Johns Hopkins University Press, 1956.

Tacitus

Annals Jackson, John, trans. *Tacitus. Annals: Books* 13–16. Loeb Classical Library, Harvard University Press, 1937.

Germania Hutton, M., and W. Peterson, trans. *Tacitus. Agricola. Germania. Dialogue on Oratory.* Rev. R. M. Ogilvie, E. H. Warmington, and Michael Winterbottom. Loeb Classical Library, Harvard University Press, 2014.

Terence

The Brothers Barsby, John, ed. and trans. *Terence. Phormio. The Mother-in-Law. The Brothers.* Loeb Classical Library, Harvard University Press, 2001.

The Woman of Andros Barsby, John, ed. and trans. *Terence. The Woman of Andros. The Self-Tormenter. The Eunuch.* Loeb Classical Library, Harvard University Press, 2001.

Tertullian

Apology Glover, T. R., and Gerald H. Rendall, trans. *Tertullian. Minucius Felix. Apology. De Spectaculis. Minucius Felix: Octavius*. Loeb Classical Library, Harvard University Press, 1931.

On the Soul

Holmes, Peter, trans. "A Treatise on the Soul." In *Ante-Nicene Fathers Vol. 3: Latin Christianity: Its Founder, Tertullian,* ed. Alexander Roberts, James Donaldson, and A. Cleveland Coxe. Christian Literature Publishing, 1885.

Waszink, J. H. *Quinti Septimi Florentis Tertulliani De Anima*. Meulenhoff, 1947.

Theodorus Priscianus

Rose, Valentino, ed. *Theodori Prisciani Euporiston libri III: cum physicorum fragmento et additamentis pseudo-Theodoreis*. Lipsiae, 1894.

Varro

On Agriculture Hooper, W. D., and Harrison Boyd Ash. *Cato. Varro. On Agriculture.* Loeb Classical Library, Harvard University Press, 1934.

Velleius Paterculus

History Woodman, A. J., ed. and trans. *Velleius Paterculus.* Loeb Classical Library, Harvard University Press, 2025.

INSCRIPTIONS, PAPYRI, OSTRACA, AND AMULETS

AE. *L'Année épigraphique,* https://anneeepigraphique.com/

BGU. *Aegyptische Urkunden aus den Koeniglichen Museen zu Berlin: Griechische Urkunden.* 4 vols. Weidmann, 1895–1912.

CBd. Campbell Bonner Magical Gems Database, http://cbd.mfab.hu/visitatori_salutem

CIL. Corpus Inscriptionum Latinarum, https://cil.bbaw.de/

CPG. Manca Masciadri, M., and O. Montevecchi. *Corpus Papyrorum Graecarum* 1. Tibiletti, 1984.

FD. École française d'Athènes. *Fouilles de Delphes.* Boccard, 1902.

IG. Inscriptiones Graecae, https://inscriptions.packhum.org/allregions

IGUR. Moretti, Luigi, ed. *Inscriptiones Graecae Urbis Romae*. 4 vols. in 5 parts. Bardi Edizioni, 1968–1990.

O.Florida. Bagnall, R. S., ed. "The Florida Ostraka: Documents from the Roman Army in Upper Egypt." *Greek, Roman, and Byzantine Monographs* 7, nos. 1–31 (1976).

P.Fam.Tebt. van Groningen, B. A., ed. *A Family Archive from Tebtunis.* Brill, 1950.

P.Fouad. Bataille, A., O. Guéraud, P. Jouguet, et al., eds. *Les Papyrus Fouad I.* L'Institut Francais d'Archeologie Orientale, 1939.

P.Gen. Wehrli, Cl., ed. *Les Papyrus de Genève II.* Nos. 82–177. Bibliothèque Publique et Universitaire, 1986.

P.Lond. Kenyon, F. G., and H. I. Bell, eds. *Greek Papyri in the British Museum III.* Nos. 485–1331. British Museum, 1907.

P.Mich. Michigan Papyri, https://quod.lib.umich.edu/a/apis?page=index

P.Münch. Hagedorn, U. and D., R. Hübner, and J. C. Shelton, eds. *Die Papyri der Bayerischen Staatsbibliothek München III.* Teubner, 1986.

P.Oxy. Oxyrhynchus Papyri, https://oxyrhynchus.web.ox.ac.uk/home

MODERN SOURCES

Adair, Mark J. "Plato's View of the 'Wandering Uterus.'" *Classical Journal* 91, no. 2 (1995): 153–63.

Agarwal, Sristy, Roshan Prasad, Saket Mantri, et al. "A Comprehensive Review of Intimate Partner Violence During Pregnancy and Its Adverse Effects on Maternal and Fetal Health." *Cureus* 15, no. 5 (2023): e39262.

Alfirevic, Zarko, Gillian M. L. Gyte, Anna Cuthbert, and Declan Devane. "Continuous Cardiotocography as a Form of Electronic Fetal Monitoring for Fetal Assessment During Labour." *Cochrane Database of Systematic Reviews* (2017): CD006066. https://pmc.ncbi.nlm.nih.gov/articles/PMC6464257/.

Alonso Alonso, Marîa de los Ángeles. "Medicae y obstetrices en la epigrafia latina del Imperio romano: Apuntes en torno a un análisis comparativo." *Classica et Cristiana* 6 (2011): 267–96.

Alston, Richard. "Roman Military Pay from Caesar to Diocletian." *Journal of Roman Studies* 84 (1994): 113–23.

Aubert, Jean-Jacques. "Threatened Wombs: Aspects of Ancient Uterine Magic." *Greek, Roman, and Byzantine Studies* 30 (1989): 421–49.

Bagley, Andrée Marie. "Roman Children in the Early Empire: A Distinct Epidemiological and Therapeutic Category?" Phd diss., University of Birmingham, 2016.

Bagnall, Roger S., and Rafaella Cribiore. *Women's Letters from Ancient Egypt, 300 BC–AD 800*. University of Michigan Press, 2006.

Baker, Patricia. "Soranus and the Pompeii Speculum: The Sociology of Gynaecology and Roman Perceptions of the Female Body." In *Proceedings of the Eighth Annual Theoretical Roman Archaeology Conference, Leicester* 1998, ed. Patricia Baker, Charles B. Forcey, Sophia Jundi, and Robert Witcher. Oxbow Books, 1999.

Banks, Jennifer. *Natality: Toward a Philosophy of Birth*. W. W. Norton, 2023.

Baskett, Thomas F. "Operative Vaginal Delivery—an Historical Perspective." *Best Practice & Research Clinical Obstetrics & Gynaecology* 56 (2019): 3–10.

Baumbach, Jens. "'Speak, Votives, . . . ' Dedicatory Practice in Sanctuaries of Hera." In *Le Donateur, l'offrande et la déesse*, ed. Clarisse Prêtre. Presses universitaires de Liège, 2009.

Beagon, Mary. *Roman Nature: The Thought of Pliny the Elder*. Clarendon Press, 1992.

Bernstine, Richard L., and Dwight A. Callagan. "Ultrasonic Doppler Inspection of the Fetal Heart." *American Journal of Obstetrics and Gynecology* 95, no. 7 (1966): 1001–4.

Bettini, Maurizio. *Women and Weasels: Mythologies of Birth in Ancient Greece and Rome*. Trans. Emlyn Eisenach. University of Chicago Press, 2013.

Birthtalk.org. "Laura Stavoe Speaks—Why She Wrote: 'There Is a Secret in Our Culture and It Is Not That Birth Is Painful but That Women Are Strong.'" Accessed May 20, 2025. https://birthtraumatruths.wordpress.com/2011/06/06/laura-stavoe-speaks-why-she-wrote-there-is-a-secret-in-our-culture-but-it-is-not-that-women-are-strong/.

Bisel, Sara, and Jane Bisel. "Health and Nutrition at Herculaneum: An Examination of Human Skeletal Remains." In *The Natural History of Pompeii*, ed. Wilhelmina F. Jashemski and Frederick G. Meyer. Cambridge University Press, 2002.

Björklund, Heta. "Protecting Against Child-Killing Demons: Uterus Amulets in the Late Antique and Byzantine Magical World." PhD diss., University of Helsinki, 2017.

Bliquez, Lawrence. *The Tools of Asclepius: Surgical Instruments in Greek and Roman Times*. Brill, 2014.

Blumenfeld-Kosinski, Renate. *Not of Woman Born: Representations of Caesarean Birth in Medieval and Renaissance Culture*. Cornell University Press, 1990.

Bodel, John. "Minicia Marcella: Taken Before Her Time." *American Journal of Philology* 116, no. 3 (1995): 453–60.

Bolton, Lesley. “Patience for the Little Patient: The Infant in Soranus’ *Gynaecia*.” In *Homo Patiens: Approaches to the Patient in the Ancient World,* ed. Georgia Petridou and Chiara Thumiger. Brill, 2016.

Bonner, Campbell. *Studies in Magical Amulets: Chiefly Graeco-Egyptian*. University of Michigan Press, 1950.

Boston Women’s Health Book Collective. *Women and Their Bodies: A Course.* New England Free Press, 1970.

Boston Women’s Health Book Collective. *Our Bodies, Ourselves: A Book by and for Women*. Simon and Schuster, 1973.

Bourbou, Chryssi. “The Bioarchaeology of Roman Diet.” In *The Routledge Handbook of Diet and Nutrition in the Roman World,* ed. Paul Erdkamp and Claire Holleran. Routledge, 2018.

Bourbou, Chryssi. “Life and Death at the ‘Land of the Three Lakes’: Revisiting the Non-Adults from Roman Aventicum, Switzerland (1st–3rd Century CE).” *International Journal of Paleopathology* 22 (2018): 121–34.

Bradley, Keith. “Wet-Nursing at Rome: A Study in Social Relations.” In *The Family in Ancient Rome: New Perspectives,* ed. Beryl Rawson. Cornell University Press, 1986.

Bradley, Keith. *Discovering the Roman Family: Studies in Roman Social History.* Oxford University Press, 1991.

Bradley, Keith. *Slavery and Society at Rome.* Cambridge University Press, 1994.

Bradley, Keith. “Children and Dreams.” In *Childhood, Class and Kin in the Roman World,* ed. Suzanne Dixon. Routledge, 2001.

Bradley, Mark, Victoria Leonard, and Laurence M. V. Totelin, eds. *Bodily Fluids in Antiquity.* Taylor & Francis, 2021.

Bridges, Khiara M. *Reproducing Race: An Ethnography of Pregnancy as a Site of Radicalization*. University of California Press, 2011.

Briggs, Laura. “The Race of Hysteria: ‘Overcivilization’ and the ‘Savage’ Woman in Late Nineteenth-Century Obstetrics and Gynecology.” *American Quarterly* 52.2 (2000): 246–73.

Bubb, Claire. *Dissection in Classical Antiquity: A Social and Medical History.* Cambridge University Press, 2022.

Bubb, Claire. “Ancient Conceptions of the Human Uterus: Italic Votives and Animal Wombs.” *Journal of the History of Medicine and Allied Sciences* 79 no. 2 (2024): 101–14.

Bushnell, Britta. *Transformed by Birth: Cultivating Openness, Resilience, and Strength for the Life-Changing Journey from Pregnancy to Parenthood.* Sounds True, 2020.

Butler, Judith. *Bodies That Matter: On the Discursive Limits of "Sex."* Routledge, 1993.

Caldwell, Lauren. *Roman Girlhood and the Fashioning of Femininity.* Cambridge University Press, 2015.

Cambron-Goulet, Mathilde, and François-Julien Côté-Remy. "Plotinus and Porphyry on Women's Legitimacy in Philosophy." In *Women's Perspectives on Ancient and Medieval Philosophy: Logic, Argumentation and Reasoning,* ed. Isabelle Chouinard, Zoe McConaughey, Aline Medeiros Ramos, and Roxane Noël. Springer, 2021.

Capasso, Luigi. *I fuggiaschi di Ercolano: Paleobiologia delle vittime dell'eruzione vesuviana del* 79 *d.C.* L'Erma di Bretschneider, 2001.

Carroll, Maureen. "Infant Death and Burial in Roman Italy." *Journal of Roman Archaeology* 24 (2011): 99–120.

Carroll, Maureen. *Infancy and Earliest Childhood in the Roman World.* Oxford Academic, 2018.

Carroll, Maureen. "Mater Matuta, 'Fertility Cults' and the Integration of Women in Religious Life in Italy in the Fourth to First Centuries BC." *Papers of the British School at Rome* 87 (2019): 1–45.

Cao, Irene. *Alimenta: Il racconto delle fonti.* Il Poligrafo, 2010.

CDC. "Births—Method of Delivery." Last modified June 5, 2025. https://www.cdc.gov/nchs/fastats/delivery.htm

Centlivres Challet, Claude-Emmanuelle. "Feeding the Roman Nursling: Maternal Milk, Its Substitutes, and Their Limitations." *Latomus* 76, no. 4 (2017): 895–909.

Clemens, Martin. "Silphium, the Ancient Contraceptive Herb Driven to Extinction." Ancient Origins, May 6, 2024. https://www.ancient-origins.net/history-ancient-traditions/silphium-002268.

Cleveland Clinic. "Breech Baby." Last modified April 4, 2024. https://my.clevelandclinic.org/health/diseases/21848-breech-baby.

Cobb, Stephanie L., ed. *The Passion of Perpetua and Felicitas in Late Antiquity.* University of California Press, 2021.

Collman, Ryan D. *The Apostle to the Foreskin: Circumcision in the Letters of Paul.* De Gruyter, 2023.

Connell, Sophia M. "Aristotle and Galen on Sex Difference and Reproduction: A New Approach to an Ancient Rivalry." *Studies in History and Philosophy of Science* 31, no. 3 (2000): 405–27.

Connell, Sophia M. *Aristotle on Female Animals.* Cambridge University Press, 2016.

Connell, Sophia M. "Women's Medical Knowledge in Antiquity Beyond Midwifery." In *Ancient Women Philosophers: Recovered Ideas and New Perspec-*

tives, ed. Katharine R. O'Reilly and Caterina Pellò. Cambridge University Press, 2023.

Constantinou, Stavroula, and Aspasia Skouroumouni-Stavrinou. "Breast Rules: The Body of the Wet Nurse in Ancient and Early Byzantine Discourses." In *Breastfeeding and Mothering in Antiquity and Early Byzantium,* ed. Stavroula Constantinou and Aspasia Skouroumouni-Stavrinou. Routledge, 2024.

Constantinou, Stavroula, and Aspasia Skouroumouni-Stavrinou. "The Lactating Woman: Breastfeeding and Mothering in Antiquity and Early Byzantium." In *Breastfeeding and Mothering in Antiquity and Early Byzantium,* ed. Stavroula Constantinou and Aspasia Skouroumouni-Stavrinou. Routledge, 2024.

Coughlin, Sean, et al. *The Soul Is an Octopus: Ancient Ideas of Life and the Body.* Berliner Medizinhistorisches Museum der Charité. Edition Topoi, 2016.

Craig, Oliver E., Marco Biazzo, Tamsin C. O'Connell, et al. "Stable Isotopic Evidence for Diet at the Imperial Roman Coastal Site of Velia (1st and 2nd Centuries AD) in Southern Italy." *American Journal of Physical Anthropology* 139 (2009): 572–83.

Cronk, Mary. "Hands off That Breech!" *AIMS Journal* 17.1 (2005). https://www.aims.org.uk/journal/item/hands-off-that-breech.

D'Ambra, Eve. *Roman Women.* Cambridge University Press, 2007.

Daniels, Cynthia R. "Fathers, Mothers, and Fetal Harm: Rethinking Gender Difference and Reproductive Responsibility." In *Fetal Subjects, Feminist Positions,* ed. Lynn M. Morgan and Meredith Wilson Michaels. University of Pennsylvania Press, 1999.

Dasen, Véronique. "Métamorphoses de l'utérus d'Hippocrate à Ambroise Paré." *Gesnerus* 59 (2002): 167–86.

Dasen, Véronique. "Femmes à tiroir." In *Naissance et petite enfance dans l'Antiquité: Actes du colloque de Fribourg, 28 novembre–1er décembre 2001,* ed. Véronique Dasen. Academic Press, 2004.

Dasen, Véronique. "Représenter l'invisible: La vie utérine sur les gemmes magiques." In *L'Embryon humain à travers l'histoire: Images, savoirs et rites,* ed. Véronique Dasen. Infolio, 2007.

Dasen, Véronique. "'All Children Are Dwarfs': Medical Discourse and Iconography of Children's Bodies." *Oxford Journal of Archaeology* 27 (2008): 49–62.

Dasen, Véronique. "Roman Birth Rites of Passage Revisited." *Journal of Roman Archaeology* 22 (2009): 199–215.

Dasen, Véronique."Healing Images: Gems and Medicine." *Oxford Journal of Archaeology* 33, no. 2 (2014): 177–91.

Dasen, Véronique. *Le sourire d'Omphale: Maternité et petite enfance dans l'Antiquité.* Presses universitaires de Rennes, 2015.

Dasen, Véronique, and Sandrine Ducaté-Paarmann. "Hysteria and Metaphors of the Uterus." In *Images and Gender: Contributions to the Hermeneutics of Reading Ancient Art,* ed. Silvia Schroer. Academic Press, 2006.

David-Floyd, Robbie. *Birth as an American Rite of Passage.* 2nd ed. University of California Press, 2003.

Davis-Floyd, Robbie, and Christine Johnson. *Mainstreaming Midwives: The Politics of Change.* Routledge, 2006.

Daviss, Betty-Anne, Kenneth C. Johnson, and Andre B. Lalonde. "Evolving Evidence Since the Term Breech Trial: Canadian Response, European Dissent, and Potential Solutions." *Journal of Obstetrics and Gynaecology Canada* 32, no. 3 (2010): 217–24.

De Luca, Francesca. "'God Was the First Anesthetist': Obstetrics and Pain in Lisbon at the Turn of the 20th Century." *Etnográfica* 22, no. 3 (2018): 619–42.

Dean-Jones, Lesley. "The Cultural Construct of the Female Body in Classical Greek Science." In *Women's History and Ancient History,* ed. Sarah B. Pomeroy. University of North Carolina Press, 1991.

Dean-Jones, Lesley. "The Politics of Pleasure: Female Sexual Appetite in the Hippocratic Corpus." In *Discourses of Sexuality: From Aristotle to AIDS,* ed. Domna C. Stanton. University of Michigan Press, 1992.

Dean-Jones, Lesley. *Women's Bodies in Classical Greek Science.* Oxford University Press, 1994.

Dean-Jones, Lesley. "Autopsia, Historia and What Women Know: The Authority of Women in Hippocratic Gynecology." In *Knowledge and the Scholarly Medical Traditions,* ed. Donald Bates. Cambridge University Press, 1995.

Dean-Jones, Lesley. "The Cultural Construct of the Female Body in Classical Greek Science." In *Sex and Difference in Ancient Greece and Rome,* ed. Mark Golden and Peter Toohey. Edinburgh University Press, 2003.

Dean-Jones, Lesley. "The Hippocratic Physician and the Female Patient." In *The Cambridge Companion to Hippocrates,* ed. Peter Pormann. Cambridge University Press, 2018.

Delatte, Armand, and Philippe Derchain. *Les intailles magiques gréco-égyptiennes.* Éditions de la Bibliothèque nationale de France, 1964.

Demand, Nancy. *Birth, Death, and Motherhood in Classical Greece.* Johns Hopkins University Press, 1994.

Dixon, Suzanne. *The Roman Mother.* University of Oklahoma Press, 1988.

Donnison, Jean. *Midwives and Medical Men: A History of the Struggle for the Control of Childbirth.* Routledge, 1977.

Dova, Stamatia. "Lactation Cessation and the Realities of Martyrdom in *The Passion of Saint Perpetua.*" *Illinois Classical Studies* 42, no. 1 (2017): 245–65.

Draycott, Jane. *Roman Domestic Medical Practice in Central Italy: From the Middle Republic to the Early Empire.* Routledge, 2019.

Drexler, Kathleen A., Johanna Quist-Nelson, and Amy B. Weil. "Intimate Partner Violence and Trauma-Informed Care in Pregnancy." *American Journal of Obstetrics and Gynecology* 4, no. 2 (2022): 100542.

duBois, Page. *Sowing the Body: Psychoanalysis and Ancient Representations of Women.* University of Chicago Press, 1988.

duBois, Page. *Slaves and Other Objects.* University of Chicago Press, 2003.

Ducaté-Paarmann, Sandrine. "Voyage à l'intérieur du corps féminin." In *L'Embryon humain à travers l'histoire: Images, savoirs et rites,* ed. Véronique Dasen. Infolio, 2007.

Duden, Barbara. *Disembodying Women: Perspectives on Pregnancy and the Unborn.* Harvard University Press, 1993.

Dupras, Tosha L., Sandra M. Wheeler, Lana Williams, and Peter Sheldrick. "Birth in Ancient Egypt: Timing, Trauma, and Triumph? Evidence from the Dakhleh Oasis." In *Egyptian Bioarcheology: Humans, Animals, and the Environment,* ed. Salima Ikram, Jessica Kaiser, and Roxie Walker. Sidestone Press, 2015.

Ecca, Giulia. "Fixing Ethical Rules for Midwives in the Early Roman Imperial Period: Soranus, 'Gynaecia' I 3–4." *Sudhoffs Archiv* 101, no. 2 (2017): 125–38.

Ehrenreich, Barbara, and Deirdre English. *Witches, Midwives, and Nurses: A History of Women Healers.* Feminist Press at CUNY, 1973.

Evans Grubbs, Judith. *Women and the Law in the Roman Empire: A Sourcebook on Marriage, Divorce and Widowhood.* Routledge, 2002.

Evans Grubbs, Judith. "The Dynamics of Infant Abandonment: Motives, Attitudes, and (Unintended) Consequences." In *The Dark Side of Childhood in Late Antiquity and the Middle Ages,* ed. Katarina Mustakallio and Christian Laes. Oxbow Books, 2011.

Faraone, Christopher A. "New Light on Ancient Greek Exorcisms of the Wandering Womb." *Zeitschrift für Papyrologie und Epigraphik* 144 (2003): 189–97.

Faraone, Christopher A. "Magical and Medical Approaches to the Wandering Womb in the Ancient Greek World." *Classical Antiquity* 30, no. 1 (2011): 1–32.

Faraone, Christopher A. *Vanishing Acts on Ancient Greek Amulets: From Oral Performance to Visual Design.* Institute of Classical Studies, 2012.

Faraone, Christopher A. *The Transformation of Greek Amulets in Roman Imperial Times.* University of Pennsylvania Press, 2018.

Federici, Silvia. *Caliban and the Witch: Women, the Body, and Primitive Accumulation.* Autonomedia, 2004.

Felton, Debbie. "Witches, Disgust, and Anti-Abortion Propaganda in Imperial Rome." In *The Ancient Emotion of Disgust,* ed. Donald Lateiner and Dimos Spatharas. Oxford Academic, 2016.

Fett, Sharla M. "Consciousness and Calling: African American Midwives at Work in the Antebellum South." In *New Studies in the History of American Slavery,* ed. Edward E. Baptist and Stephanie M.H. Camp. University of Georgia Press, 2006.

Feucht, Erika M. "Motherhood in Pharaonic Egypt." In *Women in Antiquity: Real Women Across the Ancient World,* ed. Stephanie Lynn Budin and Jean MacIntosh Turfa. Routledge, 2016.

Filippini, Nadia M. *Pregnancy, Delivery, Childbirth: A Gender and Cultural History from Antiquity to the Test Tube in Europe.* Trans. Clelia Boscolo. Routledge, 2021.

Finnigan, Sheena. "Working Moms: Motherhood, Occupation, and Status in Roman Italy, ca. 100 BCE–150 CE." PhD diss., University of Wisconsin-Madison, 2022.

Fischbein, Stuart James, and Rixa Freeze. "Breech Birth at Home: Outcomes of 60 Breech and 109 Cephalic Planned Home and Birth Center Births." *BMC Pregnancy Childbirth* 18 (2018): 397.

Flemming, Rebecca. *Medicine and the Making of Roman Women: Gender, Nature, and Authority from Celsus to Galen.* Oxford University Press, 2000.

Flemming, Rebecca. "The Pathology of Pregnancy in Galen's Commentaries on the *Epidemics.*" *Bulletin of the Institute of Classical Studies* Supplement 77 (2002): 101-12.

Flemming, Rebecca. "Women, Writing and Medicine in the Classical World." *Classical Quarterly* 57, no. 1 (2007): 257–79.

Flemming, Rebecca. "Demiurge and Emperor in Galen's World of Knowledge." In *Galen and the World of Knowledge,* ed. Christopher Gill, Tim Whitmarsh, and John Wilkins. Cambridge University Press, 2009.

Flemming, Rebecca. "Gendering Medical Provision in the Cities of the Roman West." In *Women and the Roman City in the Latin West,* ed. Emily Hemelrijk and Greg Woolf. Brill, 2013.

Flemming, Rebecca. "The Invention of Infertility in the Classical Greek World: Medicine, Divinity, and Gender." *Bulletin of the History of Medicine* 87, no. 4 (2013): 565–90.

Flemming, Rebecca. "Wombs for the Gods." In *Bodies of Evidence: Ancient Anatomical Votives Past, Present and Future,* ed. Jane Draycott and Emma-Jayne Graham. Routledge, 2017.
Flemming, Rebecca. "Fertility Control in Ancient Rome." *Women's History Review* 30, no. 6 (2021): 896–914.
Flemming, Rebecca. "One Seed, Two Seed, Three Seed? Reassessing the Fluid Economy of Ancient Generation." In *Bodily Fluids in Antiquity,* ed. Mark Bradley, Victoria Leonard, and Laurence Totelin. Routledge, 2021.
Flemming, Rebecca, and Laurence M. V. Totelin, eds. *Medicine and Markets in the Graeco-Roman World and Beyond: Essays on Ancient Medicine in Honour of Vivian Nutton.* Classical Press of Wales, 2020.
Fox, Sarah, and Margeret Brazier. "The Regulation of Midwives in England, c.1500–1902." *Medical Law International* 20, no. 4 (2020): 308–38.
Frankfurter, David, ed. *Guide to the Study of Ancient Magic.* Brill, 2019.
Fraser, Gertrude Jacinta. *African American Midwifery in the South: Dialogues of Birth, Race and Memory.* Harvard University Press, 1998.
Freidin, Anna Bonnell. "Well-Born: The Ancient History of Making the Best Babies." *Eidolon,* 2016. https://eidolon.pub/well-born-the-ancient-history-of-making-the-best-babies-e396e2c2d6b7.
Freidin, Anna Bonnell. "The Birthday Present: Censorinus' De Die Natali." *Journal of Roman Studies* 110 (2020): 141–66.
Freidin, Anna Bonnell. "Carrying Risk in Antiquity and the Present." The Immanent Frame, September 11, 2020. https://tif.ssrc.org/2020/09/11/carrying-risk-in-antiquity-and-the-present/.
Freidin, Anna Bonnell. "Animal Wombs: The Octopus and the Uterus in Graeco-Roman Culture." *Classical Philology* 116 (2021): 76–101.
Freidin, Anna Bonnell. *Birthing Romans: Childbearing and Its Risks in Imperial Rome.* Princeton University Press, 2024.
Frier, Bruce W. "Natural Fertility and Family Limitation in Roman Marriage." *Classical Philology* 89, no. 4 (1994): 318–33.
Frier, Bruce W. "Roman Law and the Marriage of Underage Girls." *Journal of Roman Archaeology* 28, no. 2 (2015): 652–64.
Frier, Bruce W. "Normalizing Illegality? The Roman Jurists and Underage Marriage." In *New Directions in the Study of Women in the Greco-Roman World,* ed. Ronnie Ancona and Georgia Tsouvala. Oxford Academic, 2021.
Gardiner, Jane F. *Women in Roman Law and Society.* Indiana University Press, 1986.
Garnsey, Peter. *Cities, Peasants and Food in Classical Antiquity: Essays in Social and Economic History.* Cambridge University Press, 1998.

Garnsey, Peter. *Food and Society in Classical Antiquity.* Cambridge University Press, 1999.

Gaskin, Ina May. *Ina May's Guide to Childbirth.* Bantam, 2003.

Gellar-Goad, T. H. M. "Todd Akin, the Greek Doctor Soranus, and 'Legitimate Rape,'" *Society for Classical Studies* (blog), March 14, 2014. https://classicalstudies.org/scs-blog/t-h-m-gellar-goad/todd-akin-greek-doctor-soranus-and-legitimate-rape.

Gianni, Gaia. *All in the Family: Childhood and Fictive Kinship in Roman Society.* University of Michigan Press, 2025.

Giladi, Avner. *Muslim Midwives: The Craft of Birthing in the Premodern Middle East.* Cambridge University Press, 2015.

Glinister, Fay. "Ritual and Meaning: Contextualising Votive Terracotta Infants in Hellenistic Italy." In *Bodies of Evidence: Ancient Anatomical Votives Past, Present and Future,* ed. Jane Draycott and Emma-Jayne Graham. Routledge, 2017.

Goff, Beatrice Laura. *Symbols of Ancient Egypt in the Late Period: The Twenty-First Dynasty.* Mouton Publishers, 1979.

Goffinet, François, Marion Carayol, Jean-Michel Foidart, et al. "Is Planned Vaginal Delivery for Breech Presentation at Term Still an Option? Results of an Observational Prospective Survey in France and Belgium." *American Journal of Obstetrics and Gynecology* 194, no. 4 (2006): 1002–11.

Golden, Mark. "Did the Ancients Care When Their Children Died?" *Greece & Rome* 35, no. 2 (1988): 152–63.

Golden, Mark. "Other People's Children." In *A Companion to Families in the Greek and Roman Worlds,* ed. Beryl Rawson. Wiley-Blackwell, 2011.

Gould, Stephen J. "Male Nipples and Clitoral Ripples." *Columbia: A Journal of Literature and Art* 20 (1993): 80–96.

Gourevitch, Danielle. "Chirurgie obstétricale dans le monde romain: Césarienne et embryotomie." In *Naissance et petite enfance dans l'Antiquité: Actes de colloque de Fribourg, 28 novembre–1 décembre* 2001, ed. Véronique Dasen. Academic Press, 2004.

Gourevitch, Danielle. "Popular Medicines and Practices in Galen." In *Popular Medicine in Graeco-Roman Antiquity: Explorations,* ed. William V. Harris. Brill, 2016.

Government Accountability Office. "Midwives: Information on Births, Workforce, and Midwifery Education." April 26, 2023. https://www.gao.gov/products/gao-23-105861 .

Government of Canada. "Perinatal Health Indicators (PHI)." Last modified June 11, 2024. https://health-infobase.canada.ca/phi/data-tool/index?Dom=2&Ind=7&MS=9.

Graham, Emma-Jayne. "The Making of Infants in Hellenistic and Early Roman Italy: A Votive Perspective." *World Archaeology* 45, no. 2 (2013): 215–31.

Graham, Emma-Jayne. "Infant Votives and Swaddling in Hellenistic Italy." In *Infant Health and Death in Roman Italy and Beyond,* ed. Maureen Carroll and Emma-Jayne Graham. *Journal of Roman Archeology* Supplemental Series 96 (2014).

Graumann, Lutz A., and Manfred Horstmanshoff. "'This I Suffered in the Short Space of My Life': The Epitaph for Lucius Minicius Anthimianus (*CIG* 3272; Peek *GV* 1166)." In *Homo Patiens: Approaches to the Patient in the Ancient World,* ed. Georgia Petridou and Chiara Thumiger. Brill, 2016.

Green, Monica H. "The Transmission of Ancient Theories of Female Physiology and Disease through the Early Middle Ages." PhD diss., Princeton University, 1985.

Green, Monica H. *The Trotula: An English Translation of the Medieval Compendium of Women's Medicine.* University of Pennsylvania Press, 2001.

Green, Monica H. *Making Women's Medicine Masculine: The Rise of Male Authority in Pre-Modern Gynaecology.* Oxford University Press, 2008.

Green, Monica. "'Cliff Notes' on the Circulation of the Gynecological Texts of Soranus and Muscio in the Middle Ages," February 23, 2023. https://works.hcommons.org/records/2b5mh-ccx69.

Groff, Elisa, and Florian Steger. "The Ethics of Ancient Lactation and the Cult of the Perfect Breastfeeding Mother." *Healthcare* 11 (2023): 2941.

Gwinnett, A. John, and Leonard Gorelick. "Beads, Scarabs, and Amulets: Methods of Manufacture in Ancient Egypt." *Journal of the American Research Center in Egypt* 30 (1993): 125–32.

Hannah, Mary E., Walter J. Hannah, Sheila A. Hewson, Ellen D. Hodnett, Saroj Saigal, and Andrew R. Willan. "Planned Caesarean Section Versus Planned Vaginal Birth for Breech Presentation at Term: A Randomised Multicentre Trial." Term Breech Trial Collaborative Group. *Lancet* 356 (2000): 1375–83.

Hänninen, Marja Leena. "From Womb to Family: Rituals and Social Conventions Connected to Roman Birth." In *Hoping for Continuity: Childhood, Education and Death in Antiquity and the Middle Ages,* ed. Katarina Mustakallio, Jussi Hanska, Hanna-Leena Sainio, and Ville Vuolanto. Acta Instituti Romani Finlandiae 33 (2005): 49–60.

Hanson, Ann Ellis. "Hippocrates: 'Diseases of Women 1.'" *Signs* 1, no. 2 (1975): 567–84.

Hanson, Ann Ellis. "The Eight Months' Child and the Etiquette of Birth: Obsit Omen!" *Bulletin of the History of Medicine* 61, no. 4 (1987): 589–602.

Hanson, Ann Ellis. "Greco-Roman Gynecology." *Society for Ancient Medicine and Pharmacy: Newsletter* 17 (1989): 83–92.

Hanson, Ann Ellis. "The Medical Writers' Woman." In *Before Sexuality: The Construction of Erotic Experience in the Ancient Greek World,* ed. David M. Halperin, John J. Winkler, and Froma I. Zeitlin. Princeton University Press, 1990.

Hanson, Ann Ellis. "Continuity and Change: Three Case Studies in Hippocratic Gynecological Therapy and Theory." In *Women's History and Ancient History,* ed. Sarah B. Pomeroy. University of North Carolina Press, 1991.

Hanson, Ann Ellis. "Conception, Gestation and the Origin of Female Nature in the Corpus Hippocraticum." *Helios: Journal of the Classical Association of the Southwest* 19 (1992): 31–71.

Hanson, Ann Ellis. "A Division of Labor: Roles for Men at Greek and Roman Births." *Thamyris* 1, no. 2 (1994): 157–202.

Hanson, Ann Ellis. "Uterine Amulets and Greek Uterine Medicine." *Medicina nei Secoli Arte e Scienza* 7 (1995): 281–99.

Hanson, Ann Ellis. "Talking Recipes in the Gynaecological Texts of the Hippocratic Corpus." In *Parchments of Gender: Deciphering the Bodies of Antiquity,* ed. Maria Wyke. Oxford University Press, 1998.

Hanson, Ann Ellis. "A Hair on Her Liver Has Been Lacerated . . . " In *Aspetti della terapia nel Corpus Hippocraticum: Atti del IXe Colloque International Hippocratique, Pisa, 25–29 Settembre* 1996, ed. Ivan Garofalo, Alessandro Lami, Daniela Manetti, and Amneris Roselli. Leo S. Olschki, 1999.

Hanson, Ann Ellis. "A Long-Lived 'Quick Birther' (okytokion)." In *Naissance et petite enfance dans l'Antiquité: Actes du colloque de Fribourg,* 28 *novembre–1er décembre* 2001, ed. Véronique Dasen. Academic Press, 2004.

Hanson, Ann Ellis. "The Hippocratic *Parthenos* in Sickness and Health." In *Virginity Revisited: Configurations of the Unpossessed Body,* ed. Bonnie MacLachlan and Judith Fletcher. J. Vrin, 2007.

Hanson, Ann Ellis. "The Gradualist View of Fetal Development." In *L'Embryon: Formation et Animation,* ed. Luc Brisson, Marie-Hélène Congourdeau, and Jean-Luc Solère. J. Vrin, 2008.

Hanson, Ann Ellis, and Monica H. Green. "Soranus of Ephesus: Methodicorum Princeps." *Aufstieg und Niedergang der römischen Welt* 37, no. 2 (1994): 968–1075.

Heath, John. "Why Corinna?" *Hermes* 141 (2013): 155–70.
Hemelrijk, Emily A. *Women and Society in the Roman World: A Sourcebook of Inscriptions from the Roman West.* Cambridge University Press, 2020.
Henneberg, H., and R. J. Henneberg. "Skeletal Material from the House of C. Iulius Polybius in Pompei, 79 AD." In *La casa di Giulio Polibio: Studi interdisciplinari,* ed. A. Ciarallo and E. De Carolis. Centro Studi Arti Figurativi, 2001.
Hines, Caitlin. *Rome's Visceral Reactions: Politics and Poetics in Flesh and Blood.* University of Michigan Press, 2026.
Hirt, Marguerite. "La législation romaine et les droits de l'enfant." In *Naissance et petite enfance dans l'Antiquité: Actes du colloque de Fribourg,* 28 *novembre–1er décembre* 2001, ed. Véronique Dasen. Academic Press, 2004.
Holman, Susan. "Molded as Wax: Formation and Feeding of the Ancient Newborn." *Helios* 24, no. 1 (1997): 77–95.
Holmes, Brooke. "Proto-Sympathy in the Hippocratic Corpus." In *Hippocrate et les hippocratismes: Médecine, religion, société; Actes du XIVe colloque international hippocratique,* ed. Jacques Jouanna and Michel Zink. Académie des Inscriptions et Belles-Lettres, 2014.
Holmes, Brooke. "Let Go of Laqueur: Towards New Histories of the Sexed Body." *Eugesta: Journal on Gender Studies in Antiquity* 9 (2019): 136–75.
Hong, Yurie. "Collaboration and Conflict: Discourses of Maternity in Hippocratic Gynecology and Embryology." In *Mothering and Motherhood in Ancient Greece and Rome,* ed. Lauren Hackworth Petersen and Patricia Salzman-Mitchell. University of Texas Press, 2012.
Hopkins, Keith. *Conquerors and Slaves.* Cambridge University Press, 1978.
Huemoeller, Katharine. *The Child Follows the Womb: Gender, Reproduction, and Roman Slavery.* Yale University Press, 2026.
Hug, Angela. *Fertility, Ideology, and the Cultural Politics of Reproduction at Rome.* Brill, 2023.
Huskinson, Janet. *Roman Children's Sarcophagi: Their Decoration and Its Social Significance.* Oxford University Press, 1996.
Incollingo Rodriguez, Angela C., Stephanie M. Smieszek, Kathryn E. Nippert, and A. Janet Tomiyama. "Pregnant and Postpartum Women's Experiences of Weight Stigma in Healthcare." *BMC Pregnancy Childbirth* 20, no. 1 (2020): 499.
Irving, Jennifer. "Restituta: The Training of the Female Physician." *Melbourne Historical Journal* 40, no. 2 (2012): 45–56.
Israelowich, Ido. *Patients and Healers in the High Roman Empire.* Johns Hopkins University Press, 2015.

Jackson, Ralph. "Roman Bivalve Dilators and Celsus' 'Instrument Like a Greek Letter . . . ' (*De Med. VII, 5, 2b*)." In *Le Latin médical: La constitution d'un langage scientifique,* ed. Guy Sabbah. Université de Saint-Etienne, 1991.
Jaeggi-Richoz, Sandra. *La fabrique des bébés dans l'Antiquite.* Brepols, 2024.
Johnston, Sarah Iles. *Restless Dead: Encounters Between the Living and the Dead in Ancient Greece.* University of California Press, 2013.
Jones, W. H. S. "Ancient Roman Folk Medicine." *Journal of the History of Medicine* 12 (1957): 459–72.
Joshel, Sandra R. "Nurturing the Master's Child: Slavery and the Roman Child-Nurse." *Signs* 12, no. 1 (1986): 3–22.
Joshel, Sandra R. *Slavery in the Roman World.* Cambridge University Press, 2010.
Kaibel, George. *Epigrammata Graeca ex lapidibus conlecta.* Reimer, 1878.
Kampen, Natalie. *Image and Status: Roman Working Women in Ostia.* Gebr. Mann Verlag, 1981.
Kanta, Athanasia, Costis Davaras, and Philip P. Betancourt. *Honors to Eileithyia at Ancient Inatos: The Sacred Cave at Tsoutsouros, Crete.* INSTAP Academic Press, 2022.
Kapparis, Konstantinos A. *Abortion in the Ancient World.* Bloomsbury, 2002.
Karivieri, Arja, ed. *Life and Death in a Multicultural Harbour City: Ostia Antica from the Republic through Late Antiquity.* Acta Instituti Romani Finlandiae, 2020.
Keenleyside, Anne, Henry Schwarcz, Lea Stirling, and Nejib Ben Lazreg. "Stable Isotopic Evidence for Diet in a Roman and Late Roman Population from Leptiminus, Tunisia." *Journal of Archaeological Science* 36 (2009): 51–63.
Ker, James. *The Ordered Day: Quotidian Time and Forms of Life in Ancient Rome.* Johns Hopkins University Press, 2023.
Killgrove, Kristina. "Bioarchaeology in the Roman Empire." In *Encyclopedia of Global Archaeology,* ed. Jeffery A. Becker and Alison Barclay. Springer, 2013.
Killgrove, Kristina. "Pregnant Women and Fetuses Among Vesuvius' Victims, Archaeologists Reveal." *Forbes,* August 24, 2017. https://www.forbes.com/sites/kristinakillgrove/2017/08/24/pregnant-women-and-fetuses-among-vesuvius-victims-archaeologists-reveal/?sh=2a2fcc41cc33.
Killgrove, Kristina, and Robert H. Tykot. "Food for Rome: A Stable Isotope Investigation of Diet in the Imperial Period (1st–3rd Centuries AD)." *Journal of Anthropological Archaeology* 32 (2013): 28–38.
King, Helen. "Once Upon a Text: Hysteria from Hippocrates." In *Hysteria Beyond Freud,* ed. Sander L. Gilman, Helen King, Roy Porter, G. S. Rousseau, and Elaine Showalter. University of California Press, 1993.

King, Helen. "Sowing the Field: Greek and Roman Sexology." In *Sexual Knowledge, Sexual Science: The History of Attitudes to Sexuality,* ed. Roy Porter and Mikulas Teich. Cambridge University Press, 1994.

King, Helen. *Hippocrates' Woman: Reading the Female Body in Ancient Greece.* Taylor & Francis, 1998.

King, Helen. *The Disease of Virgins: Green Sickness, Chlorosis and the Problems of Puberty.* Routledge, 2003.

King, Helen. *Midwifery, Obstetrics and the Rise of Gynaecology: The Uses of a Sixteenth-Century Compendium.* Ashgate, 2007.

King, Helen. "Galen and the Widow: Towards a History of Therapeutic Masturbation in Ancient Gynaecology." *Eugesta: Journal on Gender Studies in Antiquity* 1 (2011): 205–35.

King, Helen. "Introduction." In *Blood, Sweat and Tears: The Changing Concepts of Physiology from Antiquity into Early Modern Europe,* ed. Manfred Horstmanshoff, Helen King, and Claus Zittel. Brill, 2012.

King, Helen. "Motherhood and Health in the Hippocratic Corpus." *Dossier: Mères et maternités en Grèce ancienne.* Éditions de l'École des hautes études en sciences sociales, 2013.

King, Helen. *The One-Sex Body on Trial: The Classical and Early Modern Evidence.* Ashgate, 2013.

King, Helen. "Risky Business: Pregnancy, Birth and Death in Roman Times." Review of Anna Bonnell Freidin, *Birthing Romans: Childbearing and Its Risks in Imperial Rome. Times Literary Supplement,* January 17, 2025.

Kleiner, Diana. "Family Ties: Mothers and Sons in Elite and Non-Elite Roman Art." In *I Claudia II: Women in Roman Art and Society,* ed. Diana Kleiner and Susan Matheson. University of Texas Press, 2000.

Koortbojian, Michael. *Myth, Meaning, and Memory on Roman Sarcophagi.* University of California Press, 1995.

Kottek, Samuel S. "Caesarean Section in the Talmud: A Renewed Examination of a Historical Enigma." In *Female Bodies and Female Practitioners,* ed. Lennart Lehmhaus. Mohr Siebeck, 2023.

Kusukawa, Sachiko. *Anatomy and the World of Books.* Reaktion Books, 2024.

Laes, Christian. "The Educated Midwife in the Roman Empire: An Example of Differential Equations." In *Hippocrates and Medical Education: Selected Papers Read at the XIIth International Hippocrates Colloquium, Universiteit Leiden, 24–26 August* 2005, ed. Manfred Horstmanshoff. Brill, 2010.

Laes, Christian. *Children in the Roman Empire: Outsiders Within.* Cambridge University Press, 2011.

Laes, Christian. "Midwives in Greek Inscriptions in Hellenistic and Roman Antiquity." *Zeitschrift für Papyrologie und Epigraphik* 176 (2011): 154–62.

Laes, Christian. "Infants Between Biological and Social Birth in Antiquity: A Phenomenon of the 'Longue Durée.'" *Historia: Zeitschrift für Alte Geschichte* 63, no. 3 (2014): 364–83.

Laes, Christian. "Conception, Birth, and the 'Crucial' First Days." In *Disabilities and the Disabled in the Roman World,* ed. Christian Laes. Cambridge University Press, 2018.

Laes, Christian. "Women, Children, and Food." In *The Routledge Handbook of Diet and Nutrition in the Roman World,* ed. Paul Erdkamp and Claire Holleran. Routledge, 2018.

Laes, Christian. "Amitae and Materterae in Latin Inscriptions: A Contribution to the Study of the Roman Family." *Arctos: Acta philologica Fennica* 57 (2024): 103–55.

Laes, Christian, Chris Goodey, and M. Lynn Rose, eds. *Disabilities in Roman Antiquity: Disparate Bodies A Capite Ad Calcem.* Brill, 2013.

Laqueur, Thomas. *Making Sex: Body and Gender from the Greeks to Freud.* Harvard University Press, 1990.

Laurence, Ray. *Roman Archaeology for Historians.* Taylor & Francis, 2012.

Lawrence, Thea. "Breastmilk, Breastfeeding and the Female Body in Early Imperial Rome." In *Bodily Fluids in Antiquity,* ed. Mark Bradley, Victoria Leonard, and Laurence M. V. Totelin. Taylor & Francis, 2021.

Lay, Mary M. *The Rhetoric of Midwifery: Gender, Knowledge, and Power.* Rutgers University Press, 2000.

Lehmhaus, Lennart. "Re-reading Gynaecology in the Ancient World—a Transcultural and Interdisciplinary Survey." In *Female Bodies and Female Practitioners,* ed. Lennart Lehmhaus. Mohr Siebeck, 2023.

Lewis, Mary E. "Disease and Trauma in the Children from Roman Britain." In *The Oxford Handbook of the Archaeology of Childhood,* ed. Sally Crawford, Dawn M. Hadley, and Gillian Shepherd. Oxford University Press, 2018.

Lillis, Julia Kelto. *Virgin Territory: Configuring Female Virginity in Early Christianity.* University of California Press, 2022.

Lillis, Julia Kelto. "Late Ancient Christians and the Rise of Medically Perceptible Virginity." In *Female Bodies and Female Practitioners,* ed. Lennart Lehmhaus. Mohr Siebeck, 2023.

Lloyd, G. E. R. *Science, Folklore, and Ideology: Studies in the Life Sciences in Ancient Greece.* Cambridge University Press, 1983.

Lloyd, G. E. R. "Galen's Un-Hippocratic Case-Histories." In *Galen and the World of Knowledge,* ed. Christopher Gill, Tim Whitmarsh, and John Wilkins. Cambridge University Press, 2009.

Larsson Lovén, Lena. "People at Work in Ostia." In *Life and Death in a Multicultural Harbour City: Ostia Antica from the Republic through Late Antiquity,* ed. Arja Karivieri. Acta Instituti Romani Finlandiae, 2020.

Marino, Katherine. "Setting the Womb in Its Place—Toward a Contextual Archaeology of Graeco-Egyptian Uterine Amulets." PhD diss., Brown University, 2010.

Martin, Dale B. "Contradictions of Masculinity: Ascetic Inseminators and Menstruating Men in Greco-Roman Culture." In *Generation and Degeneration: Tropes of Reproduction in Literature and History from Antiquity through Early Modern Europe,* ed. Valeria Finucci and Kevin Brownlee. Duke University Press, 2001.

Marx-Wolf, Heidi. "Living Plants, Dead Animals, and Other Matters: Embryos and Demons in Porphyry of Tyre." *Preturnature* 7, no. 1 (2018): 1–26.

Marx-Wolf, Heidi. "Religion, Medicine, and Health." In *A Companion to Religion in Late Antiquity,* ed. Josef Lössl and Nicholas J. Baker-Brian. Wiley-Blackwell, 2018.

Mastrocinque, Attilio. *Les intailles magiques du département des Monnaies, Médailles et Antiques.* Éditions de la Bibliothèque nationale de France, 2014. https://doi.org/10.4000/books.editionsbnf.1182.

Mathieu, Nicolas. *L'Epitaphe et la mémoire: Parenté et identité sociale dans les Gaules et Germanies romaines.* Rennes University Press, 2011.

Mattern, Susan P. *Galen and the Rhetoric of Healing.* Johns Hopkins University Press, 2008.

Mattern, Susan P. *The Prince of Medicine: Galen in the Roman Empire.* Oxford University Press, 2013.

Mattern, Susan P. "Panic and Culture: Hysterike Pnix in the Ancient Greek World." *Journal of the History of Medicine and Allied Sciences* 70, no. 4 (2014): 491–515.

McDaniel, Spencer. "No, the Ancient Romans Didn't Overharvest Silphium to Extinction Because It Was a Highly Effective Contraceptive." *Tales of Times Forgotten* (blog), January 4, 2020. https://talesoftimesforgotten.com/2020/01/04/no-the-ancient-romans-didnt-overharvest-silphium-to-extinction-because-it-was-a-highly-effective-contraceptive/

McGinn, Thomas A. J. *Prostitution, Sexuality, and the Law in Ancient Rome.* Oxford University Press, 1998.

McGinn, Thomas A.J. "Roman Children and the Law." In *Childhood and Education in the Classical World,* ed. Judith Evans Grubbs and Tim G. Parkin. Oxford University Press, 2013.

McGregor, Deborah Kuh. *From Midwives to Medicine: The Birth of American Gynecology.* Rutgers University Press, 1998.

Michel, Simone. *Die magischen Gemmen im Britischen Museum.* British Museum Press, 2001.

Miller, Kassandra J. *Time and Ancient Medicine: How Sundials and Water Clocks Changed Medical Science.* Oxford University Press, 2023.

Milnor, Kristina. *Gender, Domesticity, and the Age of Augustus: Inventing Private Life.* Oxford University Press, 2005.

Mistry, Zubin. *Abortion in the Early Middle Ages, c.* 500–900. York Medieval Press, 2015.

Morgan, Lynn Marie, and Meredith W. Michaels, eds. *Fetal Subjects, Feminist Positions.* University of Pennsylvania Press, 1999.

Moore, Alison. "Hearth and Home: The Burial of Infants Within Romano-British Domestic Contexts." *Childhood in the Past* 2 (2009): 33–54.

Moss, Candida. *God's Ghost Writers: Enslaved Christians and the Making of the Bible.* Hachette, 2024.

Muehlberger, Ellen. "Perpetual Adjustment: The Passion of Perpetua and Felicity and the Entailments of Authenticity." *Journal of Early Christian Studies* 30, no. 3 (2022): 313–42.

Mulder, Tara. "The Hippocratic Oath in Roe v. Wade." Eidolon, March 16, 2016. https://eidolon.pub/the-hippocratic-oath-in-roe-v-wade-ded59eedfd8f.

Mulder, Tara. "Adult Breastfeeding in Ancient Rome." *Illinois Journal of Classical Studies* 42, no. 1 (2017): 227–43.

Mulder, Tara. "Female Trouble in Terence's Hecyra: Rape-Pregnancy Plots and the Absence of Abortion in Roman Comedy." *Helios* 46, no. 1 (2019): 35–56.

Mulder, Tara. "Flabby Flesh and Foetal Formation: Body Fluidity and Foetal Sex Differentiation in Ancient Greek Medicine." In *Bodily Fluids in Antiquity,* ed. Mark Bradley, Victoria Leonard, and Laurence M. V. Totelin. Routledge, 2021.

Muir, Steven, and Laurence M. V. Totelin. "Medicine and Disease." In *A Cultural History of Women in Antiquity,* ed. Janet H. Tulloch. Bloomsbury, 2013.

Muraca, Giulia M., Laura E. Ralph, Penny Christensen, et al. "Maternal and Neonatal Trauma During Forceps and Vacuum Delivery Must Not Be Overlooked." *BMJ* 383 (2023): e073991.

Musgrove, Caroline. "Oribasius' Woman: Medicine, Christianity, and Society in Late Antiquity." PhD diss., Queen's College, University of Cambridge, 2017.

Muza, Sharon. "The Miles Circuit." Sharonmuza.com, accessed May 27, 2025. http://sharonmuza.com/miles-circuit-positioning-baby/.

Nardi, Enzo. *Procurato aborto nel mondo greco romano.* A. Giuffrè, 1971.

Nasrallah, Laura Salah. *Ancient Christians and the Power of Curses: Magic, Aesthetics, and Justice.* Cambridge University Press, 2024.

Nelson, Maggie. *The Argonauts.* Greywolf Press, 2015.

Neri, I., G. Airola, G. Contu, G. Allais, F. Facchinetti, and C. Benedetto. "Acupuncture plus Moxibustion to Resolve Breech Presentation: A Randomized Controlled Study." *The Journal of Maternal-Fetal & Neonatal Medicine* 15, no. 4 (2004): 247–52.

Nguyen, Misa. "Science and Medicine." In *A Cultural History of Pregnancy and Childbirth in Antiquity (500 BCE to 600 CE),* ed. Tara Mulder. Routledge, forthcoming.

Nickel, Diethard. *Untersuchungen zur Embryologie Galens.* Akademie-Verlag, 1989.

Nifosi, Ada. *Becoming a Woman and Mother in Greco-Roman Egypt: Women's Bodies, Society and Domestic Space.* Routledge, 2019.

Nutton, Vivian. "Healers in the Medical Market Place: Towards a Social History of Graeco Roman Medicine." In *Medicine in Society: Historical Essays,* ed. Andrew Wear. Cambridge University Press, 1992.

Nutton, Vivian. *Ancient Medicine,* 3rd ed. Routledge, 2024.

Oberhelman, Steven M. *Dreams, Healing, and Medicine in Greece: From Antiquity to the Present.* Ashgate, 2013.

Ogden, Daniel. *Magic, Witchcraft and Ghosts in the Greek and Roman Worlds: A Sourcebook,* 2nd ed. Oxford University Press, 2009.

Osgood, Josiah. *Turia: A Roman Woman's Civil War.* Oxford University Press, 2014.

Oudshoorn, Carolien. *The Relationship Between Roman and Local Law in the Babatha and Salome Komaise Archives: General Analysis and Three Case Studies on Law of Succession, Guardianship and Marriage.* Brill, 2007.

Owens, Deirdre Cooper. *Medical Bondage: Race, Gender, and the Origins of American Gynecology.* University of Georgia Press, 2017.

Parca, Maryline. "The Wet Nurses of Ptolemaic and Roman Egypt." *Illinois Classical Studies* 42, no. 1 (2017): 203–26.

Park, Katharine. *Secrets of Women: Gender, Generation, and the Origin of Human Dissection.* Zone Books, 2006.

Park, Katharine. "Managing Childbirth and Fertility in Medieval Europe." In *Reproduction: Antiquity to the Present Day,* ed. Nick Hopwood, Rebecca Flemming, and Lauren Kassell. Cambridge University Press, 2018.

Parkin, Tim. *Demography and Roman Society.* Johns Hopkins University Press, 1992.

Parkin, Tim. "The Demography of Infancy and Early Childhood in the Ancient World." In *The Oxford Handbook of Childhood and Education in the Classical World,* ed. Judith Evans Grubbs and Tim Parkin. Oxford University Press, 2013.

Patey, Andrea M., Janet A. Curran, Ann E. Sprague, et al. "Intermittent Auscultation Versus Continuous Fetal Monitoring: Exploring Factors That Influence Birthing Unit Nurses' Fetal Surveillance Practice Using Theoretical Domains Framework." *BMC Pregnancy Childbirth* 17 (2017): 320.

Pedrucci, Giulia. "Mothers for Sale: The Case of the Wet Nurse in the Ancient Greek and Roman World: An Overview." *Arenal* 27, no. 1 (2020): 127–40.

Pedrucci, Giulia. "On the Use of Breast Milk and Menstrual Blood in the Greek and Roman Worlds." In *Ancient Magic: Then and Now,* ed. Atillio Mastrocinque, Joseph E. Sanzo, and Marianna Scapini. Franz Steiner Verlag, 2020.

Penniman, John David. *Raised on Christian Milk: Food and the Formation of the Soul in Early Christianity.* Yale University Press, 2017.

Perry, Matthew J. *Gender, Manumission, and the Roman Freedwoman.* Cambridge University Press, 2013.

Phang, Sara Elise. *The Marriage of Roman Soldiers (13 B.C.–A.D. 235): Law and Family in the Imperial Army.* Brill, 2001.

Pollaro, Paul, and Paul Robertson. "Reassessing the Role of Anthropogenic Climate Change in the Extinction of Silphium." *Frontiers in Conservation Science* 2 (2022).

Pomeroy, Sarah B. *The Murder of Regilla: A Case of Domestic Violence in Antiquity.* Harvard University Press, 2007.

Porter, Amber J. "Compassion in Soranus' *Gynecology* and Caelius Aurelianus' *On Chronic Diseases.*" In *Homo Patiens: Approaches to the Patient in the Ancient World,* ed. Georgia Petridou and Chiara Thumiger. Brill, 2016.

Powell, Lindsay, Rebecca C. Redfern, Andrew R. Millard, and Darren R. Gröcke. "Infant Feeding Practices in Roman London: Evidence from Isotropic Analysis." In *Infant Health and Death in Roman Italy and Beyond,* ed. Maureen Carroll and Emma-Jayne Graham. *Journal of Roman Archaeology* Supplemental Series 96 (2014): 89–110.

Prowse, Tracy L., Henry P. Schwarcz, Shelley R. Saunders, Roberto Macchiarelli, and Luca Bondioli. "Isotopic Evidence for Age-Related Variation in Diet from Isola Sacra, Italy." *American Journal of Physical Anthropology* 128 (2005): 2–13.

Rawson, Beryl. "Family Life Among the Lower Classes at Rome in the First Two Centuries of the Empire." *Classical Philology* 61, no. 2 (1966): 71–83.

Rawson, Beryl. *Children and Childhood in Roman Italy.* Oxford University Press, 2003.

Renberg, Gil H. *Where Dreams May Come: Incubation Sanctuaries in the Graeco-Roman World.* Brill, 2017.

Ricciardetto, Antonio, and Danielle Gourevitch. "The Cost of a Baby: How Much Did It Cost to Hire a Wet-Nurse in Roman Egypt?" Trans. Laurence M. V. Totelin. In *Medicine and Markets in the Graeco-Roman World and Beyond: Essays in Honour of Vivian Nutton,* ed. Laurence M. V. Totelin and Rebecca Flemming. Classical Press of Wales, 2020.

Rich, Adrienne. *Of Woman Born: Motherhood as Experience and Institution.* W. W. Norton, 1976.

Richlin, Amy. *Arguments with Silence: Writing the History of Roman Women.* University of Michigan Press, 2014.

Riddle, John M. *Contraception and Abortion from the Ancient World to the Renaissance.* Harvard University Press, 1992.

Riddle, John M. *Eve's Herbs: A History of Contraception and Abortion in the West.* Harvard University Press, 1997.

Riddle, John M. "Folk Tradition and Folk Medicine: Recognition of Drugs in Classical Antiquity." *Pharmacy in History* 55, no. 2/3 (2013 [1987]): 64–87.

Ripat, Pauline. "Roman Women, Wise Women, and Witches." *Phoenix* 70 (2016): 104–28.

Rocca, Julius. "Pneuma as a Holistic Concept in Galen." In *Holism in Ancient Medicine and Its Reception,* ed. Chiara Thumiger. Brill, 2020.

Romero, Irene Mañas, and José Nicolás Saiz López. "Pueri Nascentes: Rituals, Birth, and Social Recognition in Ancient Rome." In *Ages and Abilities: The Stages of Childhood and their Social Recognition in Prehistoric Europe and Beyond,* ed. Katharina Rebay-Salisbury and Doris Pany-Kucera. Archaeopress, 2020.

Rothe, Ursula. "Der Grabstein der Severina Nutrix aus Köln: Eine neue Deutung." *Germania* 89 (2011): 191–214.

Rothman, Barbara Katz. *In Labor: Women and Power in the Birthplace.* Rev. ed. W. W. Norton, 1991.

Rousselle, Aline. "Observation féminine et idéologie masculine: Le corps de la femme d'après les médecins grecs." *Annales: Histoire, sciences sociales 35e année* 5 (1980): 1089–115.

Rowlandson, Jane. *Women and Society in Greek and Roman Egypt: A Sourcebook*. Cambridge University Press, 1998.

Sage-Femme Collective. *Natural Liberty: Rediscovering Self-Induced Abortion Methods*. Sage-Femme, 2008.

Salvo, Irene. "Owners of Their Own Bodies: Women's Magical Knowledge and Reproduction in Greek Inscriptions." In *Women's Ritual Competence in the Greco-Roman Mediterranean,* ed. Matthew Dillon, Esther Eidinow, and Lisa Maurizio. Routledge, 2016.

Šašel Kos, Marjeta. *Pre-Roman Divinities of the Eastern Alps and Adriatic.* Narodni muzej Slovenije, 1999.

Scarfo, Barbara. "Pregnancy, Childbirth, and Primary Care-Givers in Ancient Rome." PhD diss., McMaster University, 2020.

Schofield, Roger. "Did the Mothers Really Die? Three Centuries of Maternal Mortality in 'The World We Have Lost.'" In *The World We Have Gained: Histories of Population and Social Structure; Essays Presented to Peter Laslett on His Seventieth Birthday,* ed. Lloyd Bonfield, Richard Smith, and Keith Wrightson. Blackwell, 1986.

Scott, Calloway. "Gender in the Temple: Women's Ailments in the Epidaurian Miracle Cures." *Classical Antiquity* 37, no. 2 (2018): 321–50.

Schultz, Celia E. *Women's Religious Activity in the Roman Republic.* University of North Carolina Press, 2006.

Scullin, Sarah. "'She's Only a 4': The Objectification of Birthing Bodies." Eidolon, December 12, 2016. https://eidolon.pub/shes-only-a-4-f534333fb298.

Sears, Darlene. "The Impact of the Spinning Babies Method on Labor Duration and Delivery Outcome." *Walden Dissertations and Doctoral Studies* (2023): 13765.

Sharrock, Alison. "Ovid and the Discourses of Love: The Amatory Works." In *The Cambridge Companion to Ovid,* ed. Philip Hardie. Cambridge University Press, 2002.

Sherwin-White, Susan M. *Ancient Kos: An Historical Study from the Dorian Settlement to the Imperial Period.* Vandenhoek and Ruprecht, 1978.

Simkin, Penny, and Melissa Cheney. *The Birth Partner: A Complete Guide to Childbirth for Dads, Partners, Doulas, and Other Labor Companions,* 5th ed. Harvard Common Press, 2018.

Simkins, Geradine. *Into These Hands: Wisdom from Midwives.* Spirituality and Health Books, 2011.

Simons, Julia. "Tuberculosis in the Greco-Roman World." PhD diss., University of Pennsylvania, 2023.

Simons, Patricia. *The Sex of Men in Premodern Europe: A Cultural History.* Cambridge University Press, 2011.

Singer, P. N., and Ralph M. Rosen, eds. *The Oxford Handbook of Galen.* Oxford University Press, 2024.

Sneed, Debby. "Disability and Infanticide in Ancient Greece." *Hesperia* 90, no. 4 (2021): 747–72.

Somerstein, Rachel. *Invisible Labor: The Untold Story of the Cesarean Section.* Ecco, 2024.

Southon, Emma. *Agrippina: The Most Extraordinary Woman of the Roman World.* Pegasus Books, 2019.

Southwell-Wright, William. "Perceptions of Infant Disability in Roman Britain." In *Infant Health and Death in Roman Italy and Beyond,* ed. Maureen Carroll and Emma-Jayne Graham. *Journal of Roman Archaeology* Supplemental Series 96 (2014): 111–30.

Sparreboom, Anna. "Wet-Nursing in the Roman Empire." In *Infant Health and Death in Roman Italy and Beyond,* ed. Maureen Carroll and Emma-Jayne Graham. *Journal of Roman Archaeology* Supplemental Series 96 (2014): 145–58.

Spieser, Cathie. "Meskhenet et les sept Hathors en Égypte ancienne." In *Des Fata aux fées: Regards croisés de l'Antiquité à nos jours,* ed. Martine Hennard Dutheil de la Rochère and Véronique Dasen. Université de Lausanne, Études de Lettres, 2011.

Sutton, Jean, and Pauline Scott. *Understanding and Teaching Optimal Foetal Positioning.* Birth Concepts, 1995.

Tatarkiewicz, Anna. *The "Cursus Laborum" of Roman Women: Social and Medical Aspects of the Transition from Puberty to Motherhood.* Bloomsbury, 2023.

Tatarkiewicz, Anna. "Spaces and Practitioners." In *A Cultural History of Pregnancy and Childbirth in Antiquity (500 BCE to 600 CE),* ed. Tara Mulder. Routledge, forthcoming.

Tieleman, Teun. "Galen and the Stoics, or: The Art of Not Naming." In *Galen and the World of Knowledge,* ed. Christopher Gill, Tim Whitmarsh, and John Wilkins. Cambridge University Press, 2009.

Tomlin, Roger S. O. "Special Delivery: A Graeco-Roman Gold Amulet for Healthy Childbirth." *Zeitschrift für Papyrologie und Epigraphik* 167 (2008): 219–24.

Totelin, Laurence M. V. *Hippocratic Recipes: Oral and Written Transmission of Pharmacological Knowledge in Fifth- and Fourth-Century Greece.* Brill, 2009.

Totelin, Laurence M. V. "Eating of Curds and Whey: Rennet in Ancient Medicine." The Recipes Project, July 16, 2013. https://recipes.hypotheses.org/1898.
Totelin, Laurence M. V. "Whose Fault Is it Anyway? Plant Infertility in Antiquity." In *The Palgrave Handbook of Infertility in History,* ed. Gayle Davis and Tracey Loughran. Palgrave Macmillan, 2017.
Totelin, Laurence M. V. "Animal and Plant Generation in Classical Antiquity." In *Reproduction: Antiquity to the Present Day,* ed. Nick Hopwood, Rebecca Flemming, and Lauren Kassell. Cambridge University Press, 2018.
Totelin, Laurence M. V. "Do No Harm: Phanostrate's Midwifery Practice." *Technai* 11 (2020): 129–43.
Totelin, Laurence M. V. "Breastmilk in the Cave and on the Arena: Early Christian Stories of Lactation in Context." In *Bodily Fluids in Antiquity,* ed. Mark Bradley, Victoria Leonard, and Laurence Totelin. Taylor & Francis, 2021.
Totelin, Laurence M. V. "Weaning and Lactation Cessation in Late Antiquity and the Early Byzantine Period: Medical Advice in Context." In *Breastfeeding and Mothering in Antiquity and Early Byzantium,* ed. Stavroula Constantinou and Aspasia Skouroumouni-Stavrinou. Routledge, 2024.
Treggiari, Susan. "Jobs for Women." *American Journal of Ancient History* 1 (1976): 76–104.
Tsatsou, Eleni. "Uterine Amulets: Amulets That Protect the Uterus or That Reinforce Erotic Desire?" In *Magical Gems in Their Context: Proceedings of the International Workshop Held at the Museum of Fine Arts, Budapest, 16–18 February 2012,* ed. Kata Endreffy, Árpád M. Nagy, and Jeffrey Spier. L'Erma di Bretschneider, 2019.
Turner, Sasha. "The Invisible Threads of Gender, Race, and Slavery." Black Perspectives, April 13, 2017. https://www.aaihs.org/the-invisible-threads-of-gender-race-and-slavery/.
Upson-Saia, Kristi, Heidi Marx, and Jared Secord. *Medicine, Health, and Healing in the Ancient Mediterranean (500 BCE–600 CE): A Sourcebook.* University of California Press, 2023.
Van Minnen, Peter. "Alexandrian Documents from the Reign of Augustus." Accessed May 27, 2025. https://classics.uc.edu/users/vanminnen/ancient_alexandria/index.html
Vistad, Ingvild, Milada Cvancarova, Berit L. Hustad, and Tore Henriksen. "Vaginal Breech Delivery: Results of a Prospective Registration Study." *BMC Pregnancy Childbirth* 13 (2013): 153.
Von Staden, Heinrich. *Herophilus: The Art of Medicine in Early Alexandria.* Cambridge University Press, 1989.

Von Staden, Heinrich. "Apud Nos Foediora Verba: Celsus' Reluctant Construction of the Female Body." In *Le latin médical: La constitution d'un language scientifique,* ed. Guy Sabbah. Publications de l'Université de Saint-Étienne, 1991.

Von Staden, Heinrich. "Women and Dirt." *Helios* 19 (1992): 7–30.

Wick, Livia. *Sumud: Birth, Oral History, and Persisting in Palestine.* Syracuse University Press, 2023.

Wilberding, James. "Porphyry and Plotinus on the Seed." *Phronesis* 53, no. 4/5 (2008): 406–32.

Wilson, Adrian. *The Making of Man-Midwifery: Childbirth in England, 1660–1770.* Routledge, 1995.

Witzke, Serena. "Violence Against Women in Ancient Rome: Ideology Versus Reality." In *The Topography of Violence in the Greco-Roman World,* ed. Werner Riess and Garret G. Fagan. University of Michigan Press, 2016.

Witkiewicz, Magdalena, Barbara Baranowska, Maria Węgrzynowska, et al. "Perinatal Outcomes and Level of Labour Difficulty in Deliveries with Right and Left Foetal Position—a Preliminary Study." *Healthcare* 12, no. 8 (2024): 864.

Westbrook, Raymond. "Vitae Necisque Potestas." *Historia: Zeitschrift für Alte Geschichte* 48, no. 2 (1999): 203–23.

Wolf, Jacqueline. *Deliver Me from Pain: Anesthesia and Birth in America.* Johns Hopkins University Press, 2009.

Wolf, Jacqueline. *Cesarean Section: An American History of Risk, Technology, and Consequence.* Johns Hopkins University Press, 2018.

Wolfarth, Joanna. *Milk: An Intimate History of Breastfeeding.* Weidenfeld & Nicolson, 2023.

Wood, Susan. "Mortals, Empresses, and Earth Goddesses: Demeter and Persephone in Public and Private Apotheosis." In *I Claudia II: Women in Roman Art and Society,* ed. Diana Kleiner and Susan Matheson. University of Texas Press, 2000.

Wood, Susan. "Literacy and Luxury in the Early Empire: A Papyrus-Roll Winder from Pompeii." *Memoirs of the American Academy in Rome* 46 (2001): 23–40.

Wood, Susan. "Women's Work and Women's Myths: Mothers and Children on Ivory Looms." *American Journal of Archaeology* 123, no. 3 (2019): 411–38.

World Health Organization. "Caesarean Section Rates Continue to Rise, amid Growing Inequalities in Access." June 16, 2021. https://www.who.int/news/item/16-06-2021-caesarean-section-rates-continue-to-rise-amid-growing-inequalities-in-access.

World Health Organization. "Maternal Mortality Ratio (per 100,000 Live Births)." Last updated April 25, 2025. https://data.who.int/indicators/i/C071DCB/AC597B1.
Wright, Jessica. *Psychiatry: Antiquity and Its Legacy*. Bloomsbury, 2025.
Wyke, Maria. "Mistress and Metaphor in Augustan Elegy." *Helios* 16 (1989): 25–47.

INDEX

Founded in 1893,
UNIVERSITY OF CALIFORNIA PRESS
publishes bold, progressive books and journals on topics in the arts, humanities, social sciences, and natural sciences—with a focus on social justice issues—that inspire thought and action among readers worldwide.

The UC PRESS FOUNDATION
raises funds to uphold the press's vital role as an independent, nonprofit publisher, and receives philanthropic support from a wide range of individuals and institutions—and from committed readers like you. To learn more, visit ucpress.edu/supportus.